Praise for *Diet for a Hot Pla[net]*

DIET FOR A HOT PLANET

DIET FOR A HOT PLANET

THE CLIMATE CRISIS AT THE END OF YOUR FORK

and

WHAT YOU CAN DO ABOUT IT

ANNA LAPPÉ

With a Foreword by Bill McKibben

BLOOMSBURY

NEW YORK · BERLIN · LONDON · SYDNEY

Published by Bloomsbury USA, New York

All papers used by Bloomsbury USA are natural, recyclable
products made from wood grown in well-managed forests.
The manufacturing processes conform to the environmental
regulations of the country of origin.

LIBRARY OF CONGRESS CATALOGING-IN-PUBLICATION DATA

Lappé, Anna, 1973–
Diet for a hot planet : the climate crisis at the end of your fork and
what you can do about it / Anna Lappé ; with a foreword by Bill
McKibben.—1st U.S. ed.
p. cm.
ISBN: 978-1-59691-659-3 (hardcover)
1. Crops and climate.   2. Food—Environmental aspects.
3. Climatic changes—Effect of human beings on.   I. Title.
S600.7.C54L37 2010
363.738'74—dc22
2010017363

First published by Bloomsbury USA in 2010
This paperback edition published in 2011

Paperback ISBN: 978-1-60819-465-0

1 3 5 7 9 10 8 6 4 2

Typeset by Westchester Book Group
Printed in the United States of America by
Quad/Graphics, Fairfield, Pennsylvania

For my mother, Frances Moore Lappé,
and my daughter, Ida Jeanette Marshall-Lappé,
and for all the mothers who came before us and
the daughters who will come after.

CONTENTS

IV. **ACTION**

Like artistic and literary movements, social movements are driven by imagination . . . Every important social movement reconfigures the world in the imagination. What was obscure comes forward, lies are revealed, memory shaken, new delineations drawn over the old maps: It is from this new way of seeing the present that hope emerges for the future . . . Let us begin to imagine the worlds we would like to inhabit, the long lives we will share, and the many futures in our hands.

—SUSAN GRIFFIN, environmental philosopher

FOREWORD

Climate change is the biggest thing human beings have ever done; nothing else even comes close. We've already managed to substantially melt the Arctic, to force epic drought, to thaw the high-altitude glaciers that water Asia and South America, all with a single degree of temperature rise. The scientists are all but unanimous in the conclusion that unless we very quickly mend our ways, we will see another five or six degrees' rise before children now in their infancy reach their old age. So we'd better mend our ways.

And as Anna Lappé demonstrates here better than anyone ever has, that means fixing not just our cars and our power plants but also our menus. It stands to reason that the quintessential human activity, agriculture, would play a role in our fate, and as she proves beyond any doubt, that role is large. Livestock alone may account for more global warming gases than automobiles; the entire industrial food system essentially insures that your food is marinated in crude oil before you eat it.

That industrial food system has rarely been more damningly described than in this book—especially the endless spin employed by an army of lobbyists to justify the unjustifiable, to spread doubt where no doubt exists, to undermine the obvious answers that common sense provides. Of course it's a bad idea for the environment for our culture to have evolved a system of monoculture and concentration, of fast food and quick profit. Bad for our bodies, too.

And bad, crucially, for our communities. But this is the hopeful point I'd like to make: A new way of eating will not only mean less greenhouse gases; it will mean more community, and that's almost certainly key to solving the other three quarters of the global warming puzzle. Consider the farmers' market, the fastest-growing part of the American food economy. It's a good idea environmentally: The tomato that travels five miles requires less petroleum than the long-distance traveler. (And tastes better. I mean, think how you feel after a journey of several thousand miles. That's how the tomato feels, too.) But the biggest difference may be in the experience of shopping.

When sociologists studied the behavior of customers at supermarkets, they found what we all know: You drop into a trance, visit the routine stations of the cross, and emerge blinking back into daylight with the same bag of stuff you had the week before. At the farmers' market, on the other hand, the average shopper has ten times as many conversations. Ten times! That's one of the reasons people like it. And in a society that's been hollowed out by access to cheap fossil fuel, in the first society on earth where people have no practical need of their neighbors for anything, that's a priceless trait. The farmers' market is the place where community can start to regrow, and hence lay the groundwork for all the other things that need doing: the new bus system, the ride-sharing network, the neighborhood wind turbine.

I remember some years ago, before it was quite fashionable, feeding my family for a year only on food from our valley in Vermont. It required new thinking about cooking—I had a more limited palette to draw on, and hence to please our palates I had to think a little harder. Which was good, but not as good as the fact that I came away from the experience with a whole roster of new friends, the farmers up and down the valley who made each day not just possible but delicious.

That's the sweet world on the other side of the ruinous system we now rely on. Getting there won't be easy—these are entrenched powers, and it will take more than individual actions to uproot them; it will take real political involvement. But food is the right place to begin. Three times a day, we're reminded of what is, and what could be. What *will* be, if we have the good sense to pay attention to Anna Lappé.

—BILL McKIBBEN

INTRODUCTION
Why This Book?

Sometimes the *Onion* really lands a headline.

Still barely into the research for this book, I stumbled on this one: "Fall Canceled After 3 Billion Seasons." Yes, you remember fall, don't you? That "classic period of the year," the *Onion* quipped, that "once occupied a coveted slot between summer and winter"?

As I was chuckling to myself, I looked out of my window to see November snow slowly drifting downward. It was true. There had been no fall this year. Here in Brooklyn, we had gone from balmy to bitter from one day to the next. If future winters are anything like this last one, daffodils will bloom in Central Park in January.

As more of us have become aware of the climate crisis and its ramifications for life as we know it, these weather reflections have come to seem all the more ominous. And as we have become more aware of the climate crisis, usually dubbed the innocuous-sounding "global warming," we have come to understand that the future will bring even greater weather extremes, possibly the loss of earth's climate as we've known it.

It seems many of us have at least one specific memory, a totem, of the way weather was. For me, it was during a winter more than fifteen years ago. My mother still lived on forty-five acres in southern Vermont in an old barn she had converted into a home—the horse stalls were her library. (The family joke: from horsesh** to bullsh**.)

It was Christmas eve and the snow had fallen in heaps. Born and raised in California, my brother and I, then in college, still regressed at the sight of snow. Decked in our warmest layers, we dashed out of the house, heading straight for an old logging trail on the property. We had a vision: our very own luge run.

The plan was simple and foolproof. My brother would dig; I would be the test pilot. It was a straightforward routine. He carved into soft snow with a red metal shovel, and I sailed down the newly created path. Where my sled flew off, he'd build up the embankment. We continued this way for hours. I would trudge up the hill. Head down the slope. Soar over the not-quite-high-enough edges. There would be more digging, more climbing.

Finally, as the sky darkened through the tall pines, we had the perfect run: a smooth ride down the mountain. All you had to do was hang on, close your eyes, and trust the banks. As night came, we ran into the house to get our flashlights so we could find our way back up the hill after slipping down the mountain sightless.

Christmas morning, my mother got up early, before the rest of us, and sailed through the white, white snow.

It has never snowed enough since in that spot in southern Vermont to repeat the adventure.

I know climate scientists tell us we have to take the long view, not look at changes just over a decade (or even a few). They also tell us we can't draw conclusions from our personal anecdotes. A sample size of one does not a crisis make. (And of course, this personal story is nothing compared with the climate-change tragedies impacting millions a year.)

But while we each may have our own story, or stories, collectively we've got more than anecdotes. We've got data. Unless you've spent the past year in a Hummer with the air conditioner on full blast, you know that those scientists who used elaborate modeling to predict climate chaos were on to something. The scientific consensus is that the climate crisis is real—and we humans are responsible.

Virtually every new report paints a more dire picture. New evidence is showing that carbon dioxide in the atmosphere has reached an eight-hundred-thousand-year high, and in mid-2009 Massachusetts Institute of Technology scientists reported that without immediate action the rise of global temperatures in this century will likely be twice as severe as estimated just six years ago.[1]

Perhaps no one feels the impact more powerfully than the farmers. My first research trip for this book took me a short distance from my home, to Glynwood, a farm and education center on 225 acres in New York's Hudson Valley. I got to sit in on a meeting for farmers with NASA's Goddard Institute for Space Studies' Dr. Cynthia Rosenzweig, a leading expert on climate change and agriculture. The farmers were sharing their own stories of change already happening on their farms and were hearing from Rosenzweig about changes yet to come.

I'll never forget the audible gasps from the two dozen New York State farmers gathered on that cold December day when Rosenzweig explained the significance of a slide glowing on the screen in front of them. Pointing to an arrow sweeping south from New York, Rosenzweig said, "If we don't drastically reduce greenhouse-gas emissions by 2080, farming in New York could feel like farming in Georgia."

"It was all projections before. It's not projections now; it's observational science," she continued, adding that we're already seeing major impacts of climate change on agriculture: droughts leading to crop loss and to soils ruined by salt accumulation, flooding that leaves soils waterlogged, longer growing seasons bringing new and more pests, and erratic weather shifting harvest seasons.

Researchers recently predicted that by 2100, higher temperatures in regions home to roughly half the world's population, stretching across Africa, India, and southern China and covering Australia, the southern United States, and northern Latin America, will see corn and rice harvests drop by as much as 40 percent.[2] And remember that grain, especially these two, provides almost half the calories human beings eat.[3]

When people think "climate change and food," many go first to exactly what Rosenzweig focused on that day: the impact of climate change on farming. I certainly did. Yet when it comes to the inverse—how the food system itself is heating the planet—a lot of us (that'd be me, too, before this book) draw a blank.

Challenged to name the human factors that promote climate change, we typically picture industrial smokestacks or oil-thirsty planes and automobiles, not Pop-Tarts or pork chops. Yet the global system producing and distributing food—from seed to plate to landfill—likely accounts for 31 percent or more of the human-caused global warming effect. According to the Food and Agriculture Organization of the United Nations' seminal 2006 report, *Livestock's Long Shadow*, the livestock sector alone is responsible for 18 percent of the world's total greenhouse gas emissions. That's more than the emissions produced by the entire global transportation system—every SUV, steamer ship, and jet plane combined.[4] (Emissions from transport represent just over 13 percent of total emissions.)[5]

Move over Hummer. Say hello to the hamburger.

Asked what we can do as individuals to help solve the climate crisis, most of us could recite these eco-mantras from memory: Change our lightbulbs! Drive less! Choose energy-efficient appliances! Insulate! Asked what we can do as a nation, most of us would probably mention promoting renewable energy and ending our dependence on fossil fuels. Few among us would point to changing the way our food is produced or the dietary choices we make. (Though this awareness, as you'll read in these pages, is starting to spread.)

Unfortunately, the dominant story line about climate change—the sectors most responsible for emissions and the key solutions to reducing those emissions—diverts us from understanding not only how the food sector is a critical part of the problem, but also, and even more important, how it can be a vital part of the much-needed solutions.

If the role of our food system in global warming comes as news to you, it's understandable. We've been getting the bulk of our information about global warming from reporting in mainstream newspapers, magazines, and documentaries. For many among us, Al Gore's 2006 Oscar-winning documentary *An Inconvenient Truth* was the wake-up call. In concert with this record-breaking film, Gore's train-the-trainer program, which coaches educators to share his presentation, has alerted tens of thousands more to the threat, but it offers little help in making the connection between climate change and the food on our plate.

Mainstream U.S. newspapers haven't been doing much better at covering the topic. Johns Hopkins University researchers analyzed climate-change coverage in sixteen leading U.S. newspapers from September 2005 through January 2008. Of the more than four thousand articles on climate change published, only 2.4 percent addressed the role of the food system, and most of those only mentioned it peripherally. Just half of 1 percent of all climate-change articles had "a substantial focus" on food and agriculture.[6]

Internationally, the focus hasn't been that different. Until recently, much of the attention from the global climate-change community and national coordinating bodies was also focused on the energy sector, on coal-fired power plants, and heavy industries—not on food and agriculture.

All this is finally starting to change.

By the second half of 2008, I was beginning to see articles covering the topic in publications that spanned from *O* magazine to the *Los Angeles Times* to *Etihad Inflight* magazine, the first publication to cover my work on this book. (I considered this a great moment of media irony, that the inflight magazine for the national airline of the United Arab Emirates—not exactly an eco-business—would be the first to cover this book on climate change.)

In September that same year, Dr. Rajendra Pachauri, the Indian economist in his second term as chairman of the United Nations Intergovernmental Panel on Climate Change (IPCC), minced no words: "In terms of immediacy of action and the feasibility of bringing about reductions in a short period of time," said Pachauri in a speech in England, choosing to eat less meat or eliminating meat entirely "is one of the most important personal choices we can make to address climate change."[7]

By the time I read Pachauri's bold call to action, I had been thinking, talking, and writing about the food-and-climate-change connection for some time, always with three questions in mind: Why does our food system play such a significant role in heating our planet? How can food and farming be part of the path toward healing the globe? And what can we do to be part of the solution? From these three questions, this book emerged . . . along with a profound sense of hope.

Here's why.

When I started exploring the food system's role in global warming, I quickly realized that, as with many other climate-change conundrums, most of the solutions are known. Yes, every day we're learning more, but the basic directions are clear.

Plus, I had already disabused myself of the idea that our global industrial food system was "working." For my previous two books, I'd had to face its failure to nurture healthy people or healthy ecosystems. Now, as I saw the food system's climate cost as well, I began to think that just maybe this crisis could provide additional motivation to usher in more sane ways of farming and eating.

As I learned about what a climate-friendly food system looks like, I learned that its methods not only reduce greenhouse-gas emissions but also help us pull carbon dioxide out of the atmosphere. With more than twice as much carbon stored in our soils than in the planet's living vegetation, turning our focus to the soil is critical.[8] I learned that implementing climate-friendly solutions—including agroecological and organic methods—creates even more beneficial ripples: preserving biodiversity, improving food security and people's health, strengthening communities, and reducing reliance on diminishing oil reserves. Plus, we create a more resilient food system, one better able to withstand the inevitable weather extremes.

In addition, looking squarely at the intersection of food and climate change offers each of us power, specific actions we can take. We eat every day. (I don't know about you, but I can't say the same for buying appliances, changing lightbulbs, or driving a car.) And possibly most exciting, the focus on food helps us see how the billions of people across the globe who still live on the land—and go by the name of farmer, rancher, pastoralist, or peasant—are no longer a "problem" to be solved, but among our great, untapped resources in the fight against climate change.

These are just some of the reasons to be hopeful. But this book isn't just about hope; it's also about how we humans have managed to make something that should nourish us—food—into one of the biggest environmental disasters of our era.

In part I, "Crisis," I share with you how the food on our plates has become such a contributor to global warming and give you a glimpse of the forces pushing us along this climate-destructive path.

In part II, "Spin," I explore why we've missed this key part of the climate-change story and how the food industry is waking up to the fact that it won't remain out of the climate crosshairs for long. In this section, I take you inside a meat-marketing shindig in Nashville; a Grocery Manufacturer Association conference in a swank Washington, D.C., Ritz-Carlton; and other industry get-togethers to share how the industry is framing the connection between the environment and its business. I give you a rundown of six plays from the industry spin book and offer some examples of how the industry is starting to capitalize on the nascent awareness of connections between the food sector and global warming.

In part III, "Hope," I head to the fields. Away from the PowerPoints and media releases, we hear about the solutions emerging from the land: from the soil, the crops, and the farmers who are cultivating a food system that is resilient, restorative, and regenerative—that pleases our sense and senses.

My hunch is that some of you might think this sounds pretty pie-in-the-sky. I've anticipated your skepticism; or, the skepticism you will soon encounter as you begin to talk with others about food and climate change. So, I share tips for confronting the main myths fomented by naysayers, focusing on several core and interlocking ones: the inevitability myth, the false-trade-off myth, the poverty myth, and the prosperity-first myth. I also tackle perhaps the two biggest myths of all: that hunger will be the price we pay if we move away from industrial agriculture and that biotech crops, not agroecological methods, hold our best hope for feeding ourselves in a climate-unstable future.

In part IV, "Action," I deliver a recipe for making change, for what we can do as citizens and eaters. You'll find seven principles for a climate-friendly diet and inspiring stories about going beyond our forks to be part of a global movement that is shifting our planet toward sustainability.

On my first research trip for this book, I got a serious dose of pop culture's take on our doomed future. Over the course of a cross-country trip to Seattle, I devoured Cormac McCarthy's postapocalyptic downer *The Road*. The next night, I stayed up late in my hotel room watching New York City disappear under ice in *The Day After Tomorrow* and Will Smith defend himself against a world gone mad from a virulent virus in *I Am Legend*. I then curled up with a stack of articles about global warming. As I read, I found all were drumming home the same message: If we don't reduce our greenhouse-gas emissions to 80 percent below 1990 levels, at the very minimum, by 2050, we're in big, big trouble. All of the authors were then quick to add that not only are we failing to come close to this fundamental task, but we're emitting *more*, not less, carbon dioxide every year.

Made me think Will Smith might not have had it so bad after all.

As I sank into these documents, I found myself getting depressed, even getting close to numb. That is, until I turned back to this project—and to food. There is real power in our forks, I've discovered. There is hope here. We feel it once we see ourselves connected to people creating food systems that are nourishing—nourishing for us and the earth. And we feel this connection in one of the most simple acts we perform every day: eating.

No, we need not feel paralyzed by the scale of this unprecedented global challenge. Indeed, by turning our sights to food, we may just find the integrating lens—and grounding source—for bringing to life the real solutions already before us.

I like fall. I've been really missing it here in New York. Now, after uncovering the power of the food system to be a player in redressing the most overwhelming of threats to our species, I think maybe, just maybe, the *Onion* found a good punch line, but not a prophecy.

HOW TO READ THIS BOOK

I wrote this book for anyone interested in the food on their plate and the sky up above. No prior knowledge of climate-change science is required.

I myself am not a scientist. I see my job as distilling insights and analysis from some of the world's best scientists to help you understand these complicated ideas. While I'm at it, I should add: I'm no farmer, either. I relied on the valuable, on-the-land experience of farmers who shared their experience with me so that I could, in turn, share it with you.

As with many nonfiction works, you can jump in and around this book wherever your curiosity takes you. Along with longer chapters, selected sections offer nuggets of info to help you understand the issues and take action. You'll also find a resource guide, containing recommended books, films, and Web sites, and a selected bibliography for further learning and ideas to take action.

In addition, the endnotes include all the obligatory info—journal names, Web sites, etc.—as well as suggested additional reading to help you dive in further.

Finally, this book, though printed on immutable paper in permanent ink—is a work in progress. I encourage you to offer suggestions, corrections, or ideas by visiting the book's Web site, www.takeabite.cc, and getting in touch.

ANNA LAPPÉ
Brooklyn, New York

DIET FOR A HOT PLANET

I
CRISIS

1

THE CLIMATE CRISIS AT THE END OF OUR FORK

PRELUDE TO A CRISIS: A TASTE OF A CLIMATE-FRIENDLY FARM

By the time I pull into Full Belly Farm, the rain has started to come down in sheets. I creep down a mud lane, past an orchard-in-waiting (it's not quite fruit season yet) toward a towering barn, a few houses, and a low-lying office. A two-hour drive east of San Francisco, Full Belly is nestled inside the Capay Valley. A flat, gently sloping depression twenty miles long and a few miles wide, Capay was created by the faulting of the surrounding ridges. Having separated from the coastal range at a glacial pace, it's now a haven to dozens of organic farms.

Lucky for me, I arrive in time for lunch. Before I get my tour of the farm's 250 acres, which will take me to the lambing sheep and acres of walnuts, fennel, broccoli, cauliflower, and some ninety other crops, I get to eat. And eat we do. Today, it's miso egg drop soup with mushrooms, freshly baked bread, hand-wrapped California rolls, and a huge salad with orange slices and goat cheese from down the road. Apparently, the feast is typical. Five days a week, the live-in staff and interns, volunteers, and often neighbors chow down on lunches like this one. Full belly, indeed.

I'm here to see firsthand what a thriving sustainable farm looks like, one that's gotten unhooked from an addiction to the fossil fuels and petroleum-based chemicals that define industrial farms. All while employing as many as sixty people and producing abundant food, every month, directly for the more than fourteen hundred families who are farm members, plus the many thousands more who find Full Belly's food through farmers' markets, restaurants, retail stores, and wholesalers.

This farm is a model of energy thoughtfulness—as opposed to energy-use recklessness. The founders are constantly looking for ways to decrease their dependence on fossil fuels, from experiments with biodiesel to the solar panels they just installed.

The farm is also a model for a thinking farm; it's a work in progress. Since they started it in 1989, the founders, husband and wife Dru Rivers and Paul Muller and Judith Redmond and her husband at the time, Raoul Adamchak, have continued to discover new ways to tap nature's wisdom. Take the sheep.

On my post-lunch tour, Rivers shows me the inner workings of the farm's complex ecosystem. We start with the ewes, and I decide there is nothing cuter than newborn lambs snuggling up to their baa'ing mothers.

The animals began as quasi pets. (Rivers likes to spin wool.) Today, they are vital to what makes the farm work so well. The two hundred sheep have gone well beyond pet status, becoming productive members of the farm. They weed and prep the soil; they fertilize. One day, they'll hang out on a just-harvested field of broccoli, eating what's left—the leaves and stems—and spreading their manure as fertilizer while they do. The next day, they'll be led out to a new and needy section of the farm.

To steer clear of soil-degrading and ecosystem-poisoning chemicals, Rivers and her co-farmers are constantly searching for innovative alternatives such as the alyssum, which they recently learned about. Sown between strawberry rows, this flowering plant attracts beneficial insects that help keep the harmful ones away—by eating them before they cause any damage.

And they keep learning. The Full Belly founders recently set up homes for owls, whose appetite for mice, rats, and gophers does wonders for rodent control. And thanks to advice from the Department of Agriculture's Cooperative Extension and the handiwork of local high school students, the crew was inspired to install nearly a dozen dwellings for bats on barns and buildings across the farm. Now, at dusk hundreds and hundreds of bats cavort through the night, devouring colossal quantities of insects that would otherwise harm the crops.

As I leave Full Belly, I get one last glimpse of Nellie, one of the farm dogs, dashing through a field on the hunt for gopher holes. With my windows rolled down, I hear the birds singing as they dart in and out of the trees. From my rearview window, I spot nine-year-old Jonas, the son of one of the farm owners, in his blue raincoat, hunched over a dirt bike, sloshing through the mud beneath the craggy walnut trees.

Navigating through the rain, I'm daydreaming about fuzzy lambs and really good soup when I turn a bend and see it: the Cache Creek Casino. The sprawling complex—casino, hotel, and parking garage—has dark windows that reflect the hovering gray clouds. My curiosity gets the best of me, and I detour into the five-story lot, pulling in between a vehicular California schizophrenia: a Hummer on one side and a Prius on the other.

As I descend onto the windowless gambling floor, those farm sounds—of buzzing bees and chirping birds, kids laughing and dogs barking—are replaced, faster than you can say, "Ante up," by the clanking and beeping and whirling of slot machines and roulette wheels. The farm's wet, refreshing rain is swapped for a haze of cigarette smoke. I don't last long.

Back in the car, I turn left onto Winner's Lane—yes, that's what those clever casino builders really named it—and drown out the on-again rain with a local radio station. A familiar tune fills the car. It's the Counting Crows' interpretation of Joni Mitchell's 1970 classic.

"Don't it always seem to go," Adam Duritz croons, "that you don't know what you got 'til it's gone / They paved paradise and put up a parking lot."

As I listen to the lyrics, I think about Rivers's husband, Muller, who grew up on his family's dairy farm until he was fifteen, when his parents could no longer keep it. The farm was the last dairy standing in San Jose. Rivers and Muller recently visited the spot. Where forty years ago there was a family farm, there is now a Kmart and a strip mall.

I turn back for one final look at the gargantuan Cache Creek Casino. Paving paradise, indeed.

THE BIG PICTURE: THE CLIMATE CRISIS AT THE END OF YOUR FORK

I started with this story, both the bummer of Cache Creek and the uplift of the farm, because as I sat down to write, I couldn't get that day out of my head. What you're about to read in this opening chapter isn't the good news; it's the bad. Yet as I wrote, my mind kept circling back to the *other* story. I kept thinking about Rivers and Redmond and about farms like Full Belly, thriving even in the face of casino sprawl. I found myself repeating the words of people you'll soon meet: farmers like

Mark Shepard in Wisconsin and food cooperative leader Seong-Hee Kim in South Korea, local-food activists like Jessica Prentice and real-food advocates like Tim Galarneau. I found myself picturing that thriving farm outside Seoul where I stood with dozens of small-scale food producers from across Southeast Asia as they regaled me with tales of their abundant, fossil-fuel-free farms.

My mind, in other words, was holding two plotlines at once. And we must. The one you'll read first concerns our climate-disrupting industrial food system. But never for a second forget that there is another story, a story that makes up much of the rest of this book. It is of a food system that is tapping nature's wisdom to heal the climate. From the rainforests of Indonesia to the erosion-marked ravines of Oaxaca, Mexico, this other food system is alive and well. It might not register on the S&P 500 or fill the shelves of Walmart, but it is building on the way that billions of people still procure their food and many more will—if together we create the conditions that will allow it. In this story, people are retrieving wisdom we'd almost lost and drawing on new break-throughs in ecological science.

Over the past ten years, I have had the opportunity to visit farms that embody this other food system, from the picturesque foothills of the Himalayas in India to a postindustrial Brooklyn neighborhood a few miles from my apartment. Visiting these farms, I sometimes had to pinch myself to remember that we are fast careening in the opposite direction—toward a largely industrialized food system, with its dead-end addiction to fossil fuels and synthetic chemicals. This industrial food system is hell-bent on bigger, faster, cheaper and has rarely had to pay attention to its true costs—to the soil and water, the welfare of the animals, the health of farmers and farmworkers, or the climate.

But increasingly, the world over, people are waking up to the real price of our industrial food system. Thanks to a plethora of popular books and films, including Eric Schlosser's *Fast Food Nation*, Michael Pollan's *The Omnivore's Dilemma*, the 2009 documentary *Food Inc.*, and scientific reports from venerable institutions like the United Nations' Food and Agriculture Organization (FAO), more and more of us are aware of the "dark side" of an industrial food system that has gone global. We're also beginning to comprehend the climate costs.

Today, as I write these words, my memories of Full Belly Farm are still so vivid I can picture the lambs clumsily taking their first steps and taste the savory miso soup. What I dubbed at the time a *sustainable* farm, I now realize is a *climate-friendly* one, a farm that taps natural systems to guarantee that we are all fed—and that our planet stays cool.

In this chapter, I want to help you understand how we've come to be the one species on the planet that has discovered not only how to make itself sick with the food it produces (think exploding rates of diet-related-diabetes and obesity), but also how to undermine the very resources on which it depends, particularly a stable climate. I'll help you draw a line between your pork chop, your Pop-Tart, and the rising mercury on the planet's thermometer, taking you through the food chain. It's a chain of events we tend to be blind to when we pull up our shopping carts to the cereal aisle to ponder whether we'll go for Special K or Honey Toasted Oats.

I want to start, though, with a healthy serving of caveats and a dash of definitions. As you read about emissions from the food system, remember that we have much to learn. Emissions from soils, for instance, differ wildly not just from farm to farm but *within* a farm. Emissions from livestock manure fluctuate dramatically depending on, for example, how and where it's stored. Across much of the globe, we also have only spotty data about many aspects of food system emissions. We will need much more investment in life cycle assessments of our food to grasp the precise foodprint of our diet choices.

Getting to Know Your Greenhouse Gases

When we hear about global warming we mainly hear about carbon dioxide emissions, for good reason. Human-caused emissions of the gas account for 76.7 percent of all man-made greenhouse gases in the atmosphere.[1] But other greenhouse gases matter, especially two: methane and nitrous oxide, both of which have a direct connection to the food chain, particularly livestock production. Though the livestock sector contributes only 9 percent of global carbon dioxide emissions, it is responsible for 37 percent of methane and 65 percent of nitrous oxide emissions.[2]

One reason these other greenhouse gases are so worrying is their effectiveness in trapping heat—just what we don't want them to do. To help simplify the climate-change conversation, these warming influences are expressed in carbon dioxide equivalence (or CO_2eq) based on the

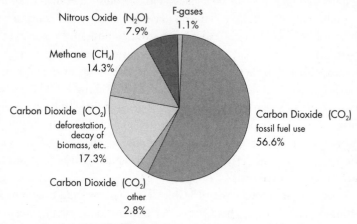

Share of Man-Made Greenhouse Gases in Total Emissions
in terms of carbon dioxide equivalence

From the International Panel on Climate Change, Fourth Assessment Report, "Synthesis Report"

global warming potential (GWP) of each gas over a one-hundred-year period. Methane, for instance, has a GWP of 23, meaning it traps heat twenty-three times more effectively than carbon dioxide over the course of a century. Nitrous oxide has a global warming potential of 296.[3]

Seems significant, right? It is. But this timescale actually downplays the impact of these gases on our atmosphere today, says Professor of Global Environmental Health at the University of California at Berkeley Kirk Smith. If you consider the GWP of methane during its first five years in the atmosphere, a tonne (metric ton) of methane turns out to be responsible for almost *one hundred times* more warming than a tonne of carbon dioxide. That's because methane breaks down much faster in the atmosphere than carbon dioxide (about eight-and-a-half years compared with many decades), so a shorter time-horizon emphasizes the greater impact of the gas. Indeed, Smith likes to call methane "carbon on steroids."[4]

You'll also hear me talk about the potential for agricultural soils to store carbon, in the form of complex organic compounds and inorganic carbonates. This process, removing carbon dioxide from the atmosphere and storing it as carbon mass in soil, is called carbon sequestration. One tonne of carbon stored in soils is equivalent to 3.66 tonnes of carbon dioxide.[5]

Key Greenhouse Gases

Main Greenhouse Gases	Global Warming Potential *relative to carbon dioxide over 100 years**	Percent of Total Emissions *expressed in carbon dioxide equivalence*
Carbon Dioxide (CO$_2$)	1	76.7%
Methane (CH$_4$)	23	14.3%
Nitrous Oxide (N$_2$O)	296	7.9%
Sulphur hexafluoride (SF$_6$)	22,800	Less than 1%
Hydrofluorocarbons (HFC)	As much as 12,500	Less than 1%
Perfluorocarbons (PFC)	As much as 9,200	Less than 1%

* Global warming potentials from IPCC, Fourth Assessment Report (2007)

Gases named under the Kyoto Protocol. The protocol established legally binding commitments from signatory governments for reduction of key greenhouse gases.

COME OUT, COME OUT, WHEREVER YOU ARE: THE MODERN FOOD SYSTEM AND GLOBAL WARMING

In 2007, the Nobel Committee awarded the Peace Prize to the IPCC and Al Gore for "their efforts to build up and disseminate greater knowledge about human-made climate change, and to lay the foundations for the measures that are needed to counteract such change."[6] About a decade earlier, the United Nations had charged the IPCC with evaluating the risk of human-caused climate change, and the panel's reports since then have synthesized the state of the science as laid out in peer-reviewed climate-change literature. By 2007, the IPCC had concluded unequivocally that concentrations in the atmosphere of the main greenhouse gases—carbon dioxide, methane, and nitrous oxide—had increased markedly as a result of human activities since

1750. And already we're seeing dramatic climate changes, with ice caps melting at twice the rate that scientists were predicting even a few years ago.

How do the various sectors in our economy rank in terms of worst offenders? According to the IPCC breakdown, 26 percent of total emissions comes from energy supply, 19 percent from industry, 17 percent from forestry, 13.5 percent from agriculture, 13 percent from transportation, 8 percent from residential and commercial buildings, and 3 percent from waste and wastewater.

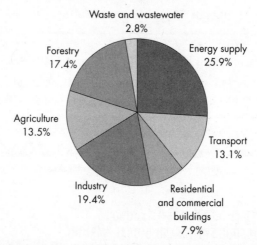

Breakdown of Emissions by Sector
in terms of carbon dioxide equivalence

From the International Panel on Climate Change, Fourth Assessment Report, "Synthesis Report"

So where's food?

You couldn't be blamed for assuming that the food chain, at most, contributes just 13.5 percent of total emissions—that would be the agriculture pie slice. Hiding in the IPCC breakdown, though, are the ways in which the food system is connected to climate change within *nearly every sector of our economy*. Peel the onion of this pie—while you excuse the mixed metaphor—and you'll see that the food system is, well, everywhere.

The Food Chain and Greenhouse Gas Emissions

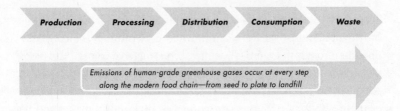

| Production | Processing | Distribution | Consumption | Waste |

Emissions of human-grade greenhouse gases occur at every step along the modern food chain—from seed to plate to landfill

Add all these slivers together—including emissions from the production and distribution of farm chemicals, from land as it's transformed to make way for crops and livestock, and from energy for factory farms and food processing—and the entire global food chain may account for roughly one third of what's heating our planet. As I mentioned in the introduction, livestock production alone is responsible for as much as 18 percent of the global warming effect.

These emissions stem from radical changes in how and where we produce food that have occurred just in the past one hundred years—and picking up pace much more recently. There's nothing "conventional" about this kind of food.

While the abrupt buildup of heat-trapping gases is brand-new, carbon dioxide, methane, and nitrous oxide are natural parts of carbon and nitrogen cycles in the food system. Since New Guineans developed taro production eight thousand years ago and the Chinese started growing rice four thousand years ago, methane has been released during food cultivation. Since ruminants like cows evolved to chomp grass, these animals have emitted methane in the natural process of digestion. The difference today is in the scope and scale of livestock production—and in crops and animals that are no longer raised within a food system that takes its cues from nature. The consequences have been dire.

In this chapter, I want to help you understand the emissions along the food chain. Though I'll primarily focus on production, which creates the bulk of agricultural and food-related emissions, I'll also trace the stages of processing, distribution, consumption, and waste, and I'll highlight how transportation adds to emissions at each of these stages.

FACTORIES IN THE FIELDS: A REVOLUTION IN HOW WE PRODUCE OUR FOOD

Trace back the roots of the global warming crisis and you'll stumble on the first Industrial Revolution, when coal mining, the construction of railroads, and rampant deforestation triggered colossal emissions of carbon dioxide into the atmosphere. As early as 1896, Swedish chemist and physicist Svante Arrhenius published the first warnings of these activities' potential consequences, including a planet getting hotter because of human-caused emissions of carbon dioxide.[7] But as we've seen, the buildup of heat-trapping gases really took off only about sixty years later. It was then, in the mid-twentieth century, that agriculture secured its place in the global warming spotlight—as we further tapped fossil fuels to expand food production, especially with the growing use of synthetic fertilizer. Fossil-fuel-based food production seemed ever more appealing after World War Two and the opening of the East Texas oil field pipeline brought oil prices down.

By the end of the Second World War, new technologies—from warplanes transformed into crop dusters to chemical weapons morphed into agricultural pesticides—were further pushing the path of industrialized food. As these technologies, bolstered by government policy, made monoculture row-crop farming cheaper and cheaper, the seed of another revolution was born: that of industrial livestock, with their massive animal feedlots.

Most observers of this transformation credit "cheap" grain with inspiring the takeoff of feedlots. But keep in mind that grain's low cost, making profitable its conversion into feed, reflected, and still does, a world of extreme poverty. If the billions of people living primarily on grain have little money to make their need felt as demand in the marketplace, grain can *look* really cheap—especially when its price doesn't reflect the costs of environmental damage.

Together with other dramatic changes in our global food system, these radical and recent shifts have turned the food and farming system, which could, as you'll learn, be a force mitigating climate change, into a key force fueling this crisis.

Sadly, this path could have been avoided, if we'd listened to the many who have anticipated these consequences, including American ecologist Howard Odum. Born in 1924, he witnessed the beginning of the industrial agricultural revolution and was not fooled. In 1970, he chided "industrial man [who] imagined that his progress in agricultural yields was due to new know-how in the use of the sun." No, said Odum: "This is a sad hoax, for industrial man no longer eats potatoes made from solar energy; now he eats potatoes partly made of oil."[8]

The Story of Soil: Synthetic Fertilizer and Climate Change

Today is nearly one hundred years from the day a key ingredient of industrial farming got its start. It was July 2, 1909, and chemical giant BASF sent two of its technical specialists, Carl Bosch and Alwin Mittasch, to visit the lab of Fritz Haber, a chemist at Berlin's Kaiser Wilhelm Institute. BASF had heard that Haber was on the brink of discovering a way to transform atmospheric nitrogen into ammonia, an essential component of fertilizer.

According to one account, before Haber could show off his breakthrough, a piece of essential equipment broke.[9] Haber labored through the afternoon and into the night to fix it. By then, Bosch had left in disappointment. The next day, Mittasch—who'd stuck it out—was among the first in the world to witness the landmark success. Seventy drops of ammonia a minute started to drip from Haber's invention. A handful of drops of ammonia may sound measly, but it foretold a revolution and BASF knew it. All that was now needed to do was figure out how to scale up—turn drops into tons—and we would have a detour around one of nature's seemingly insurmountable limits: soil fertility.

Since the advent of agriculture, farmers have innovated practices to build soil fertility, from rotating crops and using leguminous crops that naturally bind atmospheric nitrogen, to feeding the soils with plant and animal waste. BASF was seeking a way to industrialize nitrogen-based fertilizer production, making it no longer reliant on these natural farming methods. But this was no small feat. Despite its abundance in our atmosphere, nitrogen gas is challenging to bind into usable nitrogen; it requires just the right catalyst and enormous pressure.

With Haber's invention in his hands, Bosch, the BASF specialist, set to work on figuring out how to scale up. Fast-forward three and a half years and much experimentation later. By the winter of 1913, Bosch's design was producing hundreds of tons of ammonia for fertilizer.[10] (For

Exploding Nitrogen Production
in the second half of the twentieth century

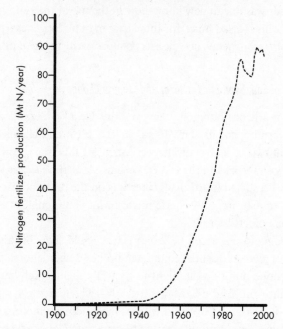

Based on graphic from Vaclav Smil, Transforming the Twentieth Century (New York: Oxford University Press, 2006)

this and other innovations, both men would go on to earn Nobel Prizes in chemistry and be credited with helping to feed a growing planet.)

The Haber-Bosch process fundamentally remade farmers' relationship to soil and agriculture's impact on climate. Since the process is so energy intensive—producing just one ton of fertilizer requires as much as thirty-three thousand cubic feet of natural gas—it locked soil fertility into a dependence on fossil fuels.[11] (The discovery had another, much darker, consequence. Ammonia isn't only useful for soils. Ammonia nitrate is also a key ingredient in explosives. So, in a strange twist, it would rewrite the First World War—prolonging the war, resulting in many more deaths. And, nearly a century later, aid the deadly tragedy in Oklahoma City. Timothy McVeigh's bomb used five thousand pounds of it.)

A few words about soil might help you grasp the consequence of what Haber and Bosch came up with. Living far from the land, many of us might think of soil as something inert that holds up plants. Wrong.

Healthy soil is alive—a handful hosts billions of living organisms, most too small for us to see. They interact with decaying roots, stems, leaves, and added composting material, such as manure, food waste, and straw. Like a sponge, this healthy organic matter retains moisture and nutrients.

The organic matter is the key. It prevents the soil from becoming solidified, so that air and water can reach the roots and so the roots can penetrate the soil. Soil's organic matter is also a source of food for bacteria, fungi, yeasts, insects, and earthworms. Without these living organisms, plants can't thrive. These tiny creatures convert unusable organic nitrogen into ammonia and nitrates that plants can use; they "fix" atmospheric nitrogen so it's available to plants and produce acids that make soil minerals accessible, too. Microorganisms also help plants take in critical nutrients, and they prey on disease organisms that might hurt the plants.

Yes, synthetic fertilizer can up yields, but it doesn't build this essential organic matter. Because synthetic fertilizer allows farming practices that don't nurture the soil—fertility is bought, not fostered—industrial farms can neglect the soil and other principles of natural farming, including crop diversity, and still see high yields.

The advent of synthetic fertilizer was just one key in the mechanization of farming that has fostered industrial-scale, energy-intensive farms on a chemical treadmill. As soils are neglected, organic matter degrades, microorganisms die, root systems weaken, all of which makes soils less able to retain water and crops more vulnerable to drought and disease and erosion, requiring ever more irrigation, pesticides . . . and fertilizer. By 2008, global production of nitrogen fertilizer had ballooned to 139.8 million tons.[12]

As a result of industrial farms' degraded soils, we're now losing topsoil in the United States many times faster than nature is making it. We've long known the consequences of lost topsoil, now we know the climate cost, too. As soils are depleted, stored carbon is released as carbon dioxide.

In addition, as nitrogen fertilizer is applied to soils, the fertilizer breaks down, releasing nitrous oxide. Globally, synthetic fertilizer use is responsible for more than three-quarters of agriculture's total nitrous oxide emissions.[13]

In addition to these emissions, consider the climate cost of fertilizer production, mostly reliant on natural gas or, in China's case, coal.

China's synthetic fertilizer industry is responsible for emitting 14.3 million tons of carbon dioxide from coal-fired power plants annually, a quarter of the world's total from fertilizer production.[14]

Also, because fertilizer inputs—potash, phosphate, nitrogen—are often manufactured or mined far from where they're used, add transportation emissions into the calculation, too. From net exporter, the United States has become a net importer of fertilizer, bringing in as much as two thirds of the nitrogen, and four fifths of the potash, our farmers use.[15] In 2007, more than half of the potash, phosphate, and ammonia came from just four countries: Canada, Russia, Belarus, and Morocco.[16] (Next time you hear corn-based ethanol advocates celebrate the energy independence we supposedly achieve with their product, remember they're handily ignoring our dependence on imports of the fertilizer ingredients and on the fossil fuel used in producing corn.)

On top of this, an estimated half of all nitrogen fertilizer applied to cornfields in the United States is not even taken up by the crop. It is lost through nitrate conversion into gas, by leaching into the soil and our waterways.[17]

Too much nitrogen has simply overwhelmed natural cycles. "We've taken the preindustrial nitrogen cycle and doubled it," said Dennis Keeney, a soil scientist who grew up on a farm in Iowa. "The system isn't set up to keep cycling that nitrogen: it just goes back out again. This shows up as acid rain, nitrates in the water, and nitrous oxide emissions."[18]

Where has this industrial model taken us?

Farmers' yields went up, increasing supply, which has pushed prices down. So farmers have had to produce still more just to scrape by. The already better off grew by squeezing out their neighbors, so that average farm size climbed steadily. In this way, the industrialization of production has played a key role in making possible an increasingly centralized farm economy—both among farmers and suppliers. And over the past century, U.S. farm policy has only tilted the playing field further to the benefit of a handful of multinational companies, chief among them grain traders ADM and Cargill. The companies are the price makers; farmers are the price takers.

Increasingly dependent on a small number of giant suppliers of agro-chemicals for their growing needs on one side, and giant grain traders to buy their product on the other, many farmers have had little choice but to follow the advice of Nixon's secretary of agriculture, Earl Butz, and "Get big or get out." And here we are today. Large farms, those with sales of at least a quarter of a million dollars—make up only 8.6 percent of total U.S. farms but account for 80 percent of total sales.[19]

Breaking free from this consolidation of power and downward cycle for farmers, the soil, and the climate means a lot of rethinking and re-making of our food system. And now's the time, for this industrial monopoly model, especially its over-production of corn, lies at the heart of two major forces driving greenhouse gas emissions from food: the livestock revolution and the explosion of processed foods.

Before going there, though, let me share with you another techno-logical innovation of the twentieth century that helped spawn this climate-destructive aberration in food production.

Chemical Soup: Agricultural Chemicals and Global Warming

Remember the German chemist Fritz Haber of fertilizer fame? His in-ventiveness with ammonia won him a Nobel Prize, but the same genius he'd applied to growing he soon applied to a quite different challenge.

On April 22, 1915, at the dawn of the First World War, the com-mander in chief of the British army cabled London with troubling news. Pilots were reporting thick yellow smoke billowing from German trenches. "What follows almost defies description," Sir John French ca-bled. "The effect of these poisonous gases was so virulent as to render the whole of the line held by the French Division . . . incapable of any action at all . . . Hundreds of men were thrown into a comatose and dying condition."[20]

French's missive was one of the first reports of chemicals used in warfare—in this case developed under Haber's direction. After the war, the use of chemicals that had been developed under wartime mandates was applied to agriculture. The synthetic pesticide, DDT, first synthe-sized in 1874, was used widely during the second half of World War Two to kill typhus-carrying lice and malarial mosquitoes. After the war, it be-came a popular tool for fending off pests on farms. A few decades later, at the end of 1972, it would be banned in the United States after Rachel Carson's *Silent Spring* popularized its toxicity to wildlife and people.

While DDT is perhaps the most widely known toxic pesticide, it is not the only one, and toxicity is not the only problem man-made pesticides pose for our planet. (Don't let the word "pesticide" fool you; the term includes herbicides, fungicides, and other substances harnessed to control pests.)

First, synthesizing these chemicals requires significant fossil fuel energy. Second, the use of chemical pesticides can erode farmers' incentives to rely on agroecological approaches for managing pests and weeds. Third, the chemical approach to farming allows farmers to plant monocultures—large swaths of land growing just one variety of crop—instead of relying on plant diversity to help address the threat of pests. Finally, keep in mind that most synthetic pesticides are petroleum-based, so factor in the fossil fuel reserves used in these chemicals. While the Environmental Protection Agency estimates that 1.2 billion pounds of active ingredient pesticides are used annually in the United States—20 percent of the global total—we can only guess at the total volume of petroleum in these pesticides since companies aren't required to divulge the "inert" ingredients in their products.

These are just some of the ways that synthetic pesticides and fertilizers have made agriculture both more susceptible to climate change and increasingly responsible for it.

The Meat of the Matter: The Livestock Revolution

Once twentieth-century agricultural innovation enabled farmers to produce industrial-scale crops, especially corn and soy, what to do with it all in a world of widespread poverty? Agribusiness soon found the answer in a massive expansion of processed foods, especially feedlot meat—itself largely a form of processed corn and soy.

Traveling to Brazil a few years ago with my mother, we had a very personal encounter with the meat revolution.

My mother has been a vegetarian since Nixon was president, *The Partridge Family* hit the little screen, and Jimi Hendrix played his final jam. I've been one on and off since I was a teen. So I suppose we could be forgiven for not knowing what we were getting ourselves into when our Brazilian interpreter took us to a classic *churrascaria* in Curitiba. When we first arrived, we thought we had entered a vegetarian's paradise. The restaurant's centerpiece was a buffet stuffed with every salad you could dream of: beet and red onion, spinach and olive, Greek salad with huge chunks of feta. We piled our plates high. It only started to dawn on us that we were missing something when our interpreter and his guest returned with empty plates.

Then the meat arrived. It came in all shapes and sizes. It came on long steel rods piercing dozens of roasted medallions. It came in vibrant red and maroon, in pink and burnt burgundy; it arrived as filet mignon, pan-roasted chicken, and pork tenderloin. The meal felt like a culinary version of the classic circus trick, but instead of clowns climbing out of an impossibly small car, our average-sized interpreter consumed a giant's portion of meat. Maybe we should have anticipated all-you-can-eat meat being served in the heart of Brazil, for the country has recently become one of the world's largest meat exporters.[21]

Today, livestock production is one of the biggest contributors to the country's greenhouse-gas emissions, both from pastures and from feed-crop production, from smallholder farmers to large-scale ranchers to multinational companies. The deforestation driven by pastureland and cropland is only one reason livestock contribute so much to global warming, as we'll see.

Globally, livestock account for as much as 18 percent of all global greenhouse-gas emissions, according to the U.N. study mentioned earlier. That figure includes almost one tenth of carbon emissions, more than one third of methane, and roughly two thirds of nitrous oxide. (Livestock is responsible for other polluting emissions as well, including two thirds of all human-made ammonia.)[22]

All told, 70 percent of all agricultural land in the world is tied up with livestock production.[23] But livestock don't need to cause such ecological harm. Traditionally and still today, in much of the world, livestock have been integrated into diverse farms and their communities, playing a range of roles: providing companionship, manure to enrich soils, muscle for farm work, and a source of protein as meat. Like those sheep on Full Belly Farm, livestock can be an integral component of sustainable systems. Well-managed livestock can even nurture the land. All that stomping and tromping helps to press seeds into the earth, fostering plant growth. The action of hooves on the ground can also break up the soil, allowing in more oxygen and improving soil quality. Today's self-described "carbon farmers" are adopting these proven practices and mimicking time-honored grazing methods to increase carbon content in the soil.[24]

But modern production practices have diverted us dangerously away from this sustainable relationship between livestock, human beings, and the farm. Indeed, today's livestock production contributes to global warming at virtually each step in the process. The consequences are colossal.

Oh No, CAFO!

Every year, for the past twenty-six, Lexington, North Carolina, has hosted a monthlong Barbecue Festival. In addition to joining in a 5K Hawg Run or a Hawg Shoot Air Rifle Tournament, you can sit back and watch a parade of pigs on bicycles. This city of twenty thousand calls itself the Barbecue Capital of the World—fitting, since it's smack-dab in the middle of a state that has become the U.S. capital of the environmental costs related to some of the nation's four-legged inhabitants: hogs, ten million of which are raised in North Carolina every year.[25]

How this state vaulted to the number-two spot, after Iowa, in hog production, captures the larger story of the transformation of the meat industry, at home and abroad, and its impact on climate.

There was nothing inevitable about North Carolina's becoming America's pig capital; the state doesn't have what economists might call natural "comparative advantage" in producing hogs. No advantage, that is, unless you count the low taxes, weak unions, lax regulation, and high poverty rate.[26] This environment appealed to pork producer Smithfield—that and the state's pressing interest in finding alternatives to its disappearing tobacco industry.

As Smithfield expanded in North Carolina in the 1980s and '90s, it transformed hog production from small-scale farming to large-scale factory operations. This transformation reflects nationwide trends. At the beginning of the twentieth century, typical hog farms were home to one hundred to two hundred hogs, mostly raised on pasture and fed grain as a supplement. By 2000, virtually all hogs were raised in confinement, and two thirds of U.S. facilities housed at least two thousand hogs.[27]

Relatively speaking, the pork industry was late to the consolidation game. By the 1990s, poultry and beef production had already concentrated into the hands of a few multinational companies, shifting control from independent producers to companies that control most aspects of the supply chain, from breeding to slaughter and processing.

In 1990, the top four beef packers controlled 72 percent of the market and the top two, nearly half. By 2007, Tyson, Cargill, Swift & Co. (now owned by Brazilian company, JBS), and National Packing Co. controlled 84.5 percent of beef packing operations. In the business of broilers (non–egg laying poultry), Pilgrim's Pride, Tyson, Perdue, and Sanderson Farms controlled 58.5 percent of the market.[28]

Today, most livestock production in the United States occurs in these factory farms, called Concentrated Animal Feeding Operations (CAFOs). CAFOs are defined by the Environmental Protection Agency (EPA) as facilities that confine animals for at least forty-five days a year and do not raise their own feed. "Large" cattle CAFOs house one thousand or more animals, and "large" hog CAFOs house twenty-five hundred or more. Poultry operations aren't technically deemed "large" until 125,000 or more birds are in confinement.[29]

By 2000, CAFOs not only reigned in the United States but also were rapidly expanding across the planet. Spreading into Europe, Japan, and the Soviet Union in the 1970s, by the late 1990s the largest meat companies were moving into "global peripheries," including emerging markets like Poland and Romania. CAFOs are increasingly common in east Asia, Latin America, and west Asia. Globally, industrial livestock production is growing twice as fast as traditional farming systems and more than six times as fast as pasture-based animal production.[30] It already accounts for nearly three quarters of global poultry production, two thirds of egg production, and nearly half of all pork.[31]

The shift from family-scale production, with animals integrated into the farm, to megascale confined feedlots has had enormous climate-change implications. First, there's the somewhat obvious energy connection: The scale and methods of industrial livestock operations depend on enormous energy inputs, including the energy required to heat and cool CAFOs, light and ventilate them, and deal with the waste. But there are a host of other ways CAFOs are costly to the planet; I detail the key ones here.

The Kernel of the Crisis: The Feed

In CAFOs, livestock are taken off pasture and traditional sources of nourishment and raised, instead, on diets of soybeans, corn, and other feedstuffs. The result?

- Globally, one third of the world's cereal harvest, including half of all corn and 90 percent of all soy, is now diverted to feed animals on factory farms.[32]

- In the United States, 80 percent of soy and as much as two thirds of our corn goes to feeding animals, not people. Nearly 50 percent goes to supplying domestic feed, and another 19 percent is exported, with much of that going to feed livestock abroad.[33]*

- More than two thirds of available agricultural land worldwide is used for animal production, from raising livestock to producing feed.[34]

- Roughly a quarter of the world's fish catch ends up as feed for livestock or farmed fish.[35]

Producing these feed crops has a serious climate toll. Environmentalists are particularly concerned about carbon dioxide released from rainforests that are destroyed to make way for pasture and cropland in hotspots like the Brazilian Amazon, one of the world's most vital carbon sinks.[36] Today, as much as three-quarters of Brazil's greenhouse gas emissions stem from deforestation, largely the result of agribusiness expansion. According to a study by Greenpeace International, most of the soybean raised today for export as feed for cattle, broilers, and hogs is being grown on deforested land. Greenpeace estimates that just three agribusiness giants, Archer Daniels Midland (ADM), Bunge, and Cargill, are responsible for financing 60 percent of this soybean production.[37] (In a response, one of the companies fingered, Cargill, claims that "nearly all" of its soy exported from Brazil is grown outside of "the Amazon biome in Mato Grosso.")[38]

Remember these names: These three companies control 80 percent of the world market for soybean processing and they are connected to many other aspects of our modern food system. ADM is the world's largest ethanol producer; Bunge is the largest fertilizer manufacturer in South America; and Cargill is among the biggest palm oil importers into the United States and a major player in the global grain market.[39]

---

* For a great film about the dominance of corn on America's farms and in its foods, check out the documentary *King Corn*.

Feed crops also depend heavily on fossil fuels to power on-farm machinery and irrigation and to produce the chemicals needed to protect against pests, stave off weeds, and foster soil fertility.[40]

Remember all those consequences of synthetic fertilizer I mentioned? Well, in the United States and Canada, half of all synthetic fertilizer is now being used to raise feed crops.[41] In the United Kingdom, the total is nearly 70 percent.[42]

Add all these factors together and half of all the energy in agriculture—including the manufacturing of fertilizers and the planting, harvesting, processing, and transportation of feed in intensive animal production—goes to producing feed, whether fish meal or crops.[43] Industrial poultry and swine together consume nearly half of all fish meal and oil.[44]

As you think about the direct and indirect emissions from feed production, also consider the staggering inefficiency of industrial livestock operations. Under industrial production, livestock returns to us humans in edible meat only a fraction of the resources it consumes. While ruminants such as cattle could naturally convert inedible-to-humans grasses into high-grade protein, feedlot cattle consume as much as sixteen pounds of grain and soy to provide us with just one pound of beef.[45] (The USDA puts the figure at seven to one.) Keep these numbers in mind the next time you hear about the wonders of our "efficient" food system.

Manure Blues

In sustainable systems, animal manure isn't a problem. It is not "waste." Instead, manure is an essential asset on the farm: It fertilizes the soil, helping to foster the pasture and forage that animals depend on as well as the crops.

In industrial livestock operations, it's a different story.

A 1995 investigative series in Raleigh, North Carolina's *News & Observer* painted a damning picture of the waste crisis triggered by the state's hog revolution:

Imagine a city as big as New York suddenly grafted onto North Carolina's Coastal Plain. Double it. Now imagine that this city has no sewage treatment plants. All the waste from 15 million inhabitants are simply flushed into open pits and sprayed onto fields. Turn those humans into hogs, and you don't have to imagine at all. It's already here.[46]

With every hog producing two to four times as much waste as the average human, by the mid-1990s hogs in North Carolina were generating as much waste as all the people living in North Carolina, California, New York, Texas, Pennsylvania, New Hampshire, and North Dakota combined.

The sheer volume of waste in industrial-scale operations is too much to cycle back through the system, a challenge made all the more difficult because CAFOs tend to be far from where feed is grown. Instead, manure from hog CAFOs is mixed with wastewater and stored as a liquid in manure "lagoons." When I hear "lagoon," I think Brooke Shields and tropical islands, not excrement. The term "cesspit" seems more apt. And these cesspits can be massive; a typical hog CAFO can be home to one that stores millions of gallons and be as large as several football fields.

In cesspits and manure holding tanks, microorganisms break down organic matter anaerobically—that is, without oxygen. As they do, they decompose and convert the manure, as well as other waste, like bedding material, into methane, carbon dioxide, and other gases. Because methane isn't soluble in water and carbon dioxide is only sparingly so, both gases enter the atmosphere as rapidly as they're generated. In contrast, in small-scale systems manure can be a beneficial addition to the farm and because it breaks down with oxygen it releases much less methane.[47]

These emissions partly explain why CAFO cesspits spell trouble, while a sustainable farm's cow patties don't. But livestock waste on CAFOs presents other big problems, too: There's the issue, for instance, of manure runoff leaching into surrounding waterways—worrisome when it's common for wastewater to include phosphorus, ammonia, pathogens, and other pollutants.[48]

As a result of the growing scale of CAFO operations, methane emissions are soaring. In just the past fifteen years, methane emissions from dairy-cow manure in the United States have jumped by half, and from pig manure, by nearly two thirds, according to data from the EPA.[49]

Thanks to CAFO cesspits, the United States has the dubious honor of being a world leader in man-made methane emissions.[50] China beats us, though, in methane emissions from manure. It's responsible for nearly one fifth of the total.[51]

Munching a Bunch: Methane and Ruminants

There's another connection between livestock and global heating: the methane released as ruminants, such as cattle, buffalo, sheep, and goats, digest. They can't help it. These animals digest by enteric fermentation, in which microbes and enzymes break down carbohydrates in the first of four stomachs, the rumen (why they're called ruminants). Think of it like an internal fermentation vat. The animals then regurgitate the "cud," re-chewing it to break it down even further. This explains why if you've ever stumbled on a field of grazing cows, they all seem to be in a constant state of chewing.

Heard any of those not-so-funny-anyway jokes about global warming and cow farts? Jokes aside, they've got it backward. Ninety percent of the methane ruminants produce comes out their *other* end, through their mouths and noses.[52]

While enteric fermentation enables ruminants to turn fibrous grasses into protein, something we humans can't do, it also contributes to their climate-change impact. Today, enteric fermentation from dairy cows and cattle on pasture and in CAFOs is a major source of methane emissions worldwide. In some countries it is the single most significant source of the gas.[53] In the United States, enteric fermentation is responsible for nearly a quarter of all methane emissions.[54] Globally, emissions from enteric fermentation constitute 27 percent of total methane. In New Zealand, 85 percent of methane emissions comes from the country's ruminants.[55] A year's worth of methane emissions from a typical Kiwi two-hundred-cow dairy herd has the same carbon dioxide equivalence, according to one estimate, as I would attain driving my Toyota Prius—if I had one—from New York to San Francisco and back forty-five times![56]

(Rice cultivation is another key source of agricultural emissions of methane—and a significant one in some developing countries. According to the IPCC, 82 percent of the world's methane emissions related to rice production came from south and east Asia.)

Out to Pasture

Livestock grazing has expanded so dramatically that today it uses a quarter of the ice-free terrestrial surface of the planet.[57] And grazing, if not well managed and at a reasonable scale, leads to soil compaction and erosion, which releases carbon stored in the soil into the atmosphere.[58] To some extent, livestock have degraded about one fifth of the world's pastures and rangelands, reports a U.N. study, and as much as three quarters in particularly dry areas.[59]

Note that for millennia, until only the last century or so, humans raised livestock using low-intensity grazing, which helps maintain soil fertility, nurturing the soils in semiarid regions. But as colonization—and in the past fifty years, World Bank and International Monetary Fund policies—pressed developing countries to industrialize farming and focus on export crops, stresses on land increased. Pastoralists were pushed off traditional grazing grounds, marginal lands were exploited, land was increasingly overgrazed—and pasture-fed livestock turned into another environmentally destructive practice.[60]

The process has been especially intense in Latin America, where nearly three quarters of formerly forested land in the Amazon has been reduced to pasture. (Feed crops cover much of the remainder.)[61] Indeed, pressures on land from livestock, for feed or pasture, have been the largest factor in Latin America's deforestation, and it's picking up its pace. Greenpeace researchers estimate that 79.5 percent of deforested land in the Amazon is now being used for cattle ranching, with the final products destined for markets in the European Union.[62]

The Real Population Boom

All the environmental impacts of livestock I've described so far are compounded by their sheer number. We see a lot of hand-wringing about the *human* population boom, but it pales in comparison to livestock's population explosion.

In 1965, eight billion livestock were alive at any given moment; ten billion were slaughtered annually. Today, thanks in part to CAFOs, whose heavy dosing of growth-promoting antibiotics and fattening on feed spur growth and thus shorten lives, twenty billion livestock animals are alive at any one time, and more than fifty-six billion are slaughtered for human consumption annually, not including fish and seafood.[63] Compare these staggering figures with human population growth over this same period: In 1965, 3.3 billion people called earth home; today, 7 billion do. In other words, there are nearly eight times as many animals slaughtered each year for food as there are humans on the planet—and the livestock population, especially poultry, is growing at rates much faster than ours.

Biodiversity Bungle

If you're with me so far, there should be no mystery about why livestock play a starring, startling role in the heating of our planet. But, it turns out, this sudden livestock revolution has not only exacerbated global warming; it has also made us more vulnerable to it.

As livestock production spreads, it undermines the very biodiversity of the flora and fauna we need more than ever to cope with climate change. Livestock now make up 88 percent, by volume, of all wild and domesticated animals combined. Pigs make up 39 percent of this total volume; poultry, 26 percent; and cattle, 23 percent.[64] Their breeding for human consumption has focused on just a few species of these animals, further diminishing biodiversity.

Plus, as feed-crop production spreads, so does a similar homogeneity. Corn, by weight, is the world's most significant crop, and soy ranks fourth—a dominance that will only increase as CAFOs do. As we face a climate-uncertain future, biodiversity is our best insurance policy. We are only beginning to learn about which crop and animal varieties might be the most resilient and best adapted to coming climate conditions. Undermine this biodiversity; undermine food security.

In addition, as small-scale farmers are squeezed out of production, losing market share to the mega-operations, the planet loses another kind of diversity: the agricultural knowledge living in farmers around the world of the unsung ways to farm in harmony with nature.

The Pringles Problem: Processed Foods and the Planet

Large agribusiness companies understand one thing for sure: Processing is profitable. The margin on Pringles sure beats what's possible selling potatoes. Customers are willing to pay four dollars a pound for a product that's only 40 percent potatoes and 60 percent fillers, when they could buy a pound of potatoes for a dollar. Even "classics" like Coca-Cola, which first entered the market in 1886, have received a twentieth-century, processed-foods face-lift. After the 1970s invention of high-fructose corn syrup provided a sweet (and cheap) alternative to sugar, Coke switched its formula. By the mid-1980s, sugar was out; corn was in.[65]

Even old standbys like fruits and vegetables are now mainly delivered after serious processing. By 1999, half of all vegetables bought in the United States were canned, frozen, or dried, and nearly half of the fruit we consumed was in the form of juice.[66] And as I've just described the vast majority of the meat in our refrigerators—from the bacon to the burgers—came from animals raised on factory farms, in close confinement and fed on diets that include genetically modified corn and soybeans.

Typical supermarket shelves are now lined with processed products bursting with multisyllabic ingredients like high-fructose corn syrup and preservatives and additives. Each step required to make these processed foods, and their multitude of ingredients, adds to the climate-change toll. Compared with whole fruits and vegetables, legumes and grains, processed foods require more energy to be produced—from the chemical fertilizers needed to grow the corn-based sweeteners to the synthetic compounds used to ensure that Twinkies stay moist; from freezing, canning, drying, and packaging the products to making the additives and preservatives. In particular, processed-foods ingredients like palm oil carry with them a high emissions toll.

Plus, chances are, the more processed the product you're eating, the less you will know, or be able to know, about the ingredients. I don't mean to pick on the Pop-Tart, but it's an easy target. The energy history of this breakfast classic is just one example of the climate impacts embedded in processed foods. You may be surprised to learn all that goes into making these so-thin-they-fit-into-your-toaster treats. Among the ingredients are gelatin, made from by-products of the meat and leather industries; sodium pyrophosphate, commonly used in household detergents as a water softener; monocalcium phosphate, a leavening agent typically found in bird and chicken feed; tert-butylhydroquinone (TBHQ), a preservative, also found in household varnishes and lacquers; and three different artificial colorants, including Red No. 40 (banned in

Denmark, Belgium, France, and other European Union countries because of concerns about its impact on human health). The list goes on.

To get from household-varnish ingredient and chemical additive to a tasty treat requires intensive processing, and the energy required to power and operate the manufacturing plants adds to the emissions toll of every Pop-Tart. One manufacturing plant that journalist Steve Ettlinger visited to trace Twinkie ingredients for his exposé *Twinkie, Deconstructed* almost fills one square mile. That's roughly sixteen and a half football fields, and the plant uses enough electricity to power 160,000 homes.[67]

Add in the energy required to produce the packaging to wrap the individual Pop-Tarts, the Pop-Tart boxes, and the distribution boxes they are shipped in. We must also add the emissions from transporting all the ingredients to where the product is made. Consult the *Food Technology Buyer's Guide* and you'll find twenty-eight companies to source the Pop-Tart's gelatin, from Taipei, Taiwan, to Tampa, Florida. The monocalcium phosphate? The guide lists three manufacturers, including two in China. Looking for a source of that TBHQ? Try one of sixty-one companies, twenty of which are based in China. And sodium pyrophosphate? Only one manufacturer is noted; it's in China, too.

In addition to those far-flung ingredients, it's anyone's guess exactly where the Pop-Tart's six corn-based ingredients (corn syrup, cornstarch, etc.) originate, or the leavening agents, the citric acid, and the colorings, like Blue No. 1 and Yellow No. 6.

There's still more to the climate impact of processed foods, including another facet I was blind to until I began this research: the spread of palm oil.

Trouble in Paradise

Pick up a box of Quaker Chewy Granola Bars, Pringles, or Philadelphia cream cheese, and global warming is probably pretty far from your mind. But these treats—along with a plethora of other popular products, including cosmetics, soaps, shampoos, and fabric softeners—share a common ingredient: palm oil. As the push for processed foods has skyrocketed, so has the demand for these ingredients.

In the last decade, the production of palm oil has more than doubled.[68] Today, palm is the most widely traded vegetable oil in the world, and demand is soaring in India and China.[69] This demand is coming from manufacturers of cookies and crackers, yes, but roughly half the world's supply—twenty million tons—is being diverted to fuel.[70]

Palm oil's origins trace back to west Africa, where it was produced on a small scale for local markets. In the mid-1800s, Dutch colonists introduced the oil in Java, and in the early 1900s, the British did the same in Malaysia. By 2008, 87 percent of the world's palm oil originated in Malaysia and Indonesia. As palm oil (and pulp and paper) plantations expand in these countries, the consequences for the climate are dramatic.

Here's why. To establish plantations, producers raze rainforests and drain peatlands, often forcibly taken from communities. These peatswamp forests are home to towering trees, sometimes as high as fifty meters and—below the water's surface—vast stores of peat, dead plant material accumulated over millennia. When these swamps are drained, the peat becomes exposed to air and the carbon gets oxidized, releasing carbon dioxide. Then, once dry, these lands become susceptible to fires that can burn for months on end. As Lafcadio Cortesi, forest campaign director at Rainforest Action Network, explains, "when peatland is destroyed, it's not just one hit of lost carbon. There's that big hit when you drain the peatland, but the hit is felt year after year."[71]

Though peatlands cover just 0.2 percent of the earth's surface their destruction is associated with 8 percent of total global emissions, estimates Wetland International, an advocacy group.[72] Typically, you'll see Indonesia ranked twenty-first in global emissions. Factor in carbon dioxide emissions from drained peat land and the country jumps to number three, says Wetlands International.

Peatland in just one Indonesian province, about the size of 2 percent of U.S. arable land, stores so much carbon that were it all destroyed the emissions would equal a year's total—for the entire planet.[73] Travel there and this loss will be immediately evident. On a recent trip to Indonesia, Cortesi described one four-hour drive through the heart of palm oil production: "It was like driving across Iowa, except instead of corn, you see palm—a vast green desert."

While small-scale farmers still grow some oil palm in Malaysia and Indonesia, private companies are rapidly displacing them. In Indonesia, two thirds of palm plantations are now owned by just ten companies.[74] Agribusiness giants, Archer Daniels Midland and Cargill are among the biggest purchasers. ADM is a significant investor in Wilmar, the world's largest palm oil producer.[75] Multinational Cargill is the biggest importer of palm oil into the United States where its oil ends up in the products of some big-name food and consumer-product companies—Unilever, Procter & Gamble, General Mills, to name a few.[76]

Many of the biggest players dismiss the climate concerns, arguing that the Roundtable on Sustainable Palm Oil (RSPO), established in 2004 by industry and international non-profits, is ensuring sustainable production through guidelines and certification programs.[77] While many environmental advocates would agree the roundtable is a step in the right direction, serious questions remain about who is setting standards and monitoring practices. Says RAN's Cortesi, "The RSPO faces many of the same problems other certification systems do: Who is policing them? Right now, the companies are doing it themselves."

Plus, even if there were improvements in production practices, mounting demand means climate trouble. The question we should be asking about palm oil, similar to the question to ask of cattle and corn, is not just how can we produce these foods to reduce the impact on the climate, but how much should we produce. And the answer? Says forest advocate Cortesi, "Let's not just let the biggest companies make that decision. Let's look to science. Let's have justice and rationality guide our decision making. Let's ratchet down production and global demand. Then we can talk about sustainability."

MILES TO GO BEFORE I EAT: THE REVOLUTION IN FOOD TRADE AND TRANSPORT

Herman Daly, an economist and environmentalist (an unlikely combo, I know), enjoys truth telling with an edge. The United States imports Danish butter cookies, says Daly, and Denmark imports butter cookies from the United States; "the cookies cross each other somewhere over the North Atlantic." Trade proponents celebrate this exchange as "expanding the range of consumer choice to the limit," writes Daly. "But could not those gains be had more cheaply by simply trading recipes?"[78]

We've traded food, of course, for millennia, even before Syrians were cooking with Indonesian cloves more than five thousand years ago, but figures from the last century confirm that food trade is growing faster than ever and is expected to keep surging. In the generation between

1968 and 1998, world food production increased by 84 percent, but world food trade increased at nearly twice that rate, climbing a whopping 184 percent.[79]

It's now not unusual to see Chilean grapes in grocery stores in California, Australian dairy destined for Japan, or Twinkies toted around the world. To get a gut sense of the magnitude of the fossil fuel wasted in food transport, visualize this: To transport just one year's supply of out-of-state tomatoes to just one state, New Jersey, takes enough fossil fuel to drive an 18-wheeler around the world 249 times.[80]

Globally, international trade in meat is also rapidly accelerating and with it food-related emissions. For unlike, say, potato chips, meat requires energy-intensive conditions: it needs refrigeration. Just since 1995, U.S. meat exports have soared, with pork exports jumping fourfold.[81]

Food transportation has serious global warming consequences, including the emissions of carbon dioxide and other gases from the refrigeration that's often required. Surprising to some, though, is that the amount of transport-related food-system emissions is relatively small compared with the contribution of food production. Even so, it's important to pay attention to food transport: For one thing, it is rapidly increasing, making its contribution to global warming increasingly significant. For another, many food-transport emissions would be relatively easy to address: I'll go out on a limb here and argue that a lot of this schlepping is unnecessary.

For example, before you pay more for water than gasoline, and up your personal global warming toll, put your gourmet bottled water to a test against what comes out of your kitchen faucet. Then ask yourself, do we really need to be shipping water into the States from Fiji? When Fiji water ads boasted, "FIJI, because it's not bottled in Cleveland," that city ran tests that compared it with municipal samples. It turned out that Fiji water fared worse; it contained arsenic as well as higher levels of contaminants.[82]

Or consider that the United States exported 1.9 billion pounds of beef and veal in 2008 and that same year imported 2.5 billion pounds of the same.[83] Yet have you ever met an American who could taste the difference? Sure, we might be able to detect the difference of some of this trade: a burger from Arby's might not quite stand up to Kobe beef from Japan. But mostly, we could cut back on this global meat swap and not even notice. At least our tastebuds wouldn't. And yes, in some cases, it may be a shorter ride to import food from Mexico or Canada than to tote across our big country, but in general it's safe to say that much of the explosion in global trade is not helping us; it is heating us.

In addition to the obvious emissions from the import and export of food (or bottled water), other transportation emissions are hiding within our modern food system. Consider that on those CAFOs I described, feed has to be shipped in, sometimes from halfway around the world. In the hog CAFOs in Poland that you'll soon learn about, farmers who formerly fed livestock homegrown food (or food waste) now mostly import feed, including genetically modified soybeans from Brazil. Add to this the hidden cost of toting live animals to CAFOs. In 2007, the United States imported nearly 2.5 million young cattle destined for feedlots and 10 million starter hogs from Mexico and Canada.[84]

Finally, there are other, even more hidden ways in which food transport impacts climate change. Emissions result, for example, from constructing and repairing the infrastructure—the highways, railways, and roads—that carries our food across countries and around the world.

WALMART AND THE WEATHER: THE REVOLUTION IN WHERE WE SHOP

Early one cold morning, on the way to meet farmers in Poland's Tatra Mountains, I was on the hunt for food. Our beat-up rental car turned the bend of a tiny road, following the signs for Carrefour, a sort of European Walmart, where you can buy everything from wedding rings to wallpaper and sometimes the staff even don roller skates, the better to speedily scurry down the long aisles. As we rounded the bend, we saw the vast parking lot and the throngs gripping shopping carts, waiting at attention for the sliding doors to open and the buying to begin.

Carrefour, Walmart, Tesco, Ahold . . . the list goes on. The trend of getting our food from ever-more-centralized megamarkets is taking hold globally.[85] In Latin America, for instance, before the 1980s only 10 to 20 percent of national food sales could be traced to supermarkets.[86] Today, the market share is closer to 80 percent, nearly as high a concentration as in the United States.[87] And the same pattern is emerging in other regions around the world. In China, over just five years, from 1995 to 2000, sales from Western-style supermarkets jumped more than six-fold.[88] (In contrast, during that same period we in the United

States witnessed only a 10 percent bump, maybe because our neighborhoods and strip malls are already saturated.)[89]

This trend is having staggering climate consequences, not only from moving food through supermarkets' long supply chain to their shelves but also from the open-air cooling cases typical in grocery stores—with no doors for fear of blocking eager, grabbing hands.[90] Indeed, grocery stores, food markets, and convenience stores emit more greenhouse gases per square foot of floor space than any other type of commercial building.[91]

A 2008 study by the United Kingdom's Environmental Investigation Agency (EIA) found that supermarkets were the country's largest source of hydrofluorocarbons (HFCs), greenhouse gases that are as much as ten thousand times more potent than carbon dioxide.[92] Globally, supermarkets represented nearly a quarter of the emissions of these gases, and the IPCC predicts that, unless there is a big shift in practices, these emissions will triple from 2002 to 2015.[93]

While data on HFC emissions in developing countries is spotty, the EIA's Fionnuala Walravens says she would not be surprised if they dramatically increased there in coming decades. Currently, many supermarkets in developing countries still use equipment that emits hydrochlorofluorocarbons (HCFCs), the ozone-depleting gases that the Montreal Protocol banned. "As these countries are required to phase out their use of these ozone-depleting gases in the next ten years," Walravens says, "the obvious alternative is, unfortunately, turning to global-warming HFCs."

The good news is that some countries are beginning to adopt climate-friendly policies to reduce the use of these gases. The EIA gives a shout-out to Norway and Denmark for taxing HFCs, based on their per-ton carbon-dioxide-equivalent emissions. Says Walravens, "These kinds of policies have helped the market move over to alternatives by putting a carbon cost on using HFCs." Too bad, she adds, U.K. supermarkets "have been slow to make the shift."

CHOMPING ON THE CLIMATE: THE REVOLUTION IN WHERE WE EAT

In any given month, more than half of all Americans will find themselves uttering some version of "Can I get fries with that?" In a recent survey, roughly one third of Americans polled said they'd dined at Subway, Burger King, Taco Bell, or Wendy's in the past month, a quarter had indulged at KFC, and about half had been to McDonald's.[94] In the past fifty years, we've radically changed not only what we grow, how we grow it, and where we shop, but also where we eat, adding another factor to the food system's impact on global warming.

In 1977 in the United States, only 16 percent of all meals and snacks were eaten away from home. By 1995, this number had risen to 25 percent. Between 1995 and 2000, the number of fast-food joints in Morocco jumped 20 percent; in Thailand, 40 percent. Both Indonesia and China saw a roughly 120 percent boost in Western-style fast-food outlets.[95] In just five years!

While the growth in fast food consumption—and eating out more generally—is most associated with the rising incomes of the better-off in our increasingly unequal world and, of course, with the massive amounts of advertising directed at us, these diet changes also reflect big changes in where people live, with more and more people moving to cities. Back in 1960, just one in three people globally claimed a city as their home; today, the figure teeters at half, with much of this increase in developing countries.[96] Many of the newly urbanized people in these countries were family farmers who had raised much of their own food.[97] As they are pushed into cities, fewer people are producing their own food, and fewer farmers are growing food in proximity to cities; both factors further dependency on a climate-intensive food system.

Unless we shift course, this planet-heating trend will continue. But many are challenging the trend by making rural life rewarding—from those in thousands of new rural Brazilian communities, many growing crops organically, to the inhabitants of hundreds of renewed villages in Niger who are successfully turning back the desert.[98]

Wasted

There's a final reason why the modern food system is responsible for nearly one third of global warming gases: waste. Globally, an estimated 3.6 percent of total greenhouse-gas emissions comes from waste and wastewater, mainly methane and secondarily nitrous oxide. One source is our food chain; some municipalities report that food waste makes up as much as half of what's in their landfills.[99] And in

The Climate Crisis at the End of Our Fork
an overview of emissions along the food chain

Stage	Sources of Emissions	Main Gases Released			
		Carbon Dioxide	Methane	Nitrous Oxide	Other
STAGE 1: Production	***Securing Land***				
	• Destroying forests, wetlands, and other carbon-rich environmental resources.	✱	✱	✱	
	Producing Inputs				
	• Manufacturing synthetic fertilizer	✱		✱	
	• Producing fossil-fuel based pesticides and other chemicals	✱			
	• Mining for fertilizer components	✱			
	• Producing other inputs for livestock production, including hormones and antibiotics	✱		✱	
	• Raising feed crops for livestock	✱		✱	
	• Producing silage or maintaining pasture	✱			
	• Shipping live animals to feedlots	✱			
	• Shipping agricultural chemicals to farms	✱			
	Raising Crops and Livestock				
	• Fueling on-farm machinery and irrigation systems	✱			
	• Degrading soil by abandoning techniques to add organic matter to the land and using agricultural chemicals	✱	✱	✱	

Stage	Sources of Emissions	Main Gases Released			
		Carbon Dioxide	Methane	Nitrous Oxide	Other
STAGE 1: Production (cont'd)	• Fertilizer use and overuse	✴		✴	
	• Cultivating rice		✴		
	• Enteric fermentation		✴		
	• Irrigation systems	✴			
	Raising Livestock in CAFOs				
	• Heating, cooling, powering, and otherwise maintaining livestock facilities	✴			✴
	• Waste management (e.g. manure kept in cesspits)		✴	✴	
STAGE 2: Processing	• Cooking, cooling, rendering, packaging, and other activities for processing meat, dairy, and other foods	✴			✴
STAGE 3: Distribution	• Transportation (domestic and international)	✴			✴
	• Supermarkets (refrigeration, lighting, and more)	✴			✴
STAGE 4: Consumption	• Transporting, refrigerating, preparing, cooking	✴			✴
STAGE 5: Waste	• Transporting waste (food and packaging waste), composting, anaerobic digestion, and incineration	✴	✴	✴	

Adapted from the Food Climate Research Network, a fabulous source of information about everything you ever wanted to know about food and climate change, with links to all the latest studies as well as a vibrant international listserv. Learn more at www.fcrn.org.uk

the United States, landfills are the second largest source of methane, after enteric fermentation—bigger than natural gas, bigger than coal mining, bigger than iron and steel production. Bigger than all of them.

When we think about waste, we should also count what fills our bellies with unnecessary calories. Today in the United States, we produce 3,900 calories for every man, woman, and child, more than twice as many calories as we need.[100] On average developed countries produce 3,309 calories per capita.[101] While some of these calories are explicitly wasted—they never make it to our plates—others are wasted implicitly: they're found in fast foods and junk foods that only serve to add to our waistline, not our health.

HOW DID WE GET HERE?

The climate-intensive food system I've described has taken hold globally at extraordinary speed—only in the past generation or two. But note well: just like Smithfield setting up camp in North Carolina, there is nothing inevitable, or natural—and therefore unstoppable—about this destructive revolution.

It grows from the wild assumption that we can go on indefinitely using finite fossil fuels, and that we could radically disrupt nature's regeneration—degrade and erode soil, pollute water, deforest land, and emit ever-increasing amounts of planet-heating gases—without dire consequences. It grows from rules we humans have created—often called "policies," which can sound so boring that we too often ignore them. In making these rules, global corporate wealth and power have overwhelmed the voices and values of citizens so much that we as taxpayers have even subsidized key pieces of our own undoing.

Probing policies driving the growth of CAFOs, to pick but one example, we discover how an industry that is one of our worst climate-change culprits is actually encouraged by public policies and subsidies. In the United States, livestock producers receive billions in direct payments etched into our Farm Bill, the multi-billion-dollar policy that governs food and farming in this country. From 1995 to 2006, the

Farm Bill doled out roughly four billion dollars in direct subsidies to livestock producers, mostly large-scale ones.[102]

Livestock producers benefit from the Farm Bill in indirect ways, too. Think about the payments to corn and soybean farmers. Between 2003 and 2005, corn producers received a whopping $17.6 billion in subsidies; soybean producers, another $2 billion.[103] Because feed accounts for 60 percent or more of the total cost of production for most CAFO operators, federal commodity subsidies that enable grain and soy prices to fall below the cost of production are a boon to the livestock industry.[104] Since so much corn and soy in the United States is going to feed animals, not people, let's rethink commodity subsidies as *livestock* subsidies, helping the largest meat and dairy producers.[105] Indeed, federal corn and soybean subsidies saved factory farms a total of $35 billion between 1997 and 2005, estimated researchers at the Global Development and Environment Institute at Tufts University.[106]

And after all you've read about the environmental crisis CAFOs create, note that livestock-industry lobbyists succeeded in 2002 in getting CAFOs covered under the Environmental Quality Incentives Program, originally designed to help small-scale farmers reduce pollution. By 2007, CAFOs were receiving as much as $125 million a year from this program alone, estimates a senior scientist at the Union of Concerned Scientists, Doug Gurian-Sherman.[107]

Our tax dollars also expand foreign markets for industrial meat. A Korean brouhaha over U.S. beef? Concerns in Japan about U.S. meat quality? Not to worry, we've got our USDA—and elected officials—on the case. As a U.S. senator, and a member of the Agriculture, Energy, and Veterans' Affairs committees, Ken Salazar, current secretary of the interior, stated in response to pushback from overseas consumers about U.S. beef, "Our ambassadors are stationed abroad to promote American interests . . . I . . . also want to make sure they are promoting American exports, including beef, as aggressively as they can."[108] (Note: My interests and yours seem to be equated with the National Cattlemen's Beef Association.)

Finally, the livestock industry has long benefited from a loophole in our environmental regulations, which classify CAFOs as farms, not factories. Meaning these operations, with their greenhouse-gas-spewing facilities, don't face the penalties or regulations that they should. Though rules on the books require owners to manage safely the closure of manure cesspits, for instance, many are simply abandoned, with few consequences.[109] New state and federal policies are emerging to seal this loophole, but to date there's been nothing with real teeth.

In the next chapter, I expose forces behind this massive food experiment threatening our earth. For a huge part of the challenge in front of us is actually *inside* us: It is demystifying not only how we got here, but also why we're headed where we're headed and the leverage needed to get us back on track.

WHAT HAPPENS ON THE FARM DOESN'T STAY ON THE FARM

Nearly forty years ago and several years before I was born, my mother, Frances Moore Lappé, hit on a powerful insight the old-fashioned way: in the library. It was 1971, and she'd left graduate school at UC Berkeley to pursue the root causes of the hunger epidemic seemingly exploding across the planet. As my mother burrowed into the stacks of Giannini Library, she stumbled on something unexpected. Despite the predictions of global famine we'd been hearing ever since Thomas Malthus first published his famous treatise *An Essay on the Principle of Population* in 1798, the world was producing—and still, by the way, does produce—more than enough food to feed us all, even to make us all chubby.[110]

Soon, her initial question, "Why hunger?," became "Why hunger in a world of plenty?" She came to realize that hunger persists not because of a scarcity of food, but because of a scarcity of democracy. For democracy means, at its very core, that we each have a voice, and none among us would choose to see our families and communities go hungry. For my mother, the squandering of abundance inherent in the industrialized food system, particularly in that modern-day invention the factory farm, was a powerful expression of the lack of democracy.

Over these nearly four decades, we've become even more painfully aware of the high costs of our industrial food system, persistent and spreading hunger being just one. We are well aware that we pay for this food system with lives cut short by diet-related illnesses, including heart disease and diabetes. We pay in polluted waterways, flooded with neurotoxic and endocrine-disrupting farm chemicals. We pay with the lives of workers: farmers in the fields, packers in meat-processing plants. Now, we realize we pay a climate cost as well.

2
THE SHAPE OF THINGS TO COME

A SWIFTLY TILTING PALATE

Swoosh through the sliding glass doors at Beijing International Airport and you'll be greeted by the ubiquitous green-and-white Starbucks mermaid. Head to Sayulita, Mexico, and you'll be sipping your margarita in a country that consumes more Coca-Cola-produced drinks than any other in the world—one and a half eight-ounce beverages for every man, woman, and child, every day of the year.[1] Head to Seoul and you can bet you'll stumble on an Outback Steakhouse. With a surge of this fast-food chain in the city, I got lost returning to my hotel located next to one because I was looking for the *wrong* Outback Steakhouse. There were two on my block.

You are probably aware, and have now seen the numbers, that more and more people across the planet—from Seoul to Sayulita—are eating our industrialized diet of highly processed, high-fat foods and chowing on meat and dairy from industrial-scale operations. Sure, there are still pockets of people who have never sunk their teeth into a Whopper. (In fact, Burger King even exploited these so-called Whopper virgins in a tasteless 2008 advertising campaign.) But throughout the developing world, the dietary revolution that rocked the United States over the past two generations is transforming eating habits, agricultural practices, and bodies, across the globe—change facilitated by the spread of curved yellow arches, a smiling pigtailed redhead, and a chipper Chihuahua.

The trends in meat and dairy consumption alone are staggering. The United Nations predicts that global consumption of meat will have more than doubled from 229 million tons in the early 2000s to 465 million tons by 2050; milk production will balloon from 580 million tons to more than one billion tons, particularly in developing countries.[2]

China's dairy consumption will likely account for nearly half of this growth.[3]

As I explained in the previous chapter, these global diet trends—as well as the trends toward more processed foods and more food trade, period—are intricately linked to our growing ecological foodprint. Based solely on meat- and dairy-consumption projections, the United Nations warns that the "environmental impact per unit of livestock production must be cut by half, just to avoid increasing the level of damage beyond its present level."[4] The IPCC warns that emissions from agriculture will escalate if current diet trends continue, predicting that agricultural nitrous oxide and methane emissions could increase by as much as 60 percent by 2030, relative to 1990.[5]

But as we reflect on the shape of things to come, recall that the future of food is not preordained. While these trends may *feel* inevitable, they're not. They're being coerced into existence.

To understand this fact it helps to identify key forces pushing the climate-destructive food system. In this chapter, I'll share just three of these driving forces: the construction of our appetite for climate-intensive cuisine; the expansion of control over land for intensive food production; and the spread of industrialized meat and dairy.

And remember as you read, our food future is being forged by specific policies, unquestioned assumptions, and corporate decisions—all of which you and I influence.

CONTROLLING OUR APPETITES

We often hear that these modern food-consumption trends simply reflect what people naturally want to eat and drink once markets open and prosperity increases. Like industrial agriculture itself, these diet trends are presented as unavoidable. This is certainly the sentiment of Laurence Wrixon, executive director of the International Meat Secretariat, who says, "Whether you like it or not, there's going to be rising demand for meat."[6] The implication is that any attempt to change these dietary desires would be forcing it down people's throats. As Wrixon is implying—and as we were all taught in Economics 101—the market merely responds to demand. Except, well, it doesn't.

What can a billion dollars buy you? If you're the CEO of PepsiCo, you hope it will buy you a growing chunk of the market in the world's fastest-growing consumer economy: China. During her four-day visit there in November 2008, PepsiCo head honcho Indra Nooyi announced that the company would invest a billion dollars in China as part of its "strategy to expand in emerging markets."[7] Already controlling nearly half the beverage market in China, PepsiCo will use the billion to expand its manufacturing and build up its sales force. A good chunk will also go to good old-fashioned marketing, or, as the company calls it, "brand-building initiatives."[8]

PepsiCo's billion-dollar gamble on China reminds us that desire is constructed—and food companies spend billions to construct it. In 2008, the marketing budgets of the three biggest food and beverage multinationals—PepsiCo, Coca-Cola, and McDonald's—totaled $2.4 billion, roughly equivalent to the gross domestic product (GDP) of Italy.[9] The entire food industry spends many times that amount, making it one of the largest advertising blocs in the world. That's a lot of money to convince us to buy something everyone supposedly already wants.

Execs at U.S.-based multinational companies like PepsiCo have long set their sights on market opportunities overseas. Says the *Wall Street Journal*, "For years, it has been apparent that Coke's signature cola can't grow much on its home turf anymore."[10] Indeed, today Coke gets 80 percent of its profits outside of North America, mostly from China, Mexico, and Brazil.[11] PepsiCo's Nooyi explains, "Where the market growth is spectacular, like China, India, and Russia, we are going to keep investing so that when the music stops, we have a great shot at being up there as the leader."[12]

As these companies spread out globally, they're stepping up their messaging, expanding markets through subtle persuasion and more obvious attacks on cultural traditions. As Benjamin Barber's prescient *Jihad vs. McWorld* explains, Coca-Cola is well aware that "thirst cannot be manufactured but taste can."[13] So how do you get a population to desire your product? "Consumption has to be associated with new 'needs,' new tastes, new status," writes Barber.[14] In India, the company opted for "aggressive investment" in advertising. The advertising served to pave the way for a Coke habit by undermining traditional (and healthier) ones, including that oh-so-terrible ritual of tea drinking.

THE SHAPE OF THINGS TO COME

"Getting people off . . . of tea," Barber underscores, "entails a cultural campaign."[15]

Some in the United States might think that no one, simply no one, once given a taste of Coke or cheeseburgers, would ever go back to samosas and mango lassis. But perhaps that's because our taste buds are indoctrinated early. It might seem we naturally gravitate to Froot Loops and Cap'n Crunch, but we too get a nudge from marketers. Friendly characters like SpongeBob and Tony the Tiger lure us in our early years. That's probably obvious. Less obvious is the sophistication of the persuasion: Marketers have even studied how young children perceive the world and created packaging appealing to youthful eyesight.[16] Children, research has shown, respond most to longer-wavelength colors, like reds, yellows, and oranges. What colors do you think are featured most prominently on sugary-cereal boxes?

We also have new evidence that branding can be so powerful that it actually changes how we perceive taste. Neuroscientist Read Montague conducted taste tests pitting Coke against Pepsi. In the blind test, Montague found he could tell, based on MRI observations of brain activity while participants were drinking the two sodas, that certain subjects preferred Pepsi. But once the brand names were revealed, another part of the brain kicked in. Now, some of those innately Pepsi-preferring subjects actually said that they preferred Coke.[17] Brand conditioning, it turns out, can even override taste buds!

The power of concentrated corporate wealth to create the brand—advertising pushing American-style, climate-intensive food around the globe—is certainly impressive. Yet all around the world, people are resisting. Seeing their diet-related-disease burden grow and family-scale shops and farms go under, they are pushing back. In India in 2000, I drove by whole stands of eucalyptus trees whose trunks were painted with the Pepsi logo, but I was also treated to mouthwatering local drinks by Indians who refuse to let go of the real nourishment they love. They're joining together to defend their traditions. They're embracing real food in the face of fast food.

Until now, we haven't perceived these efforts as part of addressing climate change; it's time we do.

CONTROLLING THE LAND

In early January 2009, Philippe Heilberg, a U.S. businessman who had amassed a small fortune as a Wall Street banker, bought a swath of land in southern Sudan roughly the size of Dubai.[18] Though Heilberg has no previous agricultural experience, the banker, who founded Jarch Capital to work on such land developments, believes his nearly million-acre purchase in the Sudan has "great potential for biofuels and food crops."[19] According to the *Financial Times*, Jarch is now on the hunt for partners with the expertise to develop the land—and to help it find and purchase more.[20]

Heilberg is the face of a trend: "the race," as some have called it, "to invest in overseas farmland."[21] More and more wealthy investors looking for the next best place to grow their fortunes—now that the old standbys on Wall Street are looking wobbly at best—are turning to land. Many are seeing an investment in agriculture as a safe bet, some even calling farmland the future "strategic resource that oilfields are now."[22] Some, no doubt, are assuming that as climate change worsens, agriculture and food security will be significantly affected. Yet ironically, these very investments, and the agricultural methods the developers are pushing, could actually be exacerbating the crisis by promoting climate-intensive large-scale production.

In 2008, Swedish companies Black Earth Farming and Alpcot-Agro purchased 800,000 acres and 300,000 acres of farmland in Russia respectively.[23] In 2009, Morgan Stanley reportedly bought roughly 98,000 acres in Ukraine.[24] That same year, Landkom, a British investment group, bought an estimated 2.5 million acres there as well. British hedge fund Dexion Capital recently invested $270 million in nearly 3 million acres in Australia, Russia, and South America. The list goes on.

Governments are buying up land, too. Sitting with reps of the South Korean Agriculture Department, I learn that their government has just secured land in Mongolia to produce food for South Koreans. Qatar is outsourcing food production to Pakistan's Punjab, where as many as twenty-five thousand families might be displaced because of the government's land development.[25] Saudi Arabia is planning to acquire nearly four million acres in Indonesia to produce rice to export back home.[26] And the Gulf Cooperation Council, which includes Bahrain, Kuwait, Qatar, Oman, Jordan, and the United Arab Emirates, is working on land deals in Laos, Indonesia, Vietnam, and beyond.[27] China, with 20 percent of the world's population but only 9 percent of its farmland, is getting in on the action, too. Since 2007, Chinese companies and the government have bought or leased nearly five million acres of land beyond the country's borders.[28]

This modern-day "land grab," as some refer to it, is being supported by international investors and institutions like the World Bank. According to the international nonprofit GRAIN, these entities are encouraging governments to "modify land ownership policies and practices so that foreign investors have more incentives to put money into farmland abroad."[29]

Of course, we've long had a global food system in which countries use natural resources beyond their borders to secure food for domestic consumption. European countries grew rich extracting raw materials from their colonies, whether it was gold from Peru, sugar from the Caribbean, or cotton from India. But today's land buy-up takes this dynamic to a new level—and adds a modern twist to it. Many of the governments buying up land are from resource-poor countries in the Global South. Advocates of these deals, mainly the investors themselves, say that they provide poor countries with "fresh inflows of foreign capital" needed for building rural infrastructure, including food storage and shipping facilities.[30] Developers also insist they're just turning "unused" or "underutilized" land into vibrant farmland.

Detractors' response: Unoccupied? Unused? Hardly! In many of the cases of land purchases in Africa, developers are staking claim on historically communal land. Take Ethiopia. Traditionally, as in much of the world, Ethiopia's grazing lands are not privately owned; they're community assets—a concept difficult to understand in a market economy and one conveniently sidestepped in these transactions.

Critics also charge that these purchases divert land that could be used for local consumption to large-scale plantations whose mandate is to feed populations half a world away. In her report "Global Land Grab," Alexandra Spieldoch, director of the Trade and Global Governance Program at the Institute for Agriculture and Trade Policy, argues that governments need to regulate this kind of investment.[31] Writes Spieldoch, "We need accountability and governments promoting climate-friendly production methods based on smaller-scale, diversified planting systems rather than large plantations growing one commodity for export."[32]

The other concern is that these land purchases erode local control of agricultural resources, weakening the accountability over how farmland is used. Says Oxfam Great Britain's head of research, Duncan Green, these arrangements are often "between partners with vastly unequal power."[33] Just what we don't need with the specter of climate change facing us.

While the push for industrial-scale production is real, there is another trend as well: Many governments, some for the very first time, are also developing an appreciation for sustainable food production—and for organic farming, as a potential aspect of their arsenal to respond to the climate crisis. Sitting in the bureaucratic offices of the South Korean Agriculture Department, I heard not only about those land purchases in Mongolia, but also about the department's new "green farming" initiatives, promoting organic production at the federal level for the very first time.

CONTROLLING PRODUCTION

In the summer of 2000, I traveled to the southeastern edge of Poland, where the country butts up against Slovakia to the south and Ukraine to the east. All of my father's grandparents immigrated from eastern Poland and western Russia (one by way of exile to Siberia for his radical politics), so maybe it's a genetic predisposition that propelled me to fall in love with the countryside, the pickles—and the farmers.

There for ten days, I was visiting small-scale farms connected by the International Coalition for the Protection of Polish Countryside, a citizen-led effort to preserve traditional farming. One strategy is to promote the value of small-scale farming by encouraging "farmcation" visitors like me.

I wanted to learn what made this country's relationship to agriculture so unique. While eating wild-strawberry cake and downing shots of vodka with spirited farmers, I heard about how their small-scale-farming traditions had persevered in the context of the large-scale operations that dominated most of Europe. That year, Poland, roughly the size of New Mexico, still boasted more farmers than the total remaining in the entire United States.[34]

Years later, as I explored the spread of energy-intensive food and farming around the planet, the road led me back to Poland.* It had been less than a decade, but what had happened to farmers there, especially hog farmers, portended one direction in which our food system could head: toward greater control of resources in the hands of a few multinational companies. For since my first voyage to Poland's farming communities, the country had opened its borders, joined the EU— and, in 1999, met Smithfield. The rest, as they say, is history (or the future, depending on how you look at it).

Pigs in Poland: How to Win Friends and Influence Food

The lighting isn't so good, but you can just make out that the inert objects floating in the black sludge are piglets. In the distance, you can see the Smithfield subsidiary where this waste, and loss of life, originated. The footage, from the organization Compassion in World Farming, is woven into British journalist Tracy Worcester's documentary *Pig Business*, about the incursion of Smithfield, and industrial-style livestock production, into Poland. The film, with its stories of workers intimidated and sickness among residents living near hog operations, exposes the very facilities that are so linked to the climate-change costs in our food system.

Smithfield entered Poland in 1999 with the acquisition of its first Polish subsidiary, Animex; by 2000, 8 of its 77 global subsidiaries were located there.[35] By 2004, those numbers had gone up to 20 out of 255 global subsidiaries.[36] And by 2007, the company had become, mainly through controlling interests in a number of processing operations in the country, Poland's largest pork producer.[37] Smithfield recently reported that it produced 1 million hogs in Poland in 2008; some estimate the figure is closer to 1.6 million.[38] The company's expansion there eventually landed it control over factories like the one in Zabin, north of Poznan, where the film footage was taken.

---

* I am indebted to Anna Witowska of Food & Water Watch for her assistance on this section.

When I heard that Smithfield had so successfully set up shop in Poland, I was surprised at first. I remembered my travels in the countryside and what I had learned about the country's small-scale-farmers' resilience. By the late 1990s, Poland was still largely an agricultural country, with one third of Poles still living in the countryside on small-scale farms.[39] Partly because unlike in other countries in eastern Europe, only farmland in Poland's northern and western regions had been consolidated into large estates under Communism. As recently as the early 2000s, 80 percent of private farms were still smaller than ten acres.

But farming changed after the Polish socialist state collapsed in 1989 and free market "shock therapy" worked to liberalize the Polish economy. Imported food took off, triggering a decline in food prices and farm incomes, which would weaken Polish farmers and make them more vulnerable to companies like Smithfield.

In part, it was Poland's desire to join the EU that led the country to embrace policies that would favor large-scale industrial production. Poland's "preparing the terrain for European Union accession," explains Anna Witowska, with the consumer advocacy organization Food & Water Watch, would "ultimately pave the way for Smithfield's entry into the country." For to comply with EU standards, Polish meat processors had to make significant capital investments. In effect, these slaughterhouse requirements created a barrier for the little guy, while giving the advantage to big guns like Smithfield. (Don't get me wrong. I'm all for standards, but not for regulations that don't actually address what matters—such as greenhouse-gas emissions from CAFOs—and instead tilt the playing field to benefit large producers.)[40]

Smithfield, like other foreign companies, also deployed specific strategies to gain a hold on the Polish pig market, strategies replicated by others across the planet. As we shape a vision to transition our global food system in the opposite direction, to make it part of the climate-change solution, it's helpful to grasp how a Smithfield wins friends and influences people in the food system.

Exploiting legal loopholes: Officially, foreign companies aren't allowed to own farms in Poland. No problem. Smithfield partnered with Polish companies to purchase post-Communism farms. When the company first arrived in Poland in 1999, it did so through Animex, then the country's biggest pork processor.[41] Using another Polish front company, Prima Farm, Smithfield also bought up many farms struggling to survive in the face of a flood of cheap imported meat from other EU countries.[42]

Capitalizing on subsidies: When you or I suffer a business loss, we don't expect to get paid back by the government. Now we know, though, that financial institutions don't play by the same rules we do. And in Poland, apparently hog producers don't either. Smithfield got bailed out big-time. When the company launched in Poland, it initially faced forty-three million dollars in losses, but that didn't kill the venture.[43] Through its subsidiary Animex, Smithfield got a twenty-five-million-dollar European Bank of Reconstruction and Development loan.[44] Meanwhile, says Witowska, "smaller slaughterhouses, which closed right before Poland's accession to the EU . . . were not given any help from the bank." The reason? The small-scale farmers projected an inability to comply with the EU rules, she says. (Though the bank claimed the loan agreement "has no contractual links to Smithfield's hog farming operations," the bank didn't have control over how the company spent the money.)[45]

Strengthening power through contract farming: Think "farmer" and what adjectives come to mind? Independent, resourceful, self-reliant? Those words used to be what came to my mind, too, until I learned about contract farming. Today, companies like Smithfield contract with farmers under terms the company sets. One day, you're an independent farmer, then you sign a contract, and the next day, you're taking orders. In the United States, one third of the total value of all our farm output is now produced under contract. With poultry, the amount is vastly greater; unless a U.S. farmer raises the birds under contract, there is virtually no market left to sell to. Hog production is moving in the same direction.[46]

What rights does the farmer lose? Smithfield gains the right to determine hog breeds, feed, vet care, time to market, and the price it will pay per animal—even whether to buy the pigs from the farmer at all. Typical contracts also require farmers to sign nondisclosure agreements, in which they promise to keep silent about the terms. Despite the drawbacks for farmers, many feel contract farming is the only option, and with many U.S. banks requiring contracts as the basis for loans, many feel even greater pressure to sign on the dotted line.[47]

Centralizing power through vertical integration: Vertical integration means one company controls most of the steps along the food chain: production, slaughter, processing, and marketing. Following in the footsteps of mega–meat companies like poultry giant Tyson, Smithfield has pioneered vertical integration in the hog industry and brought this trait to its Polish operations.

Shrinking the "free" in "free market": As Smithfield consolidates its power, its dominance shrinks the competitiveness of a so-called free market. When the company moved into pork production with full velocity in North Carolina, twenty-five thousand independent hog producers lost their farms. Today, in the pork industry, the top four companies control 64 percent of the market; the top two control 43 percent. As I mentioned earlier, it's not only the meat industry that's concentrated. Those top three grain traders—ADM, Bunge, and Cargill? They earn more than twice as much as the rest of the top ten combined.[48] The top three soft drink manufacturers, Coca-Cola, PepsiCo, and Dr Pepper/ Seven Up, control 89 percent of U.S. sales. "If competitive markets are defined as those where no one buyer or seller can influence the marketplace, we are rapidly moving to a global food system that is no longer predicated on competitive markets (indeed if it ever was)," say the authors of a 2008 study about power in the food system.[49]

These are just some of the tactics companies like Smithfield use to expand market share at home and abroad. Yet typically when we hear about the spread of climate-intensive farming, we're told it's happening because farmers, workers, and citizens want it. They want those jobs and more food choices at cheaper prices, don't they? But look beneath the surface and you'll see something else: The increasing control of these companies is not a response to consumer or farmer demand, nor even to populations hungry for economic development. The push is coming from multinationals themselves attempting to secure more markets and produce their products more cheaply, damn the environmental and social costs.

And it's not stopping at Poland. In 2008, Smithfield announced a one-billion-dollar investment to "revitalize the pork industry" in its

newest market: Romania.[50] Consumer advocates like Witowska argue
that Smithfield is now shifting its sights to Romania because farmers
and citizens, even elected officials, in her country are starting to speak
up against the company's impact on animal welfare, the environment,
and worker rights. Meanwhile, in Romania the "domestic pork market
is unsaturated, there is minimal opposition, and the government is offering its full support," explains Witowska.[51]

Nor is Smithfield stopping at Romania. Today, with more than 250
subsidiaries in France, the United Kingdom, China, Mexico, and Spain,
among other countries, 10 percent of Smithfield sales come from overseas operations; that figure is only increasing.[52] And Smithfield is not
the only food company with expansion plans. Read the annual reports of the world's largest meat companies and you'll discover that all
are looking overseas, particularly to China. The number-one ranked
beef producer and number-two poultry and pork producer, Tyson recently purchased a majority interest in a major chicken-processing facility and a pork-processing operation in China—and has plans for
greater expansion there.[53] In its 2007 annual report, Tyson made a
statement that could have been uttered by any one of these companies:
"A key element of Tyson's growth strategy is to build a multi-national
enterprise."[54]

THE GREAT WALL AND THE HUMMER

As reports from the United Nations warn, not only is the food system a
major factor in today's emissions, but if these patterns I've described
continue—pushing the climate-intensive American diet on populations around the world, gobbling up land for climate-intensive production, and spreading factory farming into the planet's every nook and
cranny—the food sector will become an ever-more-significant factor
in tomorrow's emissions. Yes, there is evidence of industrial-style meat
production spreading across eastern Europe, but perhaps even more
important for climate change is its spread into China.

"China is now the world's largest producer—and consumer—of
agricultural products," notes Mia MacDonald, who runs Brighter
Green, a New York City–based policy think tank.[55] Increasingly, just a

few countries dominate the exploding global meat market, all of them are moving in the direction of industrial-scale factory farming, and chief among them is China. Though China's industrial factories tend to shoulder the blame for greenhouse-gas emissions, we rarely hear about the country's meat facilities, yet these operations produce *forty* times the nitrogen and *three* times the solid waste of the nation's other factories.[56] Ponder the shape of things to come, and we have to talk about China.

In the fall of 2008, I traveled to China to visit communities who had first-hand experience of the direction of dependency and depletion and were saying yes to what they could create themselves. With new knowledge of ecological farming practices—coming in part via the development agency Heifer International—they could see the resources to tap right in their own backyards, literally. Instead of giving their power away to a distant corporation, they were building their family and community power. I'll never forget the confidence I sensed in these families, who knew that the food they were growing was healthy and so was the land it was growing in. And the changes, including those protecting the climate on this small scale, had taken only a few years.

A few days into our journey, I drove out to see a stretch of the Great Wall near Beijing with a group visiting Heifer projects. On our way, we endured a skyline of endless construction cranes and a view of the capital city's main reservoir, which had all but dried up. In sharp contrast to the sustainable communities we had just visited, we could see the speed with which the country was changing; the food system is just a part of a larger trend toward greater concentration of economic power and rapid industrialization.

In the parking lot at the base of the Simatai section of the Great Wall, looking up at the visual representation of thousands of years of history, I recalled the sustainable, small-scale farmers I had just met and the meal of homegrown food we had shared. And immediately, I contrasted these scenes with that first Starbucks I'd seen at Beijing International and the dozens of fast-food chains dotting the city's streets that I'd seen since.

I wondered if someday, maybe soon, the fascination with fast food and the push for climate-intensive farming would go the way of the Hummer, which, it seems, is becoming the dodo of the automobile world—at least here at home. I wondered whether someday soon the Chinese government and its citizens would see this style of food production as a skid off the road of real progress—and look to the methods of sustainable farming I'd seen with my own eyes in the country's rural communities as one element of the smartest path forward.

As I was standing there, in the exhaust haze of that parking lot, a bright yellow Hummer2, tinted windows and all, pulled up next to me.

I guess I had my answer—for now.

II
SPIN

3
BLINDED BY THE BITE

If we're speeding along in two directions at once—toward an ever-more-energy-dependent and energy-intensive food system *and* toward a food system that holds a key to healing our climate—why don't more of us know about either side of this story? The good *or* the bad? If tapping the food system to help address the climate crisis helps us engage the planet's people who still live close to the land, creating the added—and not-so-small—benefit of increasing food security, why don't we see this benefit, either? For isn't this, as they'd tell us in business school, the ultimate "win-win"? With the good news, and the bad, right in front of our noses, why has this story largely gone untold?

Lately, when I give public talks, I like to ask how many people have seen *An Inconvenient Truth*. Nearly everyone raises their hand, whether it's a six-hundred-person packed Seattle Town Hall or kids filling the seats in Solomon 001 at Brown University. Okay, I know, Seattleites and Brown students aren't exactly a representative sample of the population. Still, that so many have seen the doc tells us something about its influence, at least on the arguably environmentally inclined among us. But you could have been glued to the screen for all ninety-six minutes, even studied the closing credits, and be no wiser about food's role in the climate crisis.

As I said in the introduction, it's not just Al Gore who has, until recently, missed telling us about the food-climate connection. Much of the policy debate, the media coverage, even the research community, has overlooked the food and agriculture piece of the puzzle—both how it contributes to the crisis and how it holds solutions to it.

When Dr. Roni Neff and her colleagues at Johns Hopkins University, whom I mentioned earlier, analyzed climate-change coverage in sixteen of the twenty leading newspapers in the United States, they had a hunch that food and agriculture would be missing themes, but they were surprised by just how right they were. Of the 4,582 articles, letters to the editor, and op-eds on climate change that had been published from September 2005 to January 2008, only 2.4 percent addressed food and agriculture contributions.[1] The percentage that actually *focused* on meat and climate? Less than half of 1 percent.

Even at New York City's American Museum of Natural History, you could pass through the recent multiroom, multi-million-dollar climate-change exhibit and not learn much about food. Along with just two panels about how agriculture will be impacted by climate change, the exhibit included just one other mention of food: a small shout-out in the "What Can We Do?" section. An info panel did mention that livestock were responsible for 18 percent of all emissions. But it did so in the exhibit's smallest font and might not have registered for visitors who had already been pummeled with info, videos, and photos focused on typical global warming bogeymen like trains, planes, and automobiles.

To say we've missed this connection because the media and public education institutions like the Museum of Natural History haven't been covering the story begs the question: Why haven't they? As I tried to answer this question, it became pretty clear that 2008 was a banner year. Many around the world started waking up to the food–climate change connection. Citizen groups from People for the Ethical Treatment of Animals (PETA) and Greenpeace to the Humane Society of the United States and the Center for Food Safety launched campaigns about food and climate change.* Chef Laura Stec published *The Global Warming Diet* and the *Los Angeles Times* weighed in on the eat-less-meat-and-reduce-your-emissions theme. The year closed out with Elisabeth Rosenthal's December 3 *New York Times* article "As More Eat Meat, a Bid to Cut Emissions."[2] The article landed on the front page and within hours was among the top e-mailed of the day.

While the conversation may be shifting, we are still a long way from the average Jill not looking astonished when you tell her that her burger is more responsible for global warming than those fuming planes, trucks, and cars. Here are five possible reasons it's taking us so long to get the food and climate-change connection.

---

* To learn more about these campaigns, check out the resource section at the back of the book.

WHY WE MISSED IT

1. The Nature of Food

A few years ago, I was speaking to an Environmental Studies class at Eckerd College, in St. Petersburg, Florida. The campus feels more like Club Med than college, but the students were engaged despite the tropical surroundings that would have left me dreaming of coconuts and snorkeling. Before I launched into my lecture, I asked the students to reflect on their last experience of nature. What was it like? Where were they? What were they doing?

After a few moments of silence, a student raised her hand.

"I went kayaking over the weekend," she said. Another mentioned a run on the beach, and another described hanging out in a hammock between towering palm trees. Yes, let me remind you, this was Florida.

None of the other forty students said a peep. I then asked, "How many of you have eaten today?"

Every hand in the room shot up.

As it did for those Florida college kids, food feels far removed from nature for most of us. But all food has some connection to dirt—even Ding Dongs. Part of the challenge in getting people to see the connections between global warming and the food on their plate is the challenge of getting them to remember the natural source of all of our food, of reminding them that food doesn't grow in Aisle 8. In one survey conducted by Getty Images, people were asked what images they most associated with nature. Trees scored at the top. Oceans, rivers, and waterfalls came in a close second; flowers and "soaring birds" followed. But nowhere, on a list of more than a dozen images, did farms or food appear.[3]

2. Carbon-Centric

Quick, what do you think when you hear "greenhouse gas"? If you said, "Carbon dioxide," you wouldn't be alone. It's the most prevalent human-made greenhouse gas, responsible for roughly three quarters of the global warming effect. As the greenhouse gas of most serious concern, it's been the primary preoccupation of policy makers and activists who are addressing the crisis.

It makes sense that we might have this carbon bias, that our priority would be the worst climate-change offenders, like carbon-dioxide-spewing coal-fired power plants, for instance. James Hansen, who heads the NASA Goddard Institute for Space Studies, has even put his body on the line, getting arrested in a demonstration against mountaintop-removal coal mining in West Virginia recently, to publicize the urgent need to shut down all the world's coal plants within the next two decades if we are to avert climate disaster.[4]

Now that we realize both the complexity of the crisis and the seriousness of addressing it fast, we know that all sectors of society, food included, must be and can be part of the solution. We ignore these other possibilities at our peril. It's also high time to expand the focus and to stress the role of other key greenhouse gases, especially methane and nitrous oxide.

And what sector is most responsible for *those* gases? If you guessed the food system, give yourself a gold star; you've been paying attention. In the United States, agriculture contributes roughly three quarters of all nitrous oxide emissions. Globally, agriculture is responsible for nearly two thirds of methane emissions. With many times the global warming potential of carbon dioxide, methane and nitrous oxide must also be reduced if we want to ensure that global warming does not worsen.

I should also add that while some may have missed this complexity because of a carbon focus, many of us simply don't get the basics of climate change. When asked about the primary cause of increases in the earth's temperatures, only 53 percent of Americans, the lowest number among all the populations surveyed, answered correctly that it was the increased levels of carbon dioxide in the atmosphere. Nearly one third of Americans thought that global warming was caused by an "atmospheric 'ozone-hole' "; 7 percent thought it was caused by increased output from the sun, and 8 percent assumed it was because of the earth's orbit.[5] We've still got a lot of educating to do.

3. Systems, Oh My! The Complexity of Food

One bitter cold New York City day, I was grabbing a bite with climate-change-and-food expert Helene York, director of the Bon Appétit Management Company, an institutional caterer that dishes out eighty million meals a year. York is helping the company's chefs transition to more climate-friendly fare, including cutting back on beef. (As we ordered our snacks at a French-inspired café, I must admit I paused a moment wondering about the relative climate cost of my carrot-ginger soup.)

When I asked York why she thinks we've missed this plotline, she said, "When you're sitting in front of a steaming plate of macaroni and cheese, you're not picturing plumes of greenhouse gases. You're thinking: Dinner."

When we pick up our fork, it's harder to sense that rush of emissions the way we may when we hear the revving of our car engine. That may be partly because we don't associate food with the environment, but also because we rarely think about the chain of events that brings us the food on our plate.

"There is a clear line between stationary coal-combustion plants, carbon dioxide coming out of smokestacks, and global warming," climate-change expert Thomas Damassa, of the World Resources Institute, said when I asked him the same question. "With food, there are so many different components; there are so many different source points to latch on to. It's much more complicated to conceptualize, to explain, and to create policy around it." Ain't that the truth.

The categorizations that climate-change scientists create in ordering the science don't help, either. Food can become hidden. While clearly the economic sector "agriculture" is associated with food, the latter, as I've mentioned, also turns up throughout most of the rest of the categories: land-use change, transportation, waste, industrial processes, industry, and energy and heat. Just think of the examples I raised earlier, like agricultural chemicals, food-processing plants, farm machinery, heating and cooling supermarkets, refrigerated trucks. Food is there—if you squint hard enough.

4. Farmer vs. the Planet: The Ultimate Matchup?

Until recently, even within the environmental community the subject of food and climate change was nowhere close to center stage; it wasn't even in the dressing room. Part of the silence may have had to do with a historic gulf between some advocates of sustainable farming and mainstream environmentalists.

"As recently as five or ten years ago, the biodiversity and conservation community was sharply anti-agriculture," explained Sara Scherr when she talked to me from her home office. A founder of Ecoagriculture Partners, Scherr has been working in international development and agriculture for more than three decades. "If anything, there was antagonism toward farmers and agriculture."

Some of the antagonism stemmed from misperceptions. Scherr described cowriting her 2003 book *Ecoagriculture: How to Feed the World and Save Wild Biodiversity* with Jeffrey McNeely, a leading expert in biodiversity.[6] "The main thing we did for one another was to tell each other what *not* to say," she said. For example, to the environmental community, "productivity" was a dirty word—a euphemism for high-input polluting agriculture. For Scherr, an agricultural economist by training, the term was core to her thinking. For her, productivity meant simply the level of inputs relative to outputs, and a goal in agriculture is to increase productivity.

"I had to develop a whole different way of talking," said Scherr.

Until this last decade, Scherr shared, many advocates within the environmental community with whom she worked would talk about farmers as "threats; they weren't perceived as colleagues, collaborators, or stewards. They were seen as either the 'polluting, high-input industrial farmer' or the 'slash-and-burn farmer' or the 'poor farmer who goes out and clears land because they don't have any other option and therefore destroys everything in their path.' None of these farmers, as you can imagine, was looked on as an environmental caretaker.

"Certainly many environmentalists were supportive of sustainable agriculture, but still they would much rather farms simply not be there," she added.

Yet as Scherr's work has shown, and as many sustainable-agriculture proponents have long argued, farming can provide a vital source of "ecosystem services"—the wonky term for all the resources Mother Nature supplies us—including clean water, fresh air, homes for pollinators, and more. Thankfully, the notion that there is an inherent ecological divide between agriculture and the environment is being displaced by a deeper understanding of the agroecological potential of farms, the benefits of natural areas to farming communities, and the connection between sustainable farms and climate change mitigation, thanks in part to work like Scherr's.

5. Food Is Off-Limits

Finally, food might have been sidelined as a strategy to combat climate change because policy makers, and many folks like you and me, perceive the sector as untouchable. There is an understandable aversion to pushing for change that might seem like it would make food more expensive; it's politically unpalatable and morally reprehensible for many of us. Who would want to feel that they were pricing food out of reach for more people?

But will a more climate-friendly food system undermine the food security of the poor? To answer that question, we could begin by looking at how good a job the current food system is doing. Despite the fact that we produce more than enough calories globally to feed us all, nearly a billion still go hungry. (With the food-price crisis of 2007 and 2008, another 100 million people were pushed into hunger, which bloated the ranks to that number.) Even here in the United States, 36.2 million food-insecure people—roughly the population of Canada—one third of whom are children, are unsure where their next meal will come from.[7]

So will adopting a stance that includes the food system in strategies to address climate change just exacerbate the plight of the hungry? Indeed, it might do just the opposite. Acknowledging farmers as having a vital role in ecosystem services and respecting their skills in preserving biodiversity and protecting our watersheds, we would be giving new honor and support to some of the poorest people on the planet, many of whom are among the world's hungry.[8]

We need not censor our speech about food and climate change for fear we are being callous to the most vulnerable on the planet in talking about the connection. The opposite is true.

There's another reason why some people feel food is off-limits for serious discussion. Solitaire Townsend summed it up for me. I first met Townsend in the coffee line at a green-marketing conference hosted by industry rag *Advertising Age*. As we commiserated about the empty coffee urns, I started talking with the fiery founder of Futerra Sustainability Communications, a firm based in the United Kingdom and now with offices in New York City.

For more than a decade, Townsend has been advising both government and the private sector on how to communicate about climate change. When she was just starting out, she heard one refrain over and over.

"We can get people to turn off their lights," she was told, "but the one thing we absolutely can't tell people to do is change how they travel. Everybody loves their cars."

Well, that's proved to be about as true as saying we can never tell people to recycle; now you can find recycling bins everywhere from airports to shopping malls. I think about the long line of cars I saw waiting for "casual carpool" passengers this morning under the freeway in Oakland, which shoots passengers, like me, across the San Francisco Bay sans toll. Or all the friends who have dramatically changed their travel habits, like Michael from London, who decided to completely nix airplane travel, to the dismay of his stateside-bound sister. Or the tumbling market share of Hummers and the waiting lists for Priuses. Examples abound. Rethinking our travel doesn't seem as taboo as it once did.

Now what is Townsend hearing?

"People keep saying, 'Soli, you can't tell people what to eat! The one thing you can't talk about is food. It's never going to happen,'" Townsend said over our lukewarm decafs. Many people I interviewed echoed this sentiment. Thomas Damassa over at the World Resources Institute put it this way: "Food has so much to do with preference and personal choice. People are afraid to mandate from on high about what people should do." (Everyone, that is, except corporate advertisers, who are perfectly happy telling us what to eat.)

Townsend now replies to these naysayers, "Look, you said that about transportation, and we listened. Well, I'm not doing it this time. I'm sorry, I just don't believe it anymore. We're telling everyone to drive less or buy fuel-efficient cars. Transportation is far from verboten."

What's interesting is that just as I've been working on this project, I've noticed that the conversation has started to shift; it's already become much more open. Just since I met Townsend, in England alone, Compassion in World Farming hosted Dr. Rajendra Pachauri of the IPCC, who delivered that bold speech about eating less meat I mentioned earlier;[9] the country's National Health Service announced a carbon-reduction plan that included changing the menus in hospitals;[10] and a new study commissioned by the city of London analyzed reducing greenhouse-gas emissions through the food sector.[11]

I can safely say that Townsend is not advocating for the food police, but just as we've helped people understand how energy-efficient appliances, carpooling, and changing our lightbulbs can help us reduce our individual carbon footprint, we can talk about food, too—how to reduce our ecological foodprint.

HOW WE STOPPED WORRYING AND LEARNED TO LOVE CLIMATE CHANGE; OR, HOW THE FOOD INDUSTRY IGNORES, DENIES, AND EMBRACES GLOBAL WARMING

If the public and policy makers have missed this climate-change narrative, what about the food industry? Curious to know what food companies were saying (or not saying) about this theme, I dug into industry 10-Ks, those oh-so-fun-to-read yearly summaries of publicly traded company performance required by the Securities and Exchange Commission (SEC); attended food-biz gatherings; and devoured food-sector publications. The stances on food and climate change within the industry proved to be as different as the industry players themselves. From Hormel hot dogs to fair-trade chocolate, from Mountain Dew to Numi tea, from farmer-owned co-op Organic Valley to global dynamo Unilever, the food industry is far from monolithic. So it should come as no surprise that the different sectors have different communications strategies to respond to the growing awareness about food and climate change, strategies that span the spectrum: from silence to denial to embracing the message. The meat industry, for one, was squarely in the silent camp—that is, until it was forced to say something.

The Silent Treatment

I learned three things on my first trip to Nashville, Tennessee. Number one: There is an entire museum devoted to Cooter from *The Dukes of Hazzard*. Number two (and perhaps less unexpected): The local food movement is alive and well there— and I got to taste it. And number three: The meat industry and its communications experts seemed unfazed by the threat to their markets from growing concern about global warming. Or if they were, they certainly weren't talking about it in the spring of 2008.

That March, six hundred meat-industry reps descended on the Gaylord Opryland Convention Center for the annual conference of the Food Marketing Institute and the American Meat Institute. As a presenter joked from the stage, their numbers may have been significantly smaller than those of the National Religious Broadcasters, who filled most of the convention hall with their throngs of thousands, "but our booze is better." That got a rousing round of applause from the crowd of meat vendors, producers, and retailers from across the country.

Any alarm about public concern, or imminent policy, regarding greenhouse-gas emissions from their sector? Not a peep. The words "global warming" were never uttered, at least not at any of the plenary sessions or workshops I attended. (Keep in mind, this was two years after the United Nation's *Livestock's Long Shadow* was released, making clear the connections between livestock and climate change.)

The big public relations concern was a video on YouTube depicting animal abuse at a slaughterhouse in Northern California, shot with a hidden camera and now going viral. The industry's strategic communications teams were in overdrive working to repair its damaged reputation, including producing their own video of a "humane" slaughter house, said Deborah White of the Food Marketing Institute. The other communications workshops included one on how to beat back anti-meat groups, in which the presenter compared animal welfare organizations to Hezbollah and the Irish Republican Army.

Meat-industry silence on global warming was perceptible not only at the conference but also in the 10-Ks of the industry's biggest companies. Interested to see whether companies had been changing their tune about climate change, I searched filings available electronically back through the mid-1990s.[12] Did the words "global warming" or "climate change" appear anywhere? Rarely.

Since these are legal documents filed in part to explain exposure to risk, nearly every filing referred to national and international environmental regulation. Smithfield, the country's largest pork producer, remained mum except to say, in its 2007 10-K, "Hog production facilities generate significant quantities of manure, which must be managed

properly to protect public health and the environment."[13] At every
mention, companies would state that they were complying with these
regs, though many also mentioned million-dollar fines and lawsuits
incurred through infractions of these same regulations. That same
year, the company also noted fifty million dollars in assistance it gave
to preserve wetlands in eastern North Carolina and promote "environmental enhancement activities."[14] (A relatively small price tag for a region that is regularly ravaged by hurricanes, which have flooded the
state's large-scale hog facilities—and manure cesspits. In 1999, Hurricane Floyd, called the "worst disaster to hit North Carolina in modern
times" by Governor Jim Hunt, caused three billion dollars' worth of
damages, in part from flooded hog farms.[15] Hard-hit counties included
Duplin County, fifty miles south of Raleigh, home to 2.2 million hogs
and only forty-two thousand people.)[16]

The only 10-Ks I found that mentioned global warming were the
2008 filings from Hormel, Tyson, and Cagle's, and in those cases the
companies had no choice. Anti-meat organization PETA had submitted
shareholder resolutions that requested the disclosure by 2010 of "the
amount of greenhouse-gas emissions caused by individual products."[17]
(The strategy of using shareholder resolutions to force companies to
talk about climate change is not unique to PETA. In 2007, the number
of environmental resolutions before shareholders reached a record high,
spurred by demands that companies address the climate crisis.)[18] The
companies that PETA targeted urged their shareholders to vote against
the resolution.

Companies can play silent with a little more subtlety: It's the *our-
hands-are-clean* argument. For many food companies, this is a compelling tactic because they source from a multitude of suppliers; they're
not directly involved with the growing of the food. It's certainly the
stance we heard when we talked with agribusiness giant Bunge, which
has operations in thirty countries and $37.8 billion in annual sales,
about its sustainability concerns.

"We do not have huge emissions ourselves because of the work we do,"
said the company rep.[19] But, well, they do. Bunge is the world's biggest
fertilizer manufacturer, and remember all the energy required to produce
fertilizer? Bunge also produces a number of processed foods, from bottled oils to mayonnaise and margarine. And the company is among the

world's biggest wheat and corn millers as well as an oilseed and grain processor and distributor, providing meal for the livestock industry and oil for the food processing, food service and biofuel industries.

The Bunge rep did offer the ways in which the company is helping its suppliers, saying, "We help farmers to have more sustainable productions, to mitigate *their* problems. We have 90 percent no-tillage area, for example. We work with suppliers on a range of other techniques as well."

Silence, and this our-hands-are-clean spin on silence, is not the only way to play the denial game. Fomenting doubt is another.

Doubt Is Their Product

In 1969, an internal strategy document created by marketing executives from Brown & Williamson—the tobacco giant behind cigarettes like Pall Mall and Kool—offered a tip on countering the "anti-cigarette forces."[20]

"Doubt is our product," wrote the executives. "It is the best means of competing with the 'body of fact' that exists in the mind of the general public. It is also the means of establishing a controversy."[21]

This question-the-science strategy is not exclusive to the tobacco industry. Other industries have long perceived the benefits of manufacturing uncertainty. Obfuscation yields results, as epidemiologist David Michaels details in his book *Doubt Is Their Product*. It did for Big Tobacco, and it did for Big Oil in its effort to confuse the public about the science of climate change. Consider this excerpt from a leaked 2003 memo by Republican political consultant Frank Luntz on swaying popular opinion: "Voters believe that there is no consensus about global warming within the scientific community. Should the public come to believe that the scientific issues are settled, their views about global warming will change accordingly. Therefore, you need to continue to make the lack of scientific certainty a primary issue in the debate."[22]

That memo was penned in 2003, and its author was right. It would take another few years—following the release of *An Inconvenient Truth* and the honoring of the IPCC and almost-president Gore in 2007 with a Nobel Prize—before we in the United States would pass a tipping point and move from collective climate-change denial to climate-change awareness.

Now that the climate-change fight has shifted from "Is it a real threat?" to "What's causing it and what can we do about it?," industry is fighting back, again. And with everyone from editors at the *Los Angeles Times* to the two-term chair of the Nobel Prize–winning IPCC urging us to question that bite of a burger because of beef's impact on global warming, the meat industry and its surrogates are entering the fray, going beyond the silent treatment to forging doubt.

Fudging the Math

The cattlemen who made their way to Reno, Nevada, for the February 2008 Cattle Industry Annual Convention and Trade Show had a chance to witness a little doubt-mongering themselves. At their convention, among the workshops that attendees could choose from was one titled "Environmental Challenges Facing the Beef Industry."[23] After sitting through thirty-two PowerPoint slides on challenges that included the Clean Water Act and the Clean Air Act, attendees were finally shown (drumroll, please) a slide titled "Global Climate Change."

The take-home message? Don't worry. Allegations that livestock are worse emitters than transportation? Hogwash.

Said one slide, the "EPA does not indicate animal ag contributes significantly to US production of CO_2." While the United Nations claims livestock generate 18 percent of the world's global warming, the EPA says livestock only contribute 4.6 percent to our country's total greenhouse-gas emissions, explained the presenter. The PowerPoint presentation ended on a promising note (for the industry, that is) as well as an indecipherable one. The last slide said:

So far, Congress not talking about regulating animal ag
Polar bears and penguins

Your guess is as good as mine about those polar bears and penguins, but the pooh-poohing was obvious. Don't worry about that crazy United Nations; the industry is just a bit player in climate change. Your legislators aren't worried; you shouldn't be either.

This talking point isn't limited to presentations at meat conventions. A few months earlier, the National Cattlemen's Beef Association's CEO, Terry Stokes, used this same messaging in his rebuttal to a *Los Angeles Times* editorial that quoted the United Nations' 18 percent estimate.[24]

"The editorial," Stokes protested, "was riddled with incorrect statistics and misinformation."[25] And in April 2009, the Center for Consumer Freedom, a front group for the restaurant, alcohol, and tobacco industries, got into the ring in response to an *Archives of Internal Medicine* article about meat and climate change, saying that "U.S. meat production contributes a laughably tiny amount of carbon emissions to the climate-change picture."[26]

Ostensibly, Stokes, the Center for Consumer Freedom, and that guy in Reno all just want to set the record straight. "One of the most important tasks we have at NCBA," says Stokes, "is to refute misinformation spread by people with an anti-meat, anti-livestock agenda."[27]

While I would grant that PETA is not exactly what you would call "pro-meat," I think it's a stretch to argue that the editors at the *Los Angeles Times*, or Henning Steinfeld and his *Livestock's Long Shadow* coauthors over at the United Nations, are anti-meat. To Stokes, it seems, anybody critiquing the industry has an "anti-meat" agenda. "These activists will stoop to almost any level," says Stokes, "to persuade consumers to reduce or eliminate their meat consumption." The climate-change argument is just the "latest strategy of choice . . . to vilify meat consumption." Says Stokes, "This is just a sinister strategy to play on the consumers' emotions."

So what to make of Stokes's claim? Can we go on pigging out on pork chops without worry? Does the EPA's own data undermine the case that farm animals are a major contributor to greenhouse gases?[28]

First, the EPA data break out a little differently than Stokes would have you believe. The figure quoted doesn't tell us the complete story of meat in this country, and in failing to do so, it lowballs the sector's global warming impact. The percent figure includes only emissions of nitrous oxide and methane, not *all* the emissions from energy used in production, including manufacturing, intensive irrigation, and more, which eat up as much as 15 percent of total energy used in agriculture.[29] It doesn't include emissions from:

- the heating, cooling, and cleaning required by feedlots and meat-processing plants

- the production of farm chemicals and fertilizers, over half of which are used to grow animal feed crops

- toting those fertilizers and farm chemicals to our shores and our nation's fields

- from landfills, which contain our uneaten morsels of meat and meat by-products

- the distribution, transportation, or storage of meat, which can be relatively significant, since meat is energy intensive to transport and store

- the miles *we* drive to get our meat

Plus, while livestock emissions may be a relatively small percentage of our nation's overall emissions, that's in part because the United States is such a major emitter of the world's *total* greenhouse gases. Despite being home to just 4.6 percent of the world's population, we're responsible for more than 24.4 percent of the globe's emissions.[30] We are such a heavy emitter of carbon dioxide in part because of our exhaust-spewing cars. With just a fraction of the world's population, we are home to one third of the world's passenger cars.[31] While a relatively small portion— though not as small as the industry claims—of overall greenhouse-gas emissions come from livestock, this does not mean we shouldn't be concerned about it, only that we're such troublemakers in other ways. Stokes is lucky he lives in such a polluting country; by comparison, his sector comes off looking better.

What else gets Stokes riled? He charges that anti-meat activists "seem to think that land used to graze cattle could easily be converted to vegetable or grain production . . . Converting range land to crop production has serious environmental consequences of its own."[32] Stokes's dreamy-eyed version of sustainable cattle-production rangeland is not the reality for most cattle in this country, which are raised in feedlots and require as much as sixteen pounds, or more, of grain and soy to return to us a pound of beef. Plus, what he's missing is that sustainable vegetable and grain production can help us sequester carbon, providing us with a net benefit regarding emissions.

Despite these flaws in the Stokes argument, that of the presenter back in Reno, and the points parroted by the Center for Consumer Freedom, this type of commentary raises doubt among the public. That's exactly why it's a powerful tactic for those interested in diverting attention away from the devastation caused by livestock production.

Doubt undermines political will and keeps sustainable food advocates in the trenches fighting about percentage points while policy opportunities slip by.

Questioning the Science

I stumbled on another example of fostering doubt in a 2008 issue of *Environmental Health Perspectives*. In that journal, the Humane Society's Danielle Nierenberg and Gowri Koneswaran published a review article that summarizes some of the research comparing emissions from organic grass-fed beef and nonorganic grain-fed beef. Nierenberg and Koneswaran found that based on these studies, organic beef can emit as much as 40 percent fewer greenhouse gases and require 85 percent less energy than confined feedlot beef.[33] They argue that to reduce emissions from livestock—beyond demanding less of the stuff—we should steer clear of the feedlot. But their claims did not go undisputed.

In a response published in the journal, the Center for Global Food Issues' Alex Avery and Dennis Avery denounced the article as "terribly misleading."[34] The Averys contend that switching all U.S. cattle to grass would actually *increase* greenhouse-gas emissions by 282.5 billion pounds of CO_2-equivalent emissions every year—a whopping 58 percent more than if we just keep putting our climate faith in grain-fed beef.[35] Pretty confusing.

So what's the truth?

Well, first, I should point out, as Nierenberg and Koneswaran do, that they're not arguing for maintaining beef production at today's levels, whether those cows are chomping corn or grazing on grass. "If we're really serious about combating climate change, we need to reduce the overall amount of meat, egg, and dairy products we consume," Nierenberg stresses.

But for the cattle that *are* raised, the question remains: To eat grass or not to eat grass?

Reading the Averys' letter, you'd think we should go running to feedlots and praise them as downright ecological. But I dug into their calculations—and got on the phone with the authors of some of the studies they cite—and their argument rests on shaky ground. Exploring their math, I got a window into the win-through-obfuscation strategy behind the pseudoscience tossed around as fact by industrial-agriculture apologists.*

Before continuing, I should admit my own bias. I have come across the work of this father-and-son team before. My dog-eared copy of Dennis Avery's *Saving the Planet with Pesticides and Plastic* still sits on my bookshelf. I come to their allegations with a dose of skepticism. Call me a stickler for facts, but I raise my eyebrow at anyone who argues that Agent Orange, the toxic defoliant used in Vietnam, is harmless, as Avery does.[36] Or who argues that hogs prefer the confinement of feedlots; left with too much space, he claims, the mothers tend to fall on their young, killing them.[37] Still, I gave them a fair shake, but their numbers just didn't add up.

Dissecting the Argument

The Averys' argument uses seemingly complicated calculations—with enough zeros and decimal points to make your eyes glaze over—but rests on one central claim: that it takes three times more land to raise grass-fed beef than it does grain-fed cattle.[38] Factoring in the emissions caused by shifting all that land to pasture is what gets you to the conclusion that grass-fed production would increase emissions by the huge amount of 58 percent.

But the entire calculation rests on flimsy numbers. The claim that it takes three times more land to raise organic beef is based on the Averys' own analysis of a study from the Leopold Center for Sustainable Agriculture at Iowa State University.[39] Only, that study wasn't designed to estimate land-use differences between cattle systems. (It was designed to help farmers analyze the profitability of shifting to natural, grass-fed, or organic production.)[40] As Iowa State professor John Lawrence explained to me, the land required for grass-fed versus grain-fed systems will vary widely depending on where you are farming, and particularly on whether you can grow grass throughout the year. Lawrence went on to say, "Some grass-fed producers raise everything on their operation.

---

* I also discovered at least one elementary mistake. The Averys refer to Japanese beef shipped eighteen thousand miles. Well, eighteen thousand miles would be, uh, more than two thirds of the way around the world. The Averys meant to say eighteen thousand *kilometers*, but let's not sweat the small stuff.

The same can be said for grain-fed producers." Some raise their own calves, others buy them in the community, and still others ship them in from Mexico or Canada. Some feed them corn raised on their own farm; others transport feed in from long distances. "The bottom line is, it depends," said Lawrence.[41]

Where did the Averys get their estimate for the amount of feed, and therefore land to grow the feed, needed for grain-fed cattle? They used USDA crop-production data, but when I e-mailed the department, a rep there said the government doesn't collect any data on the amount of feed needed to produce these animals. "There is no way to accurately estimate the amount of feed or the type of feed the slaughter animals have consumed without access to the feedlot records, farmer records, and ranch records. The numbers you refer to were developed based on some estimates and rules of thumb that may or may not hold all the time," said the USDA rep.[42]

So the numbers used to calculate land use for both grain-fed and grass-fed cattle are flimsy. And yet this three-times-more-land-to-raise-organic-beef figure is critically important, because it is a basis of the Averys' equation.

We know the choices the Averys made for their land-use estimates, but what about the emissions per acre of land converted to raise all that grass-fed cattle? The Averys claim that each acre needed for grass-fed cattle would emit 10,400 pounds of CO_2-equivalent greenhouse gases each year. But this estimate of emissions per acre was lifted from a study that wasn't looking at land in the United States converted to pasture. I know because I asked the author.

"That figure is not based on a study of emissions of pastureland, or even of land that was converted from grain production to pastureland," explained one of the study's authors, Princeton professor Timothy Searchinger, "but of land that had been forests and other rangelands converted into cropland for biofuels."[43] Thus the figure includes losses not only of soil carbon but also of aboveground vegetation and roots. (Searchinger's was the study that stirred up so much controversy in 2008 about the wisdom of crop-based ethanol production.)[44]

The Searchinger figure, used for the Averys' purposes, highly overestimates emissions from land-use change in the United States. Why? In part because so much land here is currently used for corn-feed production; it's heavily irrigated and doused with synthetic fertilizers. It's not a net carbon sponge—indeed, it's often a net *emitter* of greenhouse gases. (In the United States, two thirds of man-made nitrous oxide emissions comes from agriculture, much of it from feed production.)[45] Last time I checked, we didn't have any carbon-rich rainforests here.

So if we're talking about converting some of the land currently used for feed production to grass-fed-beef production, emissions per acre would be significantly lower. You might even, gasp, see a *net benefit*, as well-managed grazing can help store carbon in soils.[46] In fact, when I asked the author of the one study on grass-fed production that the Averys cite whether grassland can act as a carbon sink, she explained that "this positive effect was not included in my study."[47]

What's at Steak?

Despite the Averys' attempt to take down the claims for grass-fed beef, we know that industrial livestock production produces greenhouse-gas emissions at nearly every stage in the process. Emissions occur during the production and use of nitrogen fertilizers; during the transportation of feed to factories, live animals to feedlots, and ready-for-slaughter cattle to slaughterhouses; and during the digestive process of cattle. With large-scale industrial factories, we must also contend with emissions from manure stored in cesspits. Moreover, carbon dioxide is emitted through the degradation of soils used for feed crops. And so on. Whereas grass-fed cattle save on emissions from fertilizer used in crop production and from energy used in raising, harvesting, and then transporting the crops. We also save on emissions from manure: In sustainable, grass-fed systems, manure can be a net benefit.

But the lifecycle of cattle is long and circuitous, and depending on where the cattle are raised, the emissions profiles will be dramatically different. Imagine the difference between the life of a dairy cow in wet and wintry Vermont and that of one in dry Colorado. Precisely because it's so complicated, we need more studies to help us understand the emissions at each step in the process and where the biggest opportunities for reduction lie.

But just because we need more study doesn't mean that we don't already have powerful evidence that industrial livestock production is a major greenhouse-gas emitter, or that we don't already have ways to reduce emissions by transitioning toward more organic production and less meat production overall.

The Averys' attack on grass-fed beef and the scaremongering claim that moving toward more-ecological production will actually increase emissions are part of a classic industry strategy. Win by confusion; triumph with doubt. Yes, with "CO_2-equivalent" and "kg/hectare" getting tossed around, it's easy to get confused, and that's just where the proponents of the industrial meat system want you to be: in a state called confusion.

Environmental Health Perspectives is one of the top journals in the public health field. It's ranked first among environmental science journals and second among public, environmental, and health journals. It's read in 190 countries and produced by the U.S. National Institute of Environmental Health Sciences. The publication of the Averys' letter in it legitimizes their perspective, even though you can blast a hole through their arguments. Worse, the echo chamber of their misinformation is large indeed. At a 2008 meat conference organized by the British Society of Animal Science and held in Tunisia, Danielle Nierenberg saw a PowerPoint presentation that included a slide from the Averys. "It was a stark realization that elsewhere I don't think people realize that they're not basing their research on science," she said.

So who are the Averys? You might not have heard of them, or the Center for Global Food Issues, or its parent organization, the Hudson Institute, but you may have heard of some of the sponsors and donors who help support the institute's ten-million-dollar budget.[48]

A peek into the Hudson Institute's annual report reveals dozens of companies, foundations, and individuals with direct and indirect connections to every single aspect of confinement beef production, from the production of drugs for livestock to the production of agrochemicals for feed crops, from grain trading to the trade associations that lobby on the industry's behalf.[49] Might these funding sources cast some doubt on the neutrality of the Averys' pro-feedlot position? Let's take a look.

Pharmaceutical industry: Within the Hudson Institute's donor "Trustees' Circle" is Big Pharma company Eli Lilly. You might be familiar with Eli Lilly's people-prescription drug line, including mass-market products like Prozac. The global pharmaceutical company also has a line of drugs for the livestock industry, including antibiotics, parasiticides, and anticoccidials, which fight infections in animal intestines—infections that are especially rampant among animals living in the unnatural state of cramped confinement.

Eli Lilly's animal drug line contains products like Rumensin, a cattle-feed additive; Coban, Monteban, and Maxiban, for poultry; Surmax, for swine and poultry; and Elector, a parasiticide for cattle.[50] In a sign that the company sees a future in intensive livestock production, Eli Lilly expanded its animal-pharma business in 2007 with the purchase of Ivy Animal Health. Said a company exec of the merger, "Our product lines are complementary, and together they deliver cumulative value to our beef-producing customers."[51]

The world's other major livestock drug company, Bayer (another company known for its human-pharma line), is also a Hudson Institute funder. One of the most popular drugs used in feedlots is Bayer's antibiotic Baycox, used in confinement poultry, hog, and cattle operations to boost growth and treat diseases like coccidiosis.[52] Bayer and Eli Lilly are among the largest producers of the pharmaceuticals—including antibiotics and synthetic growth hormones—that industrial livestock producers rely on to jack up growth rates and stave off disease and infection in the confined quarters of cattle feedlots. Call me crazy, but I imagine that both would have significant financial interest in the continued expansion of confinement production.

Agrochemical industry: And what about the institute's agrochemical funders? Hudson donors include PotashCorp, Syngenta Crop Protection, Pioneer Hi-Bred International, and DuPont. These companies are the major players in the market for agricultural chemicals that industrial livestock producers rely on to foster plant growth and protect against pests on monoculture feed fields.

PotashCorp is the largest fertilizer enterprise in the world, producing the three primary plant nutrients—nitrogen, phosphate, and potash.[53] With increasing demand, PotashCorp said in 2008 that its outlook was strong, and it planned to expand its potash production by 80 percent over five to seven years.[54]

The Hudson Institute also receives funding from foundations with direct ties to the agrochemical industry, including the Olin Foundation. (With the requirement to spend down all its assets within a generation, Olin made its last grants, including one to the Hudson

Institute, in 2005.)[55] The foundation was established in 1953 by the founder of the Olin Corporation. Today a *Fortune* 1000 company with thirty-six hundred employees, Olin has an ammunitions division and a chemical division, which produces, among other chemicals, potassium hydroxide and dilute sulfuric acid, ingredients widely used in fertilizers and herbicides.[56]

Feed industry: A third set of companies in the Hudson Institute funding circles are those in the business of producing or buying feed for those confined livestock the Averys are so excited about, including global grain giant Archer Daniels Midland and the genetically-modified-foods (GMO) behemoth Monsanto.* Monsanto's biggest stake in the grain-fed-cattle industry is through its seed lines of genetically modified corn and soy. The company controls roughly 39 percent of the market for all corn, a primary feed for U.S. livestock, and its GMO corn, cotton, canola, and soybeans grow on 90 percent of the global farmland devoted to genetically modified crops.[57] Until August 2008, the company was also the country's sole supplier of rBGH, the controversial synthetic growth hormone used in U.S. dairy CAFOs but banned in the EU.

In addition, the Hudson Institute receives funding from the American Feed Industry Association (AFIA), a lobby group that represents the "business, legislative and regulatory interests of the animal feed industry and its suppliers."[58] Among other successes, the AFIA was the primary organization responsible for drafting the "food disparagement law" that protects food companies from public criticism, which it lobbied into law in 1990.[59]

The association shares an office and works with another industrial-agriculture promoter: the Animal Agriculture Alliance. At the Food Marketing Institute and American Meat Institute's conference in Nashville, Philip Lobo, the alliance's communications director, warned about the "domestic terrorist" threat of groups operating under the guise of animal-welfare advocates. Along with workshops like the

---

* Genetically modified crops are alternately referred to as biotech or transgene crops or by the acronyms GM (genetically modified), GE (genetically engineered), or GMO (genetically modified organism). The alphabet soup can certainly be confusing, but the definition of GMOs need not be complicated: Biotech foods are those that have been engineered by forcing a gene, or genes, from one species into the DNA of another species for a result that would not have been possible in nature.

one I attended, "Animal Welfare and Activism: What You Need to Know," the alliance offers two-day antiterrorism trainings. It held its first in 2006, focusing on "the threats domestic terrorists, especially animal rights extremists, pose to animal-use industries and their customers."[60]

Oil industry: The Hudson Institute also receives funding from the Sarah Scaife Foundation, whose chairman is oil-and-banking mogul Richard Mellon Scaife. Scaife also serves on the board of trustees of the Heritage Foundation, a conservative think tank that itself has been a magnet for funding from the automobile, coal, oil, and chemical industries. As I've explained, the industrial meat complex is heavily dependent on fossil fuels, and in turn is a big customer for the oil industry. From the energy needed to operate the slaughterhouses to the petroleum-based chemicals used in feed production, feedlot meat is an oil man's dream.

I could go on. Even more funders of the Hudson Institute would be pleased to thwart consciousness-raising about the climate cost of feedlot meat.

The Averys' is just one example of the sort of attacks we are seeing, and can expect to see increasing, as more become aware of the food-and-climate connection.

FROM SILENT TREATMENT TO MARKET OPPORTUNITY

Like those in the meat industry, most of the rest of the several dozen food companies I researched have been silent on climate change in their 10-Ks—besides the required commentary about compliance regarding emissions—even those that have publicly taken a relatively bold stance. For instance, General Mills didn't mention climate change in its 10-Ks though the company's vice president and global sustainability officer, Gene Kahn, presented a persuasive PowerPoint about why his industry needs to look inward at its greenhouse-gas emissions at the 2008 Grocery Manufacturers Association (GMA) conference.[61]

Who *has been* talking about climate change? The chemical industry. Dow, DuPont, Syngenta. It seems they all see potential for profit. Each mentioned ways that its bottom line could benefit from changes in the climate: For instance, the industry's products could potentially find new customers dealing with virulent global-warming-induced pests. These companies also mentioned how they're working to reduce greenhouse-gas emissions.[62] Dow promoted its "lightweight plastics for automobiles and insulation for energy efficient homes and appliances."[63] DuPont noted that it's "committed to continuing to bring to market more products and services to meet new and expanded demands of a low-carbon economy."[64]

But it's not just chemical companies who are starting to see the green in going green. In 2008, Fiji water launched its latest campaign to promote its high-end water in the square bottle. (Fiji's owner, Lynda Resnick, seems to have a thing for distinctive packaging; she's also the wallet behind Pom Wonderful "in the curvy bottle.") The company announced that it was taking climate change seriously. Not only would Fiji water offset its emissions; it was going *carbon negative*.

Fiji is just one of the players in the food industry to lift the self-imposed gag order on talking about climate change. As I traveled to food-industry conferences and followed the changing commentary in food and agriculture trade journals and ad campaigns, it became apparent that some in the industry saw the climate crisis as a marketing opportunity—and they were jumping on it.

To see how the food industry was framing the issue, I looked up close at three trade publications—*Meat & Poultry*, *Food Processing*, and *Prepared Foods*—to compare what they were saying about the environment in 2003 and 2004 with what they were saying in 2008.[65] One thing became abundantly clear: Times are a-changing. In sharp contrast to the earlier years, by 2008 dozens of articles discussed green initiatives, warned about global warming, and praised sustainability leaders.

Back in 2003, the tone was a wee bit different. Then, climate change was mentioned only a handful of times. In *Meat & Poultry*, only to be denied: "It doesn't take a meteorologist to surmise that the weather has been wacky the past few years . . . But we shouldn't equate peculiar atmospheric conditions as a sign that the world's weather is out of whack. We call it natural climate variability."[66]

By 2008, the eco-tone had notably shifted. The use of terms like "sustainable," "environment," "climate change," and "green" had skyrocketed. *Food Processing* and *Prepared Foods* in particular were now talking about the environment, reflecting what editors perceived as a massive shift in the field, pushed in part by growing concern about global warming.

Climate change was being discussed as part of the broader concept of "sustainability," which food companies were seeing as a way to court customers. Even your raspberry-balsamic vinaigrette was not immune from the trend, mentioned a *Prepared Foods* writer in 2008: "As environmental consciousness sweeps the globe, pre-packaged salads and dressings have become caught up in the excitement."[67]

Editors were predicting that the trend had staying power. "Consumer and business interest in the 'green' movement is expected to grow during the next few years," wrote the editors at *Prepared Foods*.[68] On the corporate side, attention to "green" issues should remain strong, they continued, "as companies attempt to use a 'green' positioning to gain consumer loyalty and increase their sales."[69]

By the summer of 2008, *Prepared Foods* was getting downright wonky about climate change. An article expounded drink-company Guayakí and its "carbon-subtracting process," achieved through "the vast carbon sequestration that occurs in the vibrant South American rainforest, where Guayakí's organic yerba mate is sustainably harvested under the canopy of towering hardwood trees."[70]

Why the abrupt change in the narrative? Think about all that had shifted since early 2004. Al Gore's *An Inconvenient Truth* had been released, news about the climate crisis was flooding the media, and general acceptance of global warming was replacing climate-change denial. Industry observers also pointed to another cause: the bottom line. Spiking energy prices were making green initiatives cost-effective. Of all the reasons companies were going green, "saving money apparently is the greenest for many companies," wrote Bob Sperber in *Food Processing*.[71]

Plus there was the growing perception that addressing global warming was inevitable; every company would be affected, whether by imminent regulations, pushback from public opinion, or rising costs. (While the impact of global warming will be especially felt in the food sector because companies are so reliant on agricultural inputs, most of the costs may simply be passed on to the consumer. To date, companies like Nestlé have been able to increase prices in the face of rising input costs. In the wake of the 2007 global food-price crisis, and amid an international recession, the company saw its profits increase by 70 percent in 2008 over the previous year.)

Action on climate change within the food industry is also increasingly being perceived as a way to boost brand image, in part as a strategy for inoculating consumers against potential negative messages that they may hear about. Getting serious about climate change can "positively shape brand image and attract new customers," confirms Yale's Daniel Esty.[72] In the United Kingdom, where supermarkets are trying to one-up each other through public displays of environmentally friendly policy, "carbon reporting and emissions management has become a public relations battleground," writes Esty.[73]

The food industry is also identifying carbon-emissions regulations as a potential windfall. "Any company that can foresee business opportunities in influencing carbon-emissions regulation is practicing what is expected of business managers—capitalism," writes Andrew Hoffman in the *Harvard Business Review*.[74] Ignore these regulatory opportunities and your company could be "missing out on the fast-growing carbon-trading market—one that roughly tripled from $11 billion globally in 2005 to $30 billion in 2006," Hoffman says.[75] Sure, sustainability is trendy, but, as Bob Sperber says in *Food Processing* magazine, "dig deeper, and energy conservation and savings provide the real driver."[76]

Clearly, the food industry isn't monolithic: While Terry Stokes is defending his cattlemen and the American Meat Institute conference was mum on global warming, other sectors of the industry are acknowledging the climate costs of their operations while arguing that they're part of the solution—all in the same breath.

In the next two chapters, I explore what some of the biggest food companies are doing—or at least saying they're doing—to address the crisis. In "Playing with Our Food," I share tactics that industry players are using to position themselves as eco-heroes and how we can distinguish corporate spin from the real deal. In "Capitalizing on Climate Change," I highlight specific initiatives companies are pushing—and getting subsidies and tax breaks for—under the guise of climate-change solutions, ones that offer dubious benefits for the planet.

4
PLAYING WITH OUR FOOD

FROM CYNICAL TO SAVVY

In this brave new era—when business has begun to talk about sustainability—the world's largest food and agribusiness companies are beginning to get in on the conversation, as evidenced by the corporate execs who gathered on a wet and gray day in January 2008 in Washington, D.C., for the Grocery Manufacturers Association's Environmental Sustainability Summit. The GMA is the trade association for just about every big food company you've ever heard of (and even some you never have), and its summit at the Ritz-Carlton was bursting at its swank seams.[1]

Organizers said they had expected a hundred or so attendees; instead, more than six hundred showed up. EPA reps and a smattering of folks from nongovernmental organizations (NGOs) rubbed elbows with representatives of the world's largest food, beverage, and consumer-products companies: agricultural-chemical manufacturers like Dow and Monsanto, agribusiness giants like ADM and Cargill, and food and beverage giants Pepsi and Kraft.

These food-industry executives clearly saw the writing on the wall: It was only a matter of time before people started asking about the link between our carbon-intensive food system and the climate crisis; indeed, they already were. And it was only a matter of time before the industry saw capitalizing on climate policies as an opportunity. In this chapter, I explore plays from the greening playbook, dissecting each with examples ripped from comments overheard at industry conferences and from the pages of industry rags.

As you read this chapter, I worry you might become a tad cynical. (Or maybe you already are, and what you read may just confirm your skepticism.) But I don't want to make you cynical. I want to make you savvy.

Cynicism can breed fatalism; fatalism can make you wonder, "Can I really trust any company?" However, the savvy among us (and yes, I hope that's you) realize that yes, some companies *are* adopting genuinely sustainable practices, but with so many companies getting into the green game, we have to read between the lines to identify the real deal.

I want to help you learn how to sift through the hype, so that we're applauding those companies and practices that are actually driving the real results our planet needs. With this intention of indoctrinating savvy citizens, I follow the greening plays with tips for dissecting the hype, including a handy guide for evaluating eco-claims.

Before I share some of these tactics, it's important to begin at the beginning with this question: Why should food companies be responsible for greening their businesses at all?

See, maybe you've bought the line from those who believe that a company's social responsibility is solely to increase its profits, in which case you'll need some convincing that all this talk is worthwhile. Or maybe you already agree that corporations have responsibilities to the planet and the people who live on it. In which case, think of what follows as arguments to deploy next time you get into a debate with your Aunt Alice. (I, for one, have three.)

WHAT BUSINESS DO WE HAVE BEING GREEN?

Nobel Prize–winning free market economist Milton Friedman famously wrote, "Few trends could so thoroughly undermine the very foundations of our free society as the acceptance by corporate officials of a social responsibility other than to make as much money for their stockholders as possible."[2]

Henry Miller of the Hoover Institution conjures Friedman's ghost when he frets about the "billions of corporate dollars . . . now being diverted . . . according to the whims of activists who are accountable to no one but themselves and who pursue goals based, not on a desire for greater corporate efficiency or profits, but on their own vision of what is sustainable, equitable, and good for the rest of us." Miller concludes: "Neither free enterprise nor the human condition is likely to experience net benefit from companies pursuing corporate responsibility."[3]

Are we diverting precious resources and undermining "free society" when we ask—nay, demand—that corporations recognize the environment, and other social responsibilities, along with the bottom line?

While Friedman and Miller may take this position, polling (and just asking your friends) reveals that most of us believe corporations owe us some social responsibility. In the wake of the financial collapse of 2008, many have finally awoken to the dangers of a so-called free market system run amok, driven by no other values than the financial. In one 2008 poll of Brits, Americans, and French people, three quarters of Americans said they believed that businesses bore as "much responsibility for driving positive social change as governments."[4] Eighty-six percent said they believed it was "important that companies stand for something other than profitability."[5]

These might seem like obvious sentiments to you, but they don't ring true for the Friedman-ites among us. If we are going to argue that the food industry should take responsibility, and be held accountable, for its role in climate change, then we have to build a case for why it should.

We could simply argue that social responsibility is a good idea because it's good for the bottom line. That's certainly the line we heard from business in the last chapter. But I think it's stronger to develop a coherent argument for why companies, especially food companies, should be responsible beyond the "it's good for business" defense.

First, we should remind ourselves of the history of the corporation as a legal entity: The first corporations were created to undertake work needed by communities, to be a bridge accountable to the government. We should situate the modern corporation in this context, because today many corporations, including many of those in the business of food, have arguably become even more powerful than many governments, and have come to influence policy in direct and indirect ways. Today, the top ten biggest corporations have amassed more wealth than the GDPs of the poorest 146 countries combined.[6] The revenue of 2008's top ten largest S&P 500 companies combined would rank them seventh in the world if it were the GDP of a country, landing them between Italy and Russia.[7]

Most of us are familiar with this remark by onetime GM president Charles Wilson: "For years I thought that what was good for our country was good for General Motors, and vice versa."[8] But we've had enough decades of outsourcing, offshore banking, and tax dodging to know that this truism doesn't hold so true anymore.

We also know that the business community, including food companies, holds powerful influence over the public policy that governs our country, shaping our environmental-protection laws and more. In the United States, corporations spent a total of $3.3 billion on lobbying in 2008 alone.[9] Agribusiness alone doled out more than $65 million in campaign contributions. That same year, you could count roughly two dozen lobbyists on Capitol Hill for every member of Congress we had elected.[10]

Companies also owe us—the people—social responsibility because of what they get from us: They use (often for free or virtually free) our common resources and they benefit (often hugely so) from our taxpayer dollars, while giving back to us in return sometimes only a small fraction of the corporate taxes they actually owe. They also impact the environment in ways that cost us collectively, but that they don't pay for. The climate crisis is perhaps the most glaring example.

This is certainly a very abbreviated case for corporate responsibility, but we could also remind ourselves that companies don't operate outside of the values boundaries we determine as a society. We long ago agreed that companies should not employ slave or child labor, though they still might. We long ago agreed that companies should not pollute our waterways, our air, our backyards, even if they still do. And we agreed (not so long ago) that a company's actions should uphold civil rights law; companies shouldn't discriminate based on race or gender or sexual orientation. That companies have a responsibility to limit their greenhouse-gas emissions is another acknowledgment of a shared value we have agreed to as a society.

So yes, corporations have a responsibility; being "neutral" is not an option. The alternative to embracing greater environmental responsibility is doing nothing. And we now have the evidence that the "doing nothing" of the food industry is actively doing something, namely undermining our ability to feed ourselves and undermining the very basis of life on earth: a stable climate.

It seems that this sentiment—the feeling that indeed, it is fair to expect more from business than Friedman's mandate—is shared among many of us. In that 2008 survey I mentioned earlier, nearly two thirds said they related to this statement: "I have become more interested in corporations' conduct . . . over the past few years."[11]

If the number of sustainability reports produced by major companies since the mid-1990s is any indication, the business community thinks it should be addressing its role in sustainability, too. In 1992, 26 companies produced official sustainability reports; by 1996, the number had jumped to 267. By 2006, we could count 2,346.[12] For some companies, the distribution is far and wide. Syngenta, for instance, distributes twenty thousand copies of its report to NGOs, investors, employees, and government officials.[13]

But as more and more of us believe corporations have this responsibility, fewer and fewer of us are trusting that companies are actually doing their part. In a recent poll by the *Economist*, only 2 percent of those surveyed said they had "a great deal of trust in the leaders of big companies."[14] Nearly a third said they didn't trust them at all. And it's healthy not to believe everything we hear and read. As we face one of the world's biggest challenges, we need to be clear-eyed and demand real change, not just great ad copy.

We've reached a sustainability crossroads.

We are possibly coming to the end of the great trade-off illusion, says Stuart Hall of Cornell University's Johnson School of Management, the misguided notion, implicit in Friedman's criticism, that "societal concerns could only be drags on business."[15] Not only do we know that doing good can benefit the bottom line, but we have also reached the consensus that this social responsibility is not just a feel-good idea for the fringes of a company's business plan; it should be at a company's core. But we need the skills to detect when this ethic has cut to that core—and when it's just a marketing trick.

THE PLAYBOOK

You know big business is getting into the green game when food-retailing behemoth Walmart declares April 2008 "Earth Month." But it's not only mega-companies like Walmart that are declaring their green street cred. All up and down the food chain, "go green" has become a

mantra, so much so that commentaries in industry publications like
Advertising Age and *PRNews* have lamented a new trend, "green fa-
tigue": Consumers are so barraged by green, they're going numb.[16] I
would contend we're numb less from the green and more from the spin:
We want real green, not camouflage.

I certainly heard a lot of green fluff at the GMA eco-shindig.

Campbell Soup Company CEO Doug Conant quipped, "We see a
connection between nourishing lives and nourishing the environment." Coca-Cola's chairman and CEO, John Brock, proclaimed,
"Corporate responsibility is vital to us and our future. It is embodied
in everything we do. The whole concept of sustainability, that's where
we touch the world and the world touches us." According to Unilever
president Kevin Havelock, environmental stewardship "is in our
DNA." Over at the *Advertising Age* Green Conference, McDonald's
global chief marketing officer, Mary Dillon, piped in: "Our overall
DNA at McDonald's is about social responsibility and giving back to
community."

As we hear more of these green claims, we can get savvier about how
to detect strategies companies are deploying to spin themselves green
rather than actually make true green change.

The Playbook

> *Play 1: Advertise the new you*
> *Play 2: Spin the story*
> *Play 3: Deploy front groups and fig leaves*
> *Play 4: Exaggerate your transformation*
> *Play 5: Be your own police*
> *Play 6: Reward yourself*

Play 1: Advertise the New You

> LOW-CARBON IS THE NEW FAT-FREE
> —sign at the *Advertising Age* Green Conference,
> NYU Skirball Center, June 2008

Standing onstage at New York University's Skirball Center in the summer
of 2008, Mary Dillon unveiled the new "green" McDonald's logo. As it

flashed across the screen, she regaled the audience with the company's environmental commitments.

"I want people to see us as a socially responsible company," said Dillon to the several hundred *Advertising Age* Green Conference attendees. The Happy Meal, she explained, is one of their tools.

"Our Happy Meals deliver a positive message about the environment," Dillon continued. She described the McDonald's Europe Happy Meal initiative that connected consumers to "My Pledge," a customer commitment to taking eco-action; sustainability cross-promotions with blockbuster movies like *Kung Fu Panda*; and even an endangered-animal-themed Happy Meal. These initiatives sounded similar to a 2007 McDonald's campaign in Japan. There, consumers were encouraged to go online and check off items on a list of thirty-nine ways to reduce their personal greenhouse-gas emissions. Checking off such commitments as reducing their shower time by a minute or turning off their AC would reap them a coupon for a half-priced Big Mac.[17] (I imagine "skip the beef" was not on the list.) The promotion was so popular that the government Web site promoting it crashed with the deluge.[18]

Flash back a year and a half and Happy Meals had a different slant. It was August 2006, and McDonald's had just announced a partnership with automaker General Motors. The companies had teamed up to give away forty-two million "fun-fueled miniature HUMMER vehicles." With select purchases of Happy Meals or Mighty Kids Meals, boys could get the Metallic Sand H1, "a free-wheeling vehicle with a retractable winch," or the Laser Blue H2H, which "offers a truly enlightening ride."[19] (Girls had their pick of Polly Pocket fashion dolls.)

Oh, how times have changed. The irony of McDonald's having associated so recently with the gas-guzzling, ten-mile-per-gallon Hummer was clearly lost on the company in 2008.

Advertising the new face of the company doesn't change its core contradiction. For companies like McDonald's are, by design, inherently extensive greenhouse-gas emitters. McDonald's product line of high-fat, highly processed and packaged, meat-centered meals (with their driver-centric focus) has an intrinsically high eco-toll.

Advertising about-faces, like this one, are a glaring example of how companies are rebranding themselves to fit the times. Done successfully, such a rebranding, along with the other PR strategies in the playbook, can make it challenging for us mere mortals to distinguish the real green from the pseudo green. Indeed, as you'll see with this next strategy, a successful rebranding can be a powerful inoculation against public attacks.

Play 2: Spin the Story

> WHAT'S RIGHT TODAY MAY BE WRONG TOMORROW, SO PAINT
> THAT BRAND IMAGE A LITTLE MORE LOOSELY—
> MORE ABSTRACT, VALUE-LADEN AND INFO-POOR.
> —Getty Images, *Aspirational Environmentalism*

If you have a pulse, you've probably seen the BP eco-ads blanketing billboards, newspapers, magazines, and more. That's the nine-year-old campaign through which oil giant British Petroleum is rebranding itself as the eco-friendly "Beyond Petroleum." The bill for that rebranding is estimated at two hundred million dollars (and counting).[20] The benefit to the company? The windfall could be as much as three billion dollars in that sought-after "brand value."[21]

BP is the subject of just one of dozens of case studies on businesses going green (and profiting from it) that Yale's Daniel Esty and Andrew Winston share in *Green to Gold*. The free copies waiting on our seats at the GMA summit were quickly snatched up; the audience was riveted during Esty's presentation. (Maybe particularly so because his was one of the few not made available online—proprietary knowledge and all.)

In the book, Esty and Winston quote BP senior adviser Chris Mottershead, who describes the rebranding process as "painful." "It took a long time and lots of resources to get to the helios design and overall positioning," Mottershead says. "These were deeply conscious thoughts and it was a profound, long, painful process."[22] (Who would have thought developing a star-shaped sunburst logo would be "painful"?)

The real eyebrow-raising, though, should come in asking, never mind the pretty new logo, is BP really going beyond petroleum?

One analysis pegged the amount spent on the company redesign as much greater than the company's actual investment in renewable energy.[23] Yes, BP may be able to bill itself as "the largest producer of solar energy in the world," but that's partly because the sector is in its infancy.[24] The $45 million the company spent in 1999 to acquire the remaining shares it didn't already own of Solarex, a solar-energy company, is just a fraction of the $26.5 *billion* it spent buying oil company ARCO that same year.[25] And, despite a continued rollout of its "Beyond Petroleum" ad campaign, since 2007 the company has been cutting back on its renewable-energy initiatives while continuing to invest heavily in oil exploration, like the $1.5 billion it committed to an Alaskan oil field.[26]

BP's Mottershead himself admits there is no material difference between BP fuel and its competitors. "Why do people pull into a BP station versus an Exxon one?" asks Mottershead. "Because it's saying something about their aspirations and expectations for the future. It's not that the fuel that they're buying is any better."[27]

Yet BP's rebranding has been so effective that the company's reputation has remained relatively untarnished despite incidents that should have bruised it.[28] One was an explosion at BP's Texas City, Texas, refinery in March 2005. The explosion killed fifteen people, and the company was fined twenty-one million dollars for safety violations—a record high—by the U.S. Occupational Safety and Health Administration.[29] The safety violations were connected to company budget cuts.[30] And in March 2006, a BP pipeline leak dumped 267,000 gallons of oil into Alaska's Prudhoe Bay. The leak had gone undetected for five days and been caused by failing equipment that environmental advocates had earlier red-flagged for a fix.[31] Company execs countered that they had "had no reason to expect" the pipe to bust a leak.[32]

These incidents were not "accidents"; they were caused by real negligence, negligence that cost 15 people their lives, injured another 180, and caused untold damage in the bay.[33] These two incidents alone should have seriously damaged BP's reputation. How, then, to explain that they didn't?

Esty and Winston suggest that BP's newfound feel-good eco-reputation—love that helios!—may have given the company reputational leeway, what they call the "trust bank," that acted like an inoculation when these "bad things" happened.[34] The two quote a "knowledgeable observer" who says, "It was fascinating how much slack the environmental community cut BP. Their investment in being seen as good guys paid off handsomely."[35]

The food industry, like the oil industry, is skilled at inoculation messaging, and part of its success comes from the "we're one of you" pitch.

Picture an iconic Midwestern farm, and a red barn in a grassy field might come to mind, but a pagoda perched on a farm's green lawn? Or Japanese slippers sitting next to farmer boots on a porch? A camera pans across these curious shoes and out-of-place pagoda, and a voice-over begins: "As you can see, this isn't your typical Midwestern farm." The reason, we learn, lies "six thousand miles away," where a Japanese producer of specialty eggs needed feed corn produced to "precise specifications." Cut to a Japanese farmer standing in a beautiful shed, sunlight streaming between the boards of weathered wood. He looks closely at one of his eggs and unloads feed for his happily pecking poultry.

A close-up shows a Cargill logo printed across an egg.

This Illinois farmer producing feed for a Japanese farmer half a world away, and the friendship they form, is just one of the thirteen feel-good stories featured in Cargill's multimedia ad campaign "Cargill Creates." (The company calls these "case studies," though they're just, well, ads.)

Does the name Cargill mean anything to you? The company may not exactly be a household word, but it's ubiquitous in our food supply, from high-fructose corn syrup to livestock. Indeed, as the largest privately held company in the nation, Cargill has a global reach that is awe inspiring in its scope and its environmental impact.

It owns Cargill Pork and Cargill Beef, the second-largest beef processor in North America, and is one of the largest commercial cattle feeders in the United States. Along with vegetable, grain-related, and edible-oil operations, the company's subsidiary businesses include Cargill Regional Beef, Cargill Value Added Meats, Cargill Beef Argentina, Cargill Beef Australia, Cargill Meats Brazil, Cargill Meats Canada, Cargill Meats Central America, Cargill Meats Europe, Cargill Meats Thailand, Cargill Corn Milling, and Cargill Flour Mercosur.[36] Cargill controls 80 percent of the European market for soybean crushing and a similar share for animal-feed manufacturing.[37] It is the world's biggest processor, marketer, and distributor of grains, oilseeds, and other agricultural commodities, and has businesses developing a variety of industrial applications for its feed stocks.

Cargill also has ownership stake in businesses that supply its operations. It is a majority owner of Mosaic, for example, the world's largest producer of the fertilizer component phosphate and a leading miner, processor, and distributor of potash. Until October 2008, Cargill had a 50 percent stake in one of the world's biggest fertilizer-ingredient production facilities. This ownership is strategic, in part because Cargill's production is heavily reliant on synthetic fertilizer, but also because as Cargill and others expand their greenhouse-gas-intensive production into new markets, fertilizer demand (and thus price) is spiking. In 2008, Mosaic's operating earnings shot up from $101 million in 2006 to nearly $3 billion.[38]

Cargill has also set its sights on Wall Street, setting up investment and hedge funds to capitalize on the cash flow "thrown off by its grain and agricultural trading operations,"[39] including Black River Commodity Clean Energy Investment Fund; Black River Asset Management, with offices in eleven countries; and private-equity group CarVal Investors.[40] And it has set up energy-trading companies to capitalize on the erratic rise and fall of energy prices, which one could argue is being sparked partly by another sector of Cargill's own business: agrofuels.[41]

All of Cargill's operations have a serious climate-change toll, for the company is knee-deep in the energy-intensive commodity-crop and livestock production I described earlier. As one of the largest producers of soy in Brazil, for example, it has come under heavy fire for the impact of its business operations, which drive rainforest destruction and the displacement of indigenous communities.[42]

Despite this impact, and the company's reach, Cargill's name rarely appears on our supermarket shelves and wouldn't be at the tip of your tongue unless you were closely following which companies' profits soared during 2008's food-price crisis. While Haiti was burning and Bangladesh was raging in "food riots," as they were dubbed, in response to spiking food costs, Cargill scored nearly two billion dollars in record earnings in the first half of that year.[43]

The "Cargill Creates" ad campaign is an attempt to transform the company from a faceless multinational to a company that creates personal connection. It seems to be a strategy to fend off reproach by supplanting the image of an unaccountable multinational with that of a friendship-maker, a person-to-person collaborator. The messaging tactic takes its cues from industry observers like Getty Images, which urges companies to get wise to the consumer desire for "locally sourced" products, using "real people who represent and connect to the community they are being used to sell to."[44]

The "we're one of you" PR tactic is not novel, but as agribusiness and food companies come under fire for their global impact, they're cranking up the messaging. Consider the letter that Joe Holtz, the general manager of Brooklyn's Park Slope Food Coop, received within weeks of the co-op's decision to stop selling bottled water. In the letter, Nestlé's northeast account manager, Joe Bonanno, focuses on "what's good about the bottled water business." He describes the safety of bottled water, its health and hydration properties, and its efficient production. "A gallon of bottled water takes just 1.37 gallons of water to produce," writes Bonanno. (Odd, no, to think of water being used to "produce" water?) As his letter comes to a close, Bonanno writes, "As a father of two small children I'm confident that the case for bottled water is stronger than the argument against it."[45] A subtle reminder of the people, just like you and me, who populate these companies.

Reading meat-industry publications, I stumbled on another example of inoculate-through-humbleness: Perdue, the third-largest poultry company in the country, announced the groundbreaking on a project to turn the farm where the company started ninety years ago into a museum for corporate functions and an exhibit on Perdue family history.[46] While this farmhouse might be a reminder of the company's family-farm beginnings, Perdue is currently a $2.8-billion-in-sales multinational, selling forty-eight million pounds of chicken parts across forty countries annually.[47] And like its competitors, Perdue has faced many fines over the years from the U.S. government for health, safety, and environmental violations.[48]

The message, whether from Perdue, Nestlé, or Cargill, is that these companies are like us; they care about the same things we do. It's a messaging that forms another strand of the inoculation strategy. Of course, companies are made up of real people just like us. But this doesn't automatically mean that a particular company has our collective, or planetary, interest at heart when it makes decisions about expanding resource-intensive and emissions-heavy production—whether it be of bottled water, factory-farmed meat, or chemical-intensive crops.

Play 3: Deploy Front Groups and Fig Leaves

In 2008, the American Farmers for the Advancement and Conservation of Technology (AFACT) launched a response to farmers who had been publicly rejecting the use of Monsanto's synthetic growth hormone, rBGH, in dairy production and charging that the hormone was causing illnesses in cows—and potentially in humans. But this was no farmer-against-farmer fight. With a little digging, you'd discover that the group's Web site, www.itisafact.org, is registered to Susan Williams of Osborn Barr Communications, a brand-management company whose clients include Monsanto, the National Pork Board, and Michelin.[49] Despite its name, AFACT is a classic front group: It seems like a megaphone for real people—farmers, in this case—but is actually developed and funded by industry.

Those of us reading about the controversy in the media might miss this connection, though. In news coverage, front groups aren't always identified as such. In articles about the rBGH debate, AFACT is identified only occasionally with the qualification that it is "backed by Monsanto." Lisa Rathke, of the Associated Press, ran one of the first articles about the group, quoting Carrol Campbell, a Kansas dairy farmer, who is identified as the organization's cochair.[50] Rathke's article was picked up widely—from New Jersey's *Trentonian* to MSN.com to the Nashua, New Hampshire, *Telegraph* and the *Guardian*. If you read this coverage, it would be easy to miss the real story here: that a billion-dollar multinational company was concerned about citizen revolt against one of its products, which was causing lost profits and market share, and that this self-same company had created a fake organization to defend its position. As Monsanto and other corporations involved in industrial food find themselves in the crosshairs of a public concerned about climate change, it's likely that more companies will engage in this stealth play.

The trust that companies earn by voicing views through front groups can also be achieved through partnership with nonprofits that act like "fig leaves." While these organizations aren't created *by* the companies, look at their donor lists and you might find they read like a *Fortune* magazine who's who.

I'll highlight one example from Swiss agrochemical giant Syngenta.

When I asked representatives of Syngenta, the world's largest agrochemical company, about its sustainability programs, they plugged the company's work with Ducks Unlimited—"a big biodiversity" organization, they said.

Founded in 1937 by duck hunters who wanted to protect waterfowl and wetlands, Ducks Unlimited now has an annual budget of more than two hundred million dollars, more than half a million members, and a staff of more than five hundred. It helps meet that multi-million-dollar budget with donations from chemical companies like Bayer CropScience, Dow Chemical, Monsanto, and Syngenta.[51]

So what does Syngenta do for Ducks?

According to a company rep, Syngenta donates one hundred thousand dollars' worth of product annually. Recent donations include the contribution of 620 gallons (worth about twenty-one thousand dollars) of Touchdown HiTech herbicide used to control an invasive plant in the Wisconsin Fish Lake State Wildlife Area.[52] Not such a big price tag for a billion-dollar business like Syngenta, especially when you factor in its giving away its own product and getting a tax write-off for doing so.

(When I asked about the impact of the herbicide on the aquatic life in the wildlife area's waterways, the Ducks Unlimited guy said, "In order to manage some areas for waterfowl, so that there will be waterfowl to manage, you sometimes have to use chemicals. It's that simple." Only, it's not that simple.)

What's the irony here?

Syngenta is the country's largest manufacturer of the popular weed killer atrazine, used on golf courses, lawns, and on more than two thirds of the nation's corn crop.[53] Banned in Europe in 2007, atrazine has long worried environmentalists and public health advocates in the United States for its properties as both an endocrine disrupter and probable carcinogen. University of California at Berkeley professor Tyrone Hayes has studied the herbicide for years, uncovering the troubling connection between atrazine in our waterways and hermaphroditic frogs.[54] Says Hayes, "the evidence in every animal class that's been examined" is that "atrazine causes adverse biological effects."[55] New studies are further revealing the chemical's impact on humans, suggesting a link to birth defects, low birth weights, and menstrual problems.[56] (Syngenta maintains that the level of atrazine in water systems is far below a level that would cause any harm.)[57]

Adding to the irony, Syngenta also plugs its partnership with Ducks in the Chesapeake Bay region, where once "the clean waters . . . provided an ideal home for millions of migrating wildfowl, along with more than 2500 other native species," the company's Web site notes. "Over the years, however, approximately half the wetlands and associated forest-buffered streams around the Bay were lost."[58] Working with Ducks Unlimited, Syngenta says, the company is "restoring native warm-season grass buffers alongside upland ditches, streams and fields." These buffers "use up nitrogen, and prevent it from reaching groundwater."[59]

What goes unsaid is that much of that nitrogen is in fertilizer runoff from area farms, including Syngenta products. This runoff has led to a "dead zone" in the bay, spreading for hundreds of square miles, where fertilizer-induced algal blooms leave too little oxygen to support other aquatic life.

Through connections with nonprofit organizations that seem to work for the public good, companies like Syngenta can foster the patina of being sustainable, when their actual business practices might be anything but.

Play 4: Exaggerate Your Transformation

Let's head back to the GMA conference. In one of the more candid moments, a rep from the North American Millers Association spoke up in a workshop. "Joe Consumer is a lot more aware than six months ago or six years ago, but it's only going to go so far," he said. "They just want to know that the brand they trust is doing *something*. If they hear about a dead zone in the Gulf of Mexico, they know there's a problem, but they just want to know that we share these concerns and feel we're doing something about it."

This conviction that consumers will believe what they're told is seen throughout a food industry that's willing to exaggerate its transformation to earn public-opinion points on the assumption that customers won't dig beneath the surface.

In one example from the pages of Tyson's 2005 *Sustainability Report*, the meat giant highlights its June 2003 settlement of an EPA lawsuit. The EPA had charged the company with violations of the Clean Water Act at its Sedalia, Missouri, plant. Says Tyson, "The lawsuit and subsequent settlement have brought significant positive change to Tyson Foods. We have taken a hard look at our practices including those that gave rise to the dispute, and have made changes to improve our performance. We are a better company today because of it."[60]

That all sounds good: a corporation learning from its mistakes. But it's not exactly how Tyson talked about the case—and treated it—during the years it wrestled with the EPA over the charges. The EPA initiated the suit in 1999 after uncovering that the company had repeatedly and knowingly, over several years, discharged untreated wastewater from its Sedalia plant into the local watershed.[61]

In *that* year's 10-K and in each subsequent year's until the settlement, Tyson referred to the case with identical sentences ending with "The Company is presently discussing the possible resolution of this matter but neither the likelihood of an unfavorable outcome nor the amount of ultimate liability, if any, with respect to this matter can be determined at this time."[62]

So Tyson fights the lawsuit for years, eventually agreeing to a $5.5 million fine paid to the federal government, plus $1 million in damages paid to the state of Missouri and $1 million more to the Missouri Natural Resources Protection Fund, and only then its sustainability report describes the incident as a tool for corporate improvement?[63] Losing a lawsuit seems to have a way of changing your tune.

Here's another Tyson example. In the same sustainability report, the company boasts about its biodiversity conservation, pointing to thirty-five acres near a Tennessee facility that have been designated a wildlife preserve. In the spring of 2005, ten bluebird nests were installed on the property, each one fledging an average of five birds.[64] In explaining why the company cares about biodiversity, the report says, "It is important to people because we depend on other species for food, work, recreation, and the environmental conditions (clean water, air, and land) that sustain our lives."[65]

While I'm all for bluebirds, initiatives such as this are comically inconsequential compared with the company's overall environmental impacts. Consider Tyson's effect on biodiversity, while keeping in mind the vital role for biodiversity in a climate-unstable future. The uniformity of factory farming has whittled down the diversity of birds raised for consumption in this country to basically just one breed. Today, Tyson's sixty-five hundred contract farmers must rely on the company for chicks; they no longer raise their own. Plus, Tyson has been found responsible for the biodiversity-stunting pollution of its poultry operations. In a recent court ruling, for example, it was found guilty of ammonia pollution from its contract farms in Kentucky.[66]

Don't get me wrong; I'm not saying that companies can't play a role in positive transformation. This book's message is certainly that the food industry can, and should, be a partner in strategies addressing climate change. But our focus shouldn't be on the minor environmental benefits these companies might be providing; it should be on the climate impact of the bulk of their business. These efforts need to do more than *sound* good and make marginal improvements, bolstering reputations simply to inoculate companies from public furor. These efforts must actually be effective and significant. It's up to us, citizens, not to let companies off the hook for their environmental and climate-change damage, and to push for policies and increase public pressure to encourage them to become more responsible, ecological, and climate friendly.

Play 5: Be Your Own Police

At the industry conferences I attended, one of the most adored words seemed to be "voluntary"—as in voluntary monitoring and voluntary emissions reductions. "Third-party certification"? Verboten. "Government regulation"? The bogeyman.

These days you hear a lot of companies talking about how they're reducing their greenhouse-gas emissions; we'll certainly be hearing more of it. But these voluntary reduction schemes are not as impressive as they may seem.

After Deborah Louison, senior vice president of corporate affairs, presented Cadbury Schweppes's ambitious emissions-reduction plans at the 2008 GMA summit, she mentioned that the company would determine what year to "start the clock." Depending on what year it chooses, it can make its numbers look a lot better than they would with a different start-the-clock date.

Companies have other tricks for playing with the math. When I talked with the folks in Syngenta's sustainability department, they said the company has targeted a 40 percent reduction in emissions by 2012, compared with 2006. Sounds good. But look closely and you'll notice that the company bases their reductions on a ratio of emissions to operating profit, or EBIT.[67] In other words, Syngenta is committed to reducing greenhouse gas emissions only if it can make a profit doing so. And in 2008, it sure did. Between 2007 and 2008, the company's emissions shot up 40 percent, but thanks to its clever accounting, the emissions *ratio* was flat. Why? Simply because as its emissions skyrocketed so did its profits. Ka-ching. Good for Syngenta's CEO. Not so good for us.

There's another way in which Syngenta twists its emissions-reduction story. In its analysis of its carbon footprint, the company accounts for emissions from the production of its products, but it also takes credit for the emissions it alleges it's responsible for reducing. In 2006, its emissions from operations, employee travel, distribution, and other practices added up to more than one megatonne of carbon-dioxide-equivalent emissions, but the company claims these are more than offset by the potential of its products to improve crop yields and enhance soil carbon storage. While Syngenta acknowledges it doesn't have accurate data on emissions "outside our control"—from suppliers and farms—the company still asserts that those farm-level benefits outweigh the on-farm costs.

"Based on this analysis, we believe our business is making a positive contribution to tackling climate change overall," says Syngenta. In its sustainability report the company makes this point graphically.[68] A series of bars represent emissions from the stages of production in which the company is directly involved: its operations and purchased energy, its employee travel, and distribution of its products. The graphic also depicts two areas outside the direct control of the company, the theoretical emissions reductions achieved by protecting yield and not tilling the soil. In one fell hypothetical swoop, the company gives the impression that its emissions are neatly offset by these emissions savings, and though the report doesn't put any hard numbers on this positive farm-level reduction, the design makes it look like the benefits far outweigh the costs. If you've ever watched HBO's *The Wire*, this is what Deputy Rawls would call "juking the stats."

At the Cadbury Schweppes presentation, a corporate exec sitting next to me leaned over and whispered, "You can say anything you want with statistics. It's like saying the moon is half the size of the earth and twice as far." I didn't get what he meant at first; then I realized his point. Numbers tell you nothing unless they're presented in context.

To be fair, measuring direct and indirect emissions of business operations is tough. Especially in the food farming sector, there are a multitude of variables. But that's all the more reason to be sure that the standards for measurement are not unduly influenced by the industry.

Too bad we're already seeing the industry step up its lobbying around these regs.

Business leaders know what Andrew Hoffman means when, referring to regulation, he titles his *Harvard Business Review* article "If You're Not at the Table, You're on the Menu."[69] Hoffman illuminates all the levels where companies are getting into the lobbying game to determine the regulations coming down the pipeline. Companies, says Hoffman, are looking to shape policy on Regional Greenhouse Gas Initiatives, lobbying groups like the California Air Resources Board, which is developing mandatory-emissions-reporting rules (and the all-important and highly controversial methodology that companies will need to use to determine their emissions). They're also lobbying states that are developing inventories of emissions (to get their industry on or off the map, as best suits them). On a federal level, Hoffman encourages companies to lobby on one of more than "100 climate-related bills," and on an international level, to attempt to influence the U. N. framework convention on climate change.[70]

Play 6: Reward Yourself

On October 24, 2007, at an American Meat Institute conference in Chicago, the trade association announced the winners of its second annual Environmental Achievement and Recognition Awards. Smithfield's Farmland Foods, in Crete, Nebraska, got third place for Environmental Stewardship and snagged first place for Environmental Outreach to the Public.[71] The honor recognized the subsidiary's work "with the local high school to raise funds for college scholarships by recycling scrap metal and used equipment at the plant."[72]

"We do a lot of changing up in our processes," Farmland Foods' Jeff Waszgis told me, "and a lot of times we'll end up with scrap equipment." For the past couple of years, the company has been recycling those scraps and using the proceeds for scholarships. Last year, it gave ten five-hundred-dollar scholarships to students at four area high schools. To qualify, students must write an essay about the benefits of contributing to the community, and they must have parents who work at the plant. This year, the facility plans to add another high school and include other recycled products.

When I asked about the slaughterhouse's production, Waszgis explained, "We take the meat all the way through to fresh pork and smoked pork. Production-wise we're probably killing ten thousand or better a day."

The accolades from its own parent company and trade association aside, the Farmland Foods facility in Crete is not exactly a role model for environmental stewardship. The facility was the county's top polluter, responsible for four times as much toxic chemical releases, according to filings with the EPA in 2002, as the next runner-up, the region's Nestlé Purina manufacturing facility.[73] Farmland Foods is also a major source of nitrates in the region's waterways, which can cause the potentially serious illness methemoglobinemia, or blue baby syndrome.

And it doesn't seem to be improving. From 1998 to 2002, the facility's total releases of pollutants in local waterways increased by 3,197 percent, and its ammonia releases increased by 43 percent.[74] In Nebraska, the Farmland Foods plant is the fifth-largest contributor to water pollution and blood toxicants released into waterways.[75] But none of this stopped the American Meat Institute from honoring the facility with two Environmental Achievement and Recognition Awards.

Honors like this are becoming quite common. Some are internal awards: A company knights itself. Others have the aura of impartiality. The Forbes-Ethisphere Ethical Leadership Forum, for instance, presents its annual Most Ethical Companies awards. In 2008, McDonald's won highest honors among restaurants and cafés.

Wondering how you, too, could be the "most ethical"? Companies fill out an "Ethics Quotient" survey and receive a score based on their responses. Companies are judged in several categories, and "corporate responsibility" and "reputation track record" are the two most important, accounting for 40 percent of the overall score. In addition, companies that will "profit fairly from such ethical leadership business practices" earn higher points, "as ultimately only profit ensures continuance of desired institutional behavior."[76]

DECODING THE PLAYBOOK

Why should we care if a few companies are tooting their horns when they don't have much to toot about? Or that some eco-acts are being exaggerated? Aren't small shifts in the right direction better than nothing?

First, the kind of PR spins I described here often achieve what the companies hope they will: They bring consumer guard down so that we become less critical of companies whose actions might actually be ecologically suspect. Take Walmart, for example. The company has been pushing its green initiatives with fervor. But in internal meetings, former CEO Lee Scott "told Wal-Mart executives that their sustainability efforts would help protect the company's 'license to grow.' "[77] If these publicity stunts do generate warm-and-fuzzy feelings—that sought-after goodwill—without delivering substantive change, they can defuse demands for the transformative change really required.

Second, the flood of all this green-oriented campaigning—the advertising and the PR spins—clouds the field. It makes it challenging to tell the real deal from bogus action. This, in turn, makes it that much harder for us to celebrate the good guys and reward those companies that are taking the tough and needed stances.

Finally, sly advertising and slick strategies can create a new class of consumer: the cynical one. And the more cynical consumers become, the more likely they are to distrust *all* green claims, to think that no consumer decision they make holds greater consequence than any other. While eight in ten Americans believe it's important to buy from "green" companies, seven out of ten either "strongly" or "somewhat" agree that when companies call a product green, it is usually just a marketing tactic.[78]

So what to do? Throw up our hands and say we can't trust any claim? No. We can get smart about distinguishing authentic action from just greenwashing.

How to Detect the Real Deal

A man jogs through a lush rainforest as shots of palm-oil plantations and wildlife flash across the screen. A voice-over pronounces, "Malaysia's palm oil. Its trees give life and help our planet breathe."[79] The ad was paid for and sponsored by the Malaysian Palm Oil Council, founded in 1990 to spearhead the "promotional and marketing activities of Malaysian palm oil."[80] Said the council's chief exec, "We decided it was about time we gave a public-service announcement to the consumer."[81]

Or public disservice?

The United Kingdom's Advertising Standards Authority (ASA),

whose mandate is to ensure that "all advertising, wherever it appears, meets the high standards laid down in the advertising codes," determined that the ad was "likely to mislead viewers as to the environmental benefits of oil-palm plantations, compared with native rain forests."[82]

The ASA is one approach to reducing rampant greenwashing: setting up an agency to oversee the field. But it's certainly not foolproof. Rulings can take a long time. By the time the authority came down on this palm-industry ad, the spot had appeared on satellite channels across Europe, Asia, and the United States and was already off the air. The other limitation? Standards boards, like the authority, make "rulings" without teeth; regulators can't impose a fine.[83]

Norway is one major exception. There, government regulators can, and do, levy fines for false advertising. And in September 2007, regulators banned car companies from using claims such as "green," "clean," and "environmentally friendly" in their advertisements. "Cars cannot do anything good for the environment except less damage than others," commented Bente Oeverli, a senior official at the state-run Consumer Ombudsman, explaining the regs. Manufacturers risk fines if they fail to drop the buzzwords.

An approach that we are exploring here in the United States is to strengthen the guidelines on what companies can and can't claim about "greenness"—and be clearer about what being green means. And according to one poll, we want that. Fifty-nine percent of those Americans interviewed for the 2008 Green Gap Survey said they believed the government "needs to regulate the environmental messaging by companies to ensure it's accurate."[84] "Truth in advertising" is an established legal principle—so why not when it comes to truth about the health of our planet?

You might not have spent much time thinking about the United States' Federal Trade Commission (FTC), or what it does for you and me, but the one-thousand-person-large agency is responsible, in part, for making sure we're not lied to by business, prosecuting those businesses engaged in fleecing us. Part of its mandate is to protect consumers from fraudulent practices ranging from e-mail spam to spyware to mortgage swindles. (You might better know them from Do Not Call Registry fame; the FTC is the agency that set up that firewall between you and telemarketers.)

The commission is responsible for determining when marketers have stepped over the line from *persuasive* advertising to *deceptive* advertising. Determining exactly where that line is, though, can be hard. Those car ads with sexy women throwing themselves at the nerdy guy behind the wheel? We all know that a new sports car won't help you get a date, or turn you into the next George Clooney, but advertisers can get away with the implication. That paper products company that tells us it's "climate neutral"? A little tougher.

In response to the flurry of environmental claims flooding the market in the 1990s, the FTC set guidelines for acceptable, and unacceptable, claims when it comes to all things green. The 1992 *Guides for the Use of Environmental Marketing Claims* (commonly known as *The Green Guides*) was supposed to be reviewed again in 2009, but the agency bumped up its deliberation in part because of a "tsunami of green claims," says the FTC's associate director of enforcement in the Bureau of Consumer Protection, James Kohm.

"We've had our first carbon-neutral Superbowl, a carbon-neutral NASCAR race, a carbon-neutral Oscars," says Kohm. By one estimate, manufacturers launched 328 "environmentally friendly" products in 2007, up from only 5 in 2002.[85] The U.S. Patent and Trademark Office saw applications for products with the word "green" in their name more than double from 2006 to 2007. Indeed, one of 2006's words of the year in *The New Oxford American Dictionary* was "carbon neutral."

Kohm explains how the guidelines can help in response to this deluge. We're "generally concerned about two types of people and companies: those who cross the line and those who live over it," he says. The people who live over the line? "They're the ones who get up every day and try to commit fraud." Guidelines aren't very useful for them. They're not reading rules; they're breaking the law. As Kohm says, "they don't attend our conferences."[86]

He stresses that these guidelines are key to helping the "other people," those who step over the line because of competitive pressure. "Our job is to help clarify, in as many areas as possible, where that line is," he says. And with the clamor to one-up the competition in "greenness," the FTC is again getting into the fray to define environmental claims. We the public seem to want not only clarity but enforcement: Three quarters of people polled by GfK Roper said they were looking to the federal government to strengthen its enforcement of green regulations.[87] Says the FTC, "Ultimately, the issuance of national industry-wide guidance for environmental marketing claims was recognized as a way to promote truthful and substantiated advertising while providing certainty in the marketplace for both advertisers and consumers."[88]

Still under discussion as I write, the revised *Green Guides* will provide precision to the meaning behind green claims for packaging, buildings, and carbon-offset programs. All the terms we hear bandied about—"recyclable," "biodegradable," "compostable," "refillable," "environmentally friendly," "sustainable," "bio-based," "cradle-to-cradle," and "carbon neutral"—need better definitions. Some of the core principles of the guidelines follow, in a list of claims that companies should *not* make.

- *Unsubstantiated claims:* Evidence matters. Companies must be able to back up their words.

- *Unintelligible claims:* Companies should steer clear of claims that use terms consumers won't understand.

- *Open-ended claims:* One of the common claims on packaging is that it's recyclable, but being recyclable and you, Joe Consumer, actually being able to recycle the product are two different things. "Claims about recyclability must correspond to the availability of recycling facilities in the area where the claim is made," stresses Kohm.

- *Dangling comparative claims:* A company can't just say, "My beef is greener." Well, greener than what? The landmark FTC decision on this issue was in response to tobacco company Liggett & Myers's claim that "Chesterfields are milder."

- *Exaggerated features claims:* Companies shouldn't overemphasize aspects of a product that don't have any real benefit, or significance, to the consumer. An example cited by the FTC is Preparation H's hype of Bio-Dyne in advertisements back in the 1960s. Turns out the ingredient had "little or no therapeutic value."[89] (I guess American Home Product liked the sound of it?)

Kohm also stresses another core principle: It's not "necessarily what you intend to say that's important; it's what a reasonable consumer would take away from a broad claim."

Once the guidelines are set, they're just that: guides. They inform Section 5 of the FTC Act, which says that marketers can't engage in deceptive practices. As Kohm explains, "while in a legal sense you can't be sued for violating the guides, they're the commission's guidelines for compliance with Section 5."

What do companies think about the guidelines?

Some industry players warn that strict guidelines will "chill the marketplace" for green products. The American Association of Advertising Agencies, the American Advertising Federation, and the Association of National Advertisers signed a joint statement arguing that the FTC should not rush to judgment because existing guidelines on truth and accuracy in environmental claims are already effective; self-regulation already "ensures that environmental claims are not deceptive and must be substantiated"; changes could cause confusion that could chill "valuable advertising messages"; and there is scientific uncertainty about how to characterize certain claims.[90]

In the April 2008 hearings on the proposed guidelines, the FTC heard from other industry reps, like Jim Hanna, Starbucks' director of environmental impact, who described the guidelines as a "reactionary way of doing things." Plus, he predicted, companies would just come up with a new way around them. At Starbucks, Hanna said, "we're great at inventing new words"—he gave a shout-out to Frappuccino—and he essentially warned that "if you put these guidelines on existing words we'll create a new lexicon out there you have to react to again in five, ten years."[91]

Well, it's precisely the need to stay ahead of industry's fudging of green with its inventiveness that's getting the FTC deliberating.

Whom to Trust?

If the Malaysian Palm Oil Council is telling us that the industry's trees "give life and help our planet breathe," and the advertising-watchdog associations are only ready to clamp down a little on such clear propaganda, whom can we trust?

You can seek out and listen to the organizations that are working on the issue, with no strings attached to profit. You can listen to Rainforest Action Network (RAN), for instance.*

Why trust RAN? Well, first, the organization is not designed to make a profit; it was created as a nonprofit, advocacy organization to protect rainforests, communities, and the climate. Plus, it would say, its information is coming from its relationships with people on the ground and with NGO allies, and from research that's publicly available.

"We're out to influence change," says RAN's Leila Salazar-Lopez. "We're not just out there to criticize companies. We want companies to do better so that there can be social and environment change that benefits people and the climate."

Just because there are some flimsy groups that are more front than font of trustworthy information, it doesn't mean that all organizations are hucksters. Among those I turn to for unfiltered, unbiased information are the ones listed below. (See the resource section at the end of the book for more.)

- Center for Food Safety: www.centerforfoodsafety.org

- Consumers Union: www.consumersunion.org

- Union of Concerned Scientists: www.ucsusa.org

- And, you can also get background on many of the organizations and certifying bodies you will come across with the help of the hype-busting Center for Media and Democracy: www.prwatch.org

DIY Green: ID Greenwash When You See It

You don't have to just depend on the experts to detect greenwashing; you can learn some of the DIY tricks listed below. For more about

* For years I had been a long-distance admirer of Rainforest Action Network, and after beginning the research for this book, I decided to join its board of directors. I consider my work as a board member to be keeping RAN accountable to its interests: the communities where it works and the forests, people, and animals it is chartered to protect. Unlike most members of corporate leadership boards, I have no financial stake in RAN. One way to ensure that there continue to be organizations we can rely on to tell the truth is to do what we can to support them: through volunteering, joining their boards, or contributing other resources.

greenwashing and labeling, see the Greenpeace Stop Greenwash Web site at www.stopgreenwash.org. Futerra Sustainability Communications has a great greenwash guide, available at www.futerra.co.uk.

A product claiming to be the greenest thing since Ed Begley Jr.'s bamboo floors might make you raise an eyebrow. Here are key questions to ask concerning product claims and company commitments.

Product Claims

1. *Is it relevant?* It's easy to take credit for something that doesn't require any effort, like all those products that boast, "No CFCs!" That's not too challenging since CFCs, or chlorofluorocarbons, have been phased out of most large-scale applications for years and should be totally eliminated by 2020, as stipulated by the U.N. Montreal protocol. Another one of my favorite irrelevant claims is the "GMO-free" boast on foods containing only ingredients that aren't even available in genetically modified form.

2. *Is it vague?* "All-natural," "chemical free," "green" "eco." These are all vague terms with no official definition to date, though many food labels are brimming with similar environmental-sounding claims. As the FTC *Green Guides* is reformulated, we might get some clearer answers on what you can—and can't—claim about a product, as well as strict definitions. In the meantime, *Consumer Reports'* Greener Choices, at www.greenerchoices.org, is a great resource for sorting out the solid claims from the spurious ones.

3. *Is it a decoy?* Consider a processed-foods company that boasts of the ecological benefits of its organic ingredients, while producing its packages with the toxic plastics ingredient bisphenol A. What about the paper company that touts Forest Stewardship Council–certified towels, but processes the paper at highly polluting mills? These are examples of hidden trade-offs. As food companies explore ways to reduce their emissions, consumers and sustainability certifiers need to be cautious about companies emphasizing a specific environmental improvement when another aspect of their production has the greatest environmental impact. Companies should be "parsing their language when making claims to be sure they're presenting a balanced picture," says Brooke Barton, a

manager at Ceres, a national network of investors, environmental organizations, and other public interest groups working for sustainability.

Company Commitments

1. *What's the tense?* In a Dole press release from a 2008 Earth Day PR blitz, the company boasts of a promise to go carbon neutral with the emissions from its in-land transport of bananas in Costa Rica. Read the press release carefully, though, and you'll notice a bevy of words like "may," "expect," and "believe." In corporate parlance, these terms are known as "forward-looking language." At the bottom of the press release, you'll find a clause of legalese about how such words take the company off the hook for actually having to *do* any of the things it's promising to do. "The potential risks and uncertainties," reads the company's legalese, "could cause actual results to differ materially from those expressed or implied herein [and] include weather-related phenomena; . . . product and raw materials supplies and pricing; . . . economic crises and security risks in developing countries; international conflict." The implication? Don't blame us if we don't actually do any of these things.

   The "promise" is the oldest trick in the greenwashing playbook. We all know there's a difference between "Mom, I *may* clean my room this weekend" and "I *cleaned* my room." Whenever you hear a corporate commitment, do a tense check. Does the statement use terms like "expect," "believe," "intend"? If so, you have every right to remain skeptical until proven wrong.

2. *Is the commitment generous or a gimmick?* Walk into any Starbucks these days and you'll see those ubiquitous Ethos water bottles. The promotional material gives the impression that your purchase is going to help the poor, somewhere far away, access life-sustaining water. And while that is true, it may not be as true as you imagine. Of each bottle's $1.80 purchase price, only five cents goes to charity. And companies skimp on impact not only by giving mere slivers of our dollars to charity but also by imposing total giving limits. While a company may say it's donating a percentage of sales to charity, in

fine print you may learn that there's a limit to its total giving. By the time you're purchasing that box of cereal or pound of coffee, the limit may have already been reached, and none of your dollar is going to the cause.

3. *Does the context trump the commitment?* At Green Communications, a conference I attended in New York City in 2008, pinch hitter for Coca-Cola (her boss was stuck in Atlanta) Lisa Manley, environmental communications director, shared the proactive environmental steps the company is taking. A big focus? Water. "Right now we use about 2.5 liters of water to produce 1 liter of beverage," said Manley.[92] She estimated that the company uses 290 billion liters of water a year to produce 1.5 billion servings a day. Coca-Cola, said Manley, is working to get that number down. Let's say they are and they do. Let's say they can reduce water use by 25 percent. It would still mean the company is wasting water to produce, in some cases, water. Or, worse, wasting water to produce Coke, with all the auxiliary environmental and health impacts—among them, the impact of the seventeen teaspoons of sugar found in a 20-ounce bottle of Coke. All this in the context of a planet with deteriorating water resources: Agriculture uses up almost three quarters of the world's water withdrawals, and today as many as one billion people lack access to drinking water.[93]

Walmart has gotten big press for pushing green initiatives—from greater energy efficiency in its stores to reduced packaging. But what do we know about the bigger Walmart picture? To take but one example, Walmart's big-box stores are a large factor in the more than 40 percent increase since the early 1990s in the number of miles Americans typically travel to shop, as the company sets up shop far from downtown, pushing local enterprises out of business and forcing people to drive farther and farther for their shopping.[94] Just since Walmart announced its sustainability initiatives two years ago, 285 new stores have opened in the United States alone and more than one thousand around the world, says Stacy Mitchell, author of *Big-Box Swindle.* Even by "its own narrow measure," she writes, Walmart's "carbon dioxide emissions have gone up 9 percent."[95]

Context matters. When you hear a green claim, think like an

ecologist: consider the company's action in the context of its entire ecological footprint.

Sometimes it will be easy to answer the questions on this list to detect greenwashing, but only sometimes. Certainly, regulation, like strict and enforceable guidelines on product claims—what is acceptable language, and what the language means—will help. While we're pushing for this kind of regulation, we can also be more savvy consumers: learning to read between the lines and discovering whom to trust— from the NGOs with integrity to the third-party certifiers who have our best interests at heart.

5
CAPITALIZING ON CLIMATE CHANGE

The food industry is starting to sing the climate-change tune, partly because it sees the potential windfall from market opportunities created by the crisis and by the public demand for action in response to it. Big Ag may also be hedging against the possibility that the days of massive tax subsidies for commodity crops, like corn and soy, may someday end, with subsidies instead going to programs that can be painted as climate friendly.

Here I share examples of initiatives Big Ag is promoting and for which companies, and the sector as a whole, are lobbying for government support. But as you'll see, these initiatives represent Big Ag tinkering around the edges of the industrial model, capitalizing on our climate-change concerns without actually changing the underlying structure, or sustainability, of the food chain.

There is a grave danger to these strategies in that they can defuse political will to push for authentic ways in which agriculture—and the food sector more generally—can be a source of solutions. At the same time, they do little to address the root causes of the industrial food chain's environmental destruction and its climate cost.

A NEW KIND OF BIOFUEL

On January 13, 2009, Tyson, the country's largest poultry producer, and one of its partners, Syntroleum, a publicly traded U.S. fuel company, broke ground in Geismar, Louisiana, on a "renewable" diesel plant.[1] The "renewable" part of the fuel-plant story for Tyson will be its contribution of millions of pounds of factory-farm by-products, including animal fat and used "poultry litter."[2] (Poultry litter is the euphemistic term for poultry poop mixed with feathers, leftover feed, bedding, and whatever else ends up on the floor of a factory farm.)

In another match made in corporate heaven, ConocoPhillips, the world's seventh-largest oil and gas company (which raked in profits of more than fourteen billion dollars in the first three quarters of 2008), will also partner with Tyson, using its poultry, beef, and pork by-product fat to produce "cleaner burning" diesel in a new plant in Borger, Texas.[3]

Tyson claims the fuels produced will be used on military and commercial airlines and for highway transportation.[4] And according to the company, once working at full capacity, the Geismar plant will produce seventy-five million gallons of biofuels a year, equivalent to the total amount of biodiesel produced nationwide in 2005 and 10 percent of the U.S. total in 2008.[5]

And you thought you'd never have to ask, "Is this plane vegetarian?"

Tyson is not alone among agribusiness companies in capitalizing on concern about climate change. Poultry giant Perdue launched a biofuels division in 2006. Grain conglomerate Archer Daniels Midland has said it wants to position itself as "the global leader in bioenergy," with plans for "explosive growth" in the biodiesel market.[6] The list goes on. Name a big food producer—whether grain trader or meat processor—and you'll most likely find that in the past few years it has entered the fuel market, too. Or, as these companies call it, the *renewable*-fuels market, though environmentalists beg to differ.

See, something happens when your industry is no longer an invisible influence on the crisis of global warming. Sure, it means your industry can be targeted as a climate-change culprit. But it also means your industry can capitalize on the windfall—the subsidies, tax breaks, and booming carbon market—that defines our new era. For as long as you're part of the problem, why not argue that you're part of the solution—and get paid for it?

Just recently, the food industry—primarily big agricultural producers and the meat industry—has been arguing swiftly and effectively that it is already developing ways to mitigate its impact on climate change, and has been asking for big perks for doing so.

So far, though, these solutions are not necessarily reducing net emissions or addressing the root causes of the sector's lack of sustainability, or its disastrous environmental impacts. In the best cases, they are the environmental equivalent to addressing a burst carotid artery with

Band-Aids. As such, they're a dangerous distraction. While these initiatives are doing little to decrease net emissions, they're diverting critical funds, research, and attention from changes that would have a meaningful impact. In the worst cases, they're actually digging the knife in deeper, making the wound worse, increasing, not decreasing, net emissions.

Consider Tyson's "poultry litter." After it's used, and before it's shipped off to be transformed into fuel in the new plant, it is mainly manure. Along with this poultry by-product, Tyson plans to use nonedible fats and grease from its plants to create the fuel in its new diesel facilities. The technical name for this type of fuel is "coprocessed renewable diesel." It's different from biodiesel because the fuel is made by mixing crude oil with livestock fat, which is then run through a refinery.

Tyson calls it renewable; environmentalists don't.

To Tyson and other promoters of coprocessed renewable diesel, it's renewable because unlike the sources of fossil fuel, finite resources like coal and petroleum, the sources of this fuel—such as crops and animal by-products from factory farms—can be grown or harvested.

But critics argue that this fuel can only be considered renewable in the narrowest sense: by ignoring the complete life cycle of the energy production. Producing the fuel depends on the large-scale animal production that we know depletes topsoil, abuses nitrogen fertilizer, and contaminates waterways. And large-scale factory farms produce the greenhouse gas methane, as well as ammonia, hydrogen sulfide, and other nasty compounds.[7] As I discussed earlier, the inputs to grow the crops for concentrated livestock facilities are also energy intensive and emissions heavy. Feed crops like corn require huge amounts of nitrogen fertilizer, whose production often necessitates the heavy use of natural gas. And in the end? The fuel burns with emissions no cleaner than those of regular diesel.[8]

Furthermore, poultry-processing plants, where 55,000 turkeys or 125,000 chickens is considered a normal population for a large CAFO, use enormous amounts of energy themselves, from the cooling needed to maintain temperatures for the animals to the heating needed to provide a constant supply of scalding water for processing to the ventilation systems needed to regulate air circulation in the enclosed spaces.

Finally, the plants where the fuel is being processed also require additional energy inputs. "Because it is a high-temperature, high-pressure process, we expect it would take much more energy to make that conversion from biomass to liquid fuel," explains Jessica Robinson from the National Biodiesel Board about the ConocoPhillips-Tyson process.[9]

All this, and then there are the myriad environmental tolls from poultry factory farms—the source of all that "by-product." In a damning critique of the livestock sector as a whole, a two-and-a-half-year study by the Pew Commission on Industrial Farm Animal Production determined that "the rapid ascendance of [this style of production] has produced unintended and often unanticipated environmental and public health concerns."[10] Tyson itself has even admitted to multiple violations of the Clean Water Act from its plants' waste. In one recent case, the company settled with the EPA and paid a $5.5 million fine for contaminating waterways near one of its facilities over a four-year period.[11]

Yet Tyson has managed to spin its new fuel initiatives as a green alternative to dirty coal and other nonrenewable fossil fuels, and get government support—our money—for the construction of its facilities through the following avenues.

- *Low-cost bonds:* On June 19, 2008, the Louisiana State Bond Commission "without objection" authorized $100 million in tax-free bonds to help fund the construction of Tyson and Syntroleum's estimated $138 million Louisiana fuel plant.[12] The bonds, made possible through the state's share of Gulf Opportunity Zone funds, were created to help spur redevelopment in communities affected by Hurricanes Rita and Katrina. They carry an interest rate that is 25 to 30 percent lower than the market rate.[13] Plus, they're tax-exempt, meaning that the private investors who buy up the bonds and receive the interest on them don't have to pay tax on that interest. So it's a government subsidy for the buyers of the bonds and, by association, for Tyson. The subsidy that taxpayers provide allows Tyson to build the plant with some of the cheapest capital around.

- *Local development support:* In addition to the low-cost bonds, Tyson secured $400,000 from the Louisiana Economic Development Corporation. In addition, the parish that the project will call home has pledged $600,000 in sales tax rebates to assist in rail-spur construction for the site, supporting the project because it sees it as an economic driver that will create jobs in the community.[14] (The parish's only concern was whether the poultry would be slaughtered at the plant. When Tyson promised to import the poultry grease for the fuel from other facilities, the deal was sealed.)

• *Tax breaks:* The synthetic fuels could also qualify for a tax break per gallon of fuel produced.[15]

Yes, we urgently need to require CAFOs to reduce their pollution, including greenhouse-gas emissions. But as the Humane Society's Danielle Nierenberg, an animal agriculture and climate-change specialist, points out, "Fuel from farm-animal waste has the potential to perpetuate the environmental problems created by CAFOs, while giving animal agribusiness the opportunity to greenwash its unsustainable and welfare-unfriendly practices."

"Making fuel out of poop is not a silver bullet for reducing greenhouse gases from the livestock industry," says Nierenberg. "Allowing animals to graze on pasture, which can be carbon sinks that prevent carbon from being released into the atmosphere, is a better, more environmentally sustainable solution."

We need to be talking about reducing production on these kinds of factories, not tinkering at the edges.

WHAT'S THE MATTER WITH MANURE?

A few hours' drive along bumpy roads to the east of the Chinese city of Shexian, in Anhui Province, I got to see my first methane digester. It was a far cry from the digesters I would stumble on during my tour of farms in the U.S. Midwest. The digesters in China were part of the sustainability efforts of antihunger organization Heifer International.

The farmers I met showed me the latest technology they'd installed with help from Heifer: Concrete tanks were set into the ground between their fields and their homes. The farmers would add manure to

the tanks from the handful of pigs that roamed a small pen, munching
on scrap crops from the fields. As the tanks baked in the day's sun, the
manure released methane gas, which was transmitted to their homes
via small pipes.

With these simple devices, inexpensive to build, the farmers'
houses could be lit in the evenings, and their cooking stoves could be
powered by the gas. The manure left in the tanks could be harvested
again, brought from the tanks back out to the nearby fields to be used
as fertilizer.

With the help of a translator, I asked one of the farmers what difference the digester made. She answered without skipping a beat, "Before,
we used to have to use wood for fuel. We'd spend at least one month
out of every year collecting wood in the forests, leaving our families
early in the morning and not returning until late at night. We'd spend
at least another month cutting and drying the wood."

"Now we can use waste from pigs to produce biogas," she added.

Sixteen other families in the community had already installed similar biogas tanks; more were planning to install them.

The concept behind simple methane digesters, like the ones I saw in
China, is that they capitalize on the natural decomposition of manure,
which under anaerobic conditions (where there is no oxygen) releases
a gas that is about one-third carbon dioxide, two-thirds methane, and
trace amounts of other gases.[16] Digesters capture this gas and transform it into usable energy, which can be compressed into fuel or, as is
more common, used as electricity.[17] (Methane digesters can use either
animal manure, like the ones I describe here, or food wastes and agricultural residues.)

But not all digesters are created equal. The sustainable biogas tanks
I saw in China differ dramatically from the methane digester I saw in
Wisconsin at the Wild Rose Dairy.

Down a series of progressively smaller roads in the verdant valleys
cutting across western Wisconsin, Wild Rose sits on the crest of a hill surrounded by acres of row corn. Inside its two 320-foot-long metal-roofed
barns and one smaller one are 1,069 dairy cows who stand shoulder to
shoulder on slabs of concrete, their necks jutting through metal fencing.
These cows are pumped with the synthetic growth hormone rBGH and
most milked three times a day on a twenty-four-hour cycle. (As I walked
up to greet the third-generation farmer whose family has owned Wild

Rose since 1931, the outdoor thermometer was pushing ninety, and I couldn't help noticing that it was corporate swag from Monsanto, producer of Posilac, its brand of the controversial synthetic growth hormone.)

The family farmed tobacco before it converted to dairy, Wild Rose's Art Thelen explained as he showed me a photo of his family's first dairy barns on the property. Today, along with the cows, the farm grows corn and alfalfa for hay on eighteen hundred acres of tillable ground. And now, it grows electricity, too.

Wild Rose, like a handful of other CAFOs in the state, is pioneering methane digestion on a large scale.[18] Installed next to the farm's liquid-manure cesspit, Thelen's methane digester started producing electricity in earnest, twenty-four hours a day, a little more than three years ago.

Walking down to visit the cows, we could hear its hum in the distance.

Believers are convinced that methane digesters like this one are taking the dairy farm into a cleaner twenty-first century. Detractors contend that they are simply putting a shiny green finish on a fundamental flaw in livestock production: the concentration of massive waste.

Both know we've got a problem. Thelen certainly did.

His thousand-plus cows produce thirty-three thousand gallons of manure a day, enough to fill an Olympic-sized swimming pool every twenty days. Sounds like a lot, but his farm size is not uncommon in a country where confinement operations like these are typical.* Where confined poultry, cattle, hogs, and other livestock produce five hundred million tons of manure every year—three times the waste produced by human beings.[19]

And all this waste has to go somewhere.

On Wild Rose Farm, a mixture of manure and urine washes down the slanted concrete floors, where the cows spend their days, into gullies

---

* A recent Government Accountability Office (GAO) report found inadequate government tracking of CAFOs. The agency uses large dairy farms as a proxy for dairy CAFOs. Under this formula, 35 percent of the nation's dairy cattle, or 3,183,086, are on farms of 700 or more cattle. The median number of cattle on each farm is 1,200 head, a 32 percent increase since 1982. In total, there are about twelve thousand livestock CAFOs in operation. *Concentrated Animal Feeding Operations: EPA Needs More Information and a Clearly Defined Strategy to Protect Air and Water Quality from Pollutants of Concern* (Washington, DC: GAO, 2008).

that drain into a manure cesspit down the hill from the holding structures. Gravity and water do the work.

For years, Thelen began every morning passing by his manure cesspit,
which stored millions of gallons of manure. Each year, he and his team
would pump out five million gallons in the spring and another six million in the fall. Some of that manure was pumped out through a six-inch
hose, stretching as far as three miles away as well as fertilizing his fields
with fourteen thousand gallons per acre each year.

While this was a productive use of some of the manure, there was
still the problem of what happened while it sat there. First, there were
the fears of overflow from heavy rainfall. "We were scared to death of
it getting anywhere close to full," Thelen said. As we stood alongside
the manure cesspit, whose thick black surface was just a few short
feet below the ground we stood on, memories of recent flooding
throughout the state crept into my mind. Even without deluges of
rain, manure cesspits like this one leach contaminants into local
waterways.

Second, there was the other menace: emissions of methane. "I would
come out in the morning and see the lagoon covered with bubbles about
the size of my hand, just thousands and thousands of them," Thelen told
me. "When the sun would hit them—pop, pop, pop. The methane would
go up into the sky."

This is the methane I've been talking about, the gas that is such a
concern for climate change. In some states, the emissions from dairies
are particularly striking. One half of California's livestock methane
emissions comes from manure, 95 percent of which is from dairy
cattle.[20] Nationally, the combined total of emissions from dairy cattle's
enteric fermentation and manure is equivalent to 30 percent of the total for the nation's landfills.[21]

Thelen knew that the day might soon arrive when inspectors would
come to his farm with clipboards and calculators and say, "You have
this many cows and this much methane"—and he was going to have
to pay for it. So he and his partners started seeking alternatives for
their waste, and they stumbled on Microgy Cogeneration Systems, a
subsidiary of Environmental Power that develops, owns, and operates
facilities like the digester on Thelen's farm. A few phone calls later,
Wild Rose had agreed to partner with Microgy to build a digester and

sell gas to the Wisconsin-based Dairyland Power, a power-generation and -transmission cooperative.

After a tour of the milking room and the feed barns, Thelen took me out back. Beyond the main structures, with their cement floors and high ceiling fans, next to a pit of black liquid (that would be the manure), stands the gleaming methane digester. Costing $1.3 million for the Microgy tank and another $1.3 million for Dairyland's scrubber and engine, it's sixty-one feet tall and holds 750,000 gallons of manure.

Digesters like this one aren't a new phenomenon, but they've gotten a shot in the arm with growing interest in reducing methane emissions. The last time we saw a boom of digesters on dairy farms was in the 1970s; farmers installed them to combat high energy prices, but when energy prices fell again, the digesters lost favor.[22]

Advocates of digesters claim they're a win-win, reducing on-farm methane emissions while producing electricity and thereby reducing the reliance on fossil fuels. But like fuel facilities using animal by-products, methane digesters require that we take a bigger view.

Certainly, the digester is capturing some of the methane that would otherwise be emitted and turning it into usable energy, arguably decreasing the demand for non-clean sources of power. The EPA has gotten behind such methane capture, maintaining that "using biogas decreases greenhouse gas emissions, produces renewable energy, and safeguards local air and water quality."[23] The EPA and USDA's AgSTAR program "encourages the use of waste methane recovery systems on dairy and swine farms."[24]

Energy production is a big plus in Thelen's mind, too. According to his own figures, the Wild Rose plant produces enough electricity to power four hundred to six hundred houses, with his township only using 60 percent of the electricity produced on the farm; the rest is used elsewhere. "If every township had a one-thousand-cow dairy in it, we would have enough power to export to Canada," he told me.

Proponents also tout digesters for reducing solid waste produced on farms. One study of digesters found that they reduced solid waste volume by 50 to 60 percent. Sounds like a lot, right? But consider this: Manure from dairy farms is mostly liquid so reducing the solids only shrinks the total volume by a small fraction.[25]

But detractors question whether the eco-benefits of digesters outweigh the *total* costs of CAFOs—not just the climate-change toll of those methane-bubbling cesspits, but the full range of environmental, social, and animal-welfare costs that are built into a CAFO's DNA.

Mind you, these detractors aren't fringe environmental purists. In their review of industrial animal farming, the fifteen commissioners of the Pew Commission on Industrial Farm Animal Production, who include public health advocates, government officials, and esteemed scientists, conclude, "Although the benefits of methane digesters have been widely promoted, serious challenges remain when it comes to the large volumes of [industrial-farm-animal-production] waste and its components such as nitrogen, phosphorus, pathogens, arsenic, and other heavy metals."[26] As the Pew commissioners suggest, while it may be better that Wild Rose is finding new markets for its manure, the sheer volume of manure produced by CAFOs like this one poses a host of problems not redressed by digesters.

Janelle Hope Robbins of Robert Kennedy Jr.'s water advocacy group, Waterkeeper Alliance, has studied the water-quality perspective on methane digesters for a book on manure treatment. Her findings? Robbins is concerned that both inappropriate use of manure on CAFO fields and the digesters themselves can lead to higher levels of phosphorus in our soils and nitrogen in our groundwater, streams, lakes, and rivers.[27] "Anything that perpetuates the lagoon system isn't a viable solution," says Robbins. "You're still going to have the risk of overtopping, and there's still the potential for pollutants to leach out the bottom of the unlined pits—a direct route to groundwater and in many cases drinking water."[28]

Why should we care about too much phosphorus and nitrogen in our waterways? It leads to rapid and copious aquatic-plant growth, like algae blooms. As the algae die, the microorganisms that consume them also remove oxygen from the water. Water devoid of oxygen? Let's just say it's not a very welcome environment for the fish, frogs, and other animals that call water home. Robbins writes, "The long-term water quality benefits from these treatment technologies have yet to be fully evaluated, even though some companies and organizations assert great environmental improvements."[29]

She's also concerned that methane digesters on CAFOs may be poorly managed, creating the risks of nitrogen oxides produced during combustion and leaks of pathogens into the water supply, which would negate any of the technology's positive effects on water quality.[30] "There is an inherent risk in having that much manure in one location," stresses Robbins. "Concentrating waste is concentrating the risk of catastrophe."[31]

Supporters of methane digesters for CAFOs tend to downplay these risks—and play up the benefits to the farmers who use them, particularly the big cost savings. But do the farmers accrue these benefits? Yes, and no. In the case of Wild Rose, the digester was financed by Microgy and small state and federal grants. The company owns it; Wild Rose will have the opportunity to buy back the lease at the end of a ten-year contract. And while some methane digesters are used to power (and thus save money on powering) on-farm equipment, Wild Rose's digester is designed to sell all its power to the grid, with the profits going to Microgy. The farmer gets nada. But Thelen gets other benefits. He is able to sell some of the solid waste coming out of the digester as fertilizer to neighbors and he has reduced some of his own waste-management costs. Plus, Thelen says, he's "ahead of the game" in reducing his methane emissions. The big windfall, though, is going to the company, not to him.

Despite some of these benefits, the fundamental critique of methane digesters on CAFOs is that they help to sanction, indeed incentivize, large-scale confinement feedlots, in part because multi-million-dollar digesters like the one at Wild Rose can only operate with a certain volume of manure. Said Thelen, "These guys won't put them up unless you got eight hundred to nine hundred cows. And they're now saying even one thousand is too small."

When I asked his opinion on CAFO methane digesters from the farmer's-eye view, Brian Depew of the Center for Rural Affairs summed it up this way: "On some narrow basis, an eleven-hundred-head dairy CAFO with a methane digester is 'better' than one without. But I don't want to engage in that conversation because then I have already lost the core point that the CAFO shouldn't exist at all."[32] Methane digesters can become yet another justification for large-scale animal agriculture, with all the costs: the environmental degradation, the animal abuse— and the climate-change toll as well. Colleague Mark Muller over at the Institute for Agriculture and Trade Policy stressed this point: "These are all end-of-pipe solutions"; we need holistic ones.

Methane digestion can be a positive solution, but only within sustainable systems. We should instead be supporting systems that are sustainable from the get-go, systems where waste is a valuable by-product in a closed loop, where natural cycles are regenerated, not broken. To date, though, digester subsidies are mainly being handed out to huge dairy CAFOs; large-scale methane digesters have gotten much of the research dollars, too.

There's one more piece of the puzzle that concerns me. After my farm tour, I headed back to the sleepy town of Viroqua, Wisconsin, where—should you ever find yourself there—you must visit the farmers' market and check out the handmade aprons and pot holders sold by the Amish families who bring their wares every week. Coming out of the town's local food co-op with my haul of fresh produce, I noticed a petition against Dairyland Power, which buys the Wild Rose gas from Microgy. The community was opposing a Dairyland coal-ash dump that was planned for just outside of town and had prompted a heated battle. It turns out Dairyland Power has a long history in coal; only recently has the company begun to shift to "renewable" energy.[33] The poster urged concerned citizens to come out for a town meeting to protest the dump. As I read the details, I pondered the other downside of this digester: Power leaves the community; the risk stays.

III
HOPE

6
COOL FOOD: FIVE INGREDIENTS OF CLIMATE-FRIENDLY FARMING

NATURE INCLUDES US . . .
WE ARE IN IT AND ARE A PART OF IT . . .
IF IT DOES NOT THRIVE, WE CANNOT THRIVE.
—*Wendell Berry*

COOL FARMS

Mark Shepard's 106-acre farm doesn't look or feel like the CAFOs that dot our rural landscapes or the vast farming operations bi-coasters are used to seeing from thirty-five thousand feet above the Midwest. When I pull up to New Forest Farm, nestled in Wisconsin's Kickapoo Valley, eighty miles west of Madison, Shepard and his current farmer-in-training, Joseph Zarr, are hanging out on the shaded porch of a solar-powered cider house. Joseph is outstretched on an army cot, recovering from a stomach bug. Shepard is regaling him with tales of the night before, when the sound of squealing pigs awakened him at four in the morning and he dashed out to fend off some local coyotes on the attack.

As I get out of my rental car, a dog barks in the distance. A few lazy bees buzz by. The mild summer heat is cut with a slight breeze.

"Yup," Shepard jokes as he jumps up to greet me, "it's a tough day on the farm."

Going head-to-head with coyotes might sound like a big deal, but I got what Shepard was communicating. He would take a few coyotes any day over what typical farmers put up with. For Shepard, there are no weekly (or more) visits from the vet for sick livestock. No fueling up $250,000 tractors and worrying nights about the debt he incurred to pay for them. On his farm, there are no neat rows like those that cover most of our country's farmland, where acres upon acres of corn and soybeans grow, made even tidier by tons of pesticides with names like

Avenge and Marksmen that demand careful attention to avoid dangerous exposure.

In fact, nearly everything about Shepard's farm flips our modern
idea of farming on its head: Instead of undermining soil quality, New
Forest is restoring health to the soil. Instead of emitting harmful greenhouse gases, it's pulling carbon dioxide out of the atmosphere, storing
it in that healthy soil and in the farm's woody plants. Instead of taking
government pay-outs, like the megafarms that receive millions in commodity subsidies every year, Shepard doesn't receive a dime—*and* the
farm is profitable.

Instead of relying on fossil fuel for power, every building on the farm
has its own electrical generating capacity built into it; each new building becomes a new energy source. "When you build photovoltaics or
wind power into the construction of a building, it is a capital cost rather
than a monthly expense," says Shepard. "The electric bill becomes an
electric *check.*"

Shepard's practices make climate as well as eater sense (the food he's
producing is healthy for us), and his choices make business sense. His
farming methods help keep his land resilient in the face of the increasingly erratic weather that global warming will bring.

Plus, Shepard's farm—106 acres he owns and 80 more acres he
rents—grows tons of food a year: half a ton of peppers, a ton of asparagus, seven to ten tons of winter squash, a ton of hazelnuts, and chestnuts, which should increase to twenty thousand pounds in a few years.
The farm also produces two thousand gallons of cider from roughly
one thousand bushels of apples. And these figures are just Shepard's estimates for the most significant products. There are "oodles of things,"
he says, that the farm produces on a small scale, from beef and pork to
morel mushrooms.

"This isn't backyard gardening where Joe and Jane Hippie are living
in their little botanical paradise; this is a working farm, hundreds of
acres of a working farm," Shepard stresses. "This is agriculture."

Some might see this upside-down farm, and Shepard himself, as rene-
gade, but he's hardly alone in this clever, sustainable tinkering in his
fields. Indeed, Shepard is just one participant in a movement of farmers and citizen activists, scattered from the rural areas of South Korea
to the verdant valleys of Wisconsin. They are part of a long tradition of
stewardship of the land, proving we can create a sustainable and abun-

dant food system that nurtures nature and helps us fight climate change, and adapt to it, at the very same time.

LEAVING THE WUMP WORLD BEHIND

"Ever heard of *The Wump World*?" Shepard asks within minutes of my arrival. When I admit I never have, he grabs a book out of the back of a blue Oldsmobile minivan filled with buckets of hazelnuts, bins of brochures, and boxes of books. He's just gotten back from one of his regular "show-and-tell" road shows, in which he talks about what he does here on his farm and about the lesson of the Wumps.

Drawn by a Disney illustrator, the book tells the story of cute guinea-pig-like creatures who inhabit a lush land. Shepard, forty-six, wearing a baseball cap pulled over short blond hair and jeans that are caked with a respectable amount of farmer-dirt, flips through the pages. Monsters—called Pollutians and hailing from the planet Pollutus—land on the Wump world and declare they're going to improve this new land they've discovered.

He shows me page after page of detailed drawings. Improvement, we learn, means factories and smokestacks, highways and skyscrapers.

"Yes," Shepard says sarcastically, "vastly improved."

The book ends with the Pollutians heading off to find a new planet to call home, as this one has been completely trashed. (Think *Wall-E* without the computer animation.)

"We live," Shepard says as he turns away from his traveling salesman trunk, "in the Wump world."

A quick glance across the road from New Forest and you'll see just that kind of progress: row upon row of commodity corn (the stuff that looks edible but mainly gets turned into animal feed and high-fructose corn syrup), grown with tons of synthetic fertilizer. Nationally, farms like this are part of the reason why the United States has lost half of its topsoil since 1960—and why we continue to lose that precious topsoil seventeen times faster than the rate at which we're replacing it.[1]

Pointing across the road to those fields, Shepard asks rhetorically, "That's progress?"

He grew up learning firsthand about this so-called progress. Near his family home in Lancaster, Massachusetts, along the Nashua River, just north of Worcester and about an hour west of Boston, he and his childhood friends loved playing a guessing game: What color would the river be that day?

"I grew up in a toxic dump, living downstream from Dow Chemical, Foster Grant, and DuPont manufacturing operations," Shepard tells me. Along with pollutants from these factories, there were toxins from the plastics industry, which was birthed in the next town over.

"I was already convinced that the toxic mess had done its thing; agriculture was just another part of it," he says.

Are rivers that run red progress? Is turning healthy soil into pale, lifeless dirt (as Shepard keeps calling it) progress? Is changing our climate through the way we grow food progress?

Shepard doesn't think so. And this farm grew out of his search for a place to bring to life a different vision of progress: a farm that is restorative, regenerative, and resilient, that approaches farming as a knowledge-intensive practice, not a chemical-intensive one. New Forest is a farm that's connected to its community (including its customers) through a chain of values, not a chain of money-siphoning, globe-spanning, disconnected corporate middlemen.

Five Ingredients of Climate-Friendly Farming

Ingredient 1: Nature-mentored—following the real leader
Ingredient 2: Restorative—bringing the farm back to life
Ingredient 3: Regenerative—mitigating climate change on the farm
Ingredient 4: Resilient—food for the future, too
Ingredient 5: Community-empowered—promoting sustainability in economics

Ingredient 1: Nature-Mentored—Following the Real Leader

At one point in our tour, we crest a ridge, and suddenly I'm overlooking undulating fields of bush cherries, Siberian peas, apricots, cherries, kiwis, autumn olives, mulberries, blueberries, rose hips, asparagus, and hickory nuts as well as oak, apple, and chestnut trees. We stop to admire a particularly biologically diverse patch of land, about half an acre that boasts 137 species of edible plants. As we stand on the ridge, from which the farm's humming life is audible, I dig my fingers into the rich, organic soil. As I look over this landscape, I try to picture what it was all like before, when it was just rows of one plant: corn. I can't; it's unrecognizable.

But I don't need to imagine, for I can see what this all used to be. I need only look beyond the edge of the property to the corn that surrounds us. I make a comment about how different his farm looks, and is, and Shepard reminds me that the difference I see and smell, hear and touch—the buzzing bees, the rich dirt, the towering trees—has all been created in only a little more than a decade.

It's been thirteen years since Shepard started his experiment, taking over land from a farmer who considered it "junk" property, because its steep and curvy slopes meant there was no room for big rectangular fields and large tractors.

What depresses many people, once they've woken up to the damage we've done, is the assumption that it's too late, that recovery will take generations, time we don't have. But that's not necessarily the case. The speedy regeneration of soil decimated by at least four decades of chemical farming is here for me to see, because one gutsy guy believed in a farming philosophy that boils down to following nature's lead, an ecological model that asks the farmer not to control nature but to work with nature, to learn from it, imitating its genius.

"Nature doesn't do straight lines; it's all sloshing in between," Shepard says, explaining his chaotic-looking farm. It's this "sloshing" that led him to embrace such a seemingly radical biodiversity, one that is a natural mix of annuals (crops that you seed every year) and perennials (plants that thrive year after year). This means, for example, mixing annuals like acorn squash and peppers with diverse perennials, from the asparagus that can live for thirty years to the chestnut trees that have been known to survive for four thousand.

"The problem with keeping farm and forest separate in your mind is that you keep them separate on the land," Shepard says. By thinking of the farm as a whole, you manage the farm as a whole. And New Forest is a farm bursting with trees and shrubs, flowers and mushrooms, created by a farmer who plants what grows best in each nook of his land. Indeed, Shepard likes to call himself not a farmer but a population manager, "making sure everything is in balance." His job—though he doesn't call it a job—is to make sure the inhabitants of his farm get along.

Shepard's climate-friendly path owes a lot, he tells me, to two books: *Tree Crops: A Permanent Agriculture*, by J. Russell Smith, first published in 1929, and *The One-Straw Revolution*, by Masanobu Fukuoka, which first appeared in English in 1978. Smith's philosophy is that "farming should fit the land." And most land the world over couldn't stand our industrial approach—it would give out even faster than ours has, releasing its stored carbon into the atmosphere. For Smith, the agriculture practiced on most of the world's farmland can be summed up, quite simply, as a one-way progression from forest to field to plow to desert.[2]

Fukuoka, an inspections officer in the Yokohama customs bureau before his epiphany about natural farming, describes his philosophy as a search for "the natural pattern," as "do-nothing" farming, character-ized by its ease compared with the stress of industrial agriculture's harmful chemicals. For Fukuoka, and for Shepard, there is a spiritual dimension to this approach: The ultimate goal of agriculture is the cul-tivation of the human soul.

Shepard's inspiration also came from his own tinkering—and its limitations.

"I became disillusioned that even the organic foods I was eating were grown in annual fields, which means every year you've got to plow them and replant them," he says. "That's not an ecological system. Even many of the best organic farms will have a cover crop in the winter that's only two or three inches tall, and that's not a complete, intact, abundant ecosystem."

A key solution, he found, was to stop fighting nature and to work with it. Fundamental to this approach is the choice about what to plant in the first place: You grow what would thrive naturally in your bio-region. So Shepard spent his first years here researching the ecology of the area. Now he's bringing back to life the crops native to this oak sa-vanna biome.

"It's a whole family of species," he explains. "Oaks, chestnuts, and beech; apples, hazelnuts, plum, cherry, gooseberries, raspberries, grapes, and grass." The diversity that is the hallmark of his farm is a stark con-trast to the three crops—corn, soybeans, and wheat—grown across much of the Midwest.

This farming philosophy is also grounded in trust. You have to trust nature to help itself, as Shepard has done with a patch of grapevines we stumble on. Instead of spending forty thousand dollars or more an acre on building grape trellises that will age and fall apart eventually, he trellises his grapevines on pear trees. (This has an added benefit for Shepard: He only has to prune each acre once, for both crops.)

Thinking like an ecosystem also means seizing the advantages of your unique place on earth and using plants to help each other, planting trees and shrubs, for example, that rise to different heights and grow well together. *Tree Crops* author Smith calls it "two-story agriculture." At one spot, Shepard points to such an intercropping of grapes, raspberries, autumn olives, cherries, and plums. And he shows me a patch of apple trees where, in the spring, morels grow; the mushroom just loves these trees.

"Who planted that? Who plowed it? Who fertilized it? Who did the weed control, the pest control, the disease control? No one," Shepard says. Well, no one of *our* species, anyway.

So why don't most farms look like this?

Farmers have been taught that planting rows is the only way to control outcomes; that uniform crops are required in order to be planted mechanically, harvested mechanically, and maintained mechanically. Once you get into the industrial model, you get locked in; you're on the treadmill. "The reason these techniques seem to be necessary," writes Fukuoka, "is that the natural balance has been so badly upset . . . By using those techniques the land has become more and more dependent on them."[3]

"There are two kinds of control," says Shepard. "There's the straitjacket control, and then there's the keeping-your-car-on-the-road control." Shepard is not into the straitjacket. And the road he's following is a curvaceous one created by nature and embodied in his farm's horseshoe-shaped beds of asparagus and swerving plantings of chestnut trees, grapes, raspberries, and elderberries.

While many misperceive this method of farming as simplistic, or call it backward or antiscience, there's nothing simple about it. Indeed, as poet-farmer Wendell Berry writes in his introduction to a 1987 reissue of *Tree Crops*, this regenerative farming creates productivity "not by the mechanical and chemical simplifications that are associated with industrial agriculture, but by complicating the biological pattern . . . For this, great care, knowledge, and skill would be needed."[4]

A few years ago, I was visiting a row-crop farmer on the outskirts of Columbia, Missouri. After several hours of chatting in his large farmhouse kitchen about his decision to grow GM corn, his family's farming history, and the industrial practices on his thousands of acres, he said to me matter-of-factly, "*You* could farm these fields."

I laughed at the thought: a city girl born and raised, with ten years in Brooklyn under my belt. I didn't think so, and said as much.

"Well, can you read a calendar?" he asked. "That's about all it takes."

He explained that his planting and spraying schedule followed the calendar dates, not the weather, the land, or the state of the crops. It was a simplicity, of a certain kind, that is absent from these wild fields I am standing in with Shepard. Some farmers go for it thinking, probably, that the farm-by-the-corporate-book approach offers more security. Maybe, though, as farms continue to fail and GM seeds don't live up to their hype, more farmers may start to trust themselves—and nature.

Ingredient 2: Restorative—Bringing the Farm Back to Life

A few weeks before my visit to New Forest, two hydrologists came by for a tour; they couldn't believe what they saw. Shepard had been digging a twelve-foot ditch for a wind turbine he is installing to power the cider house. In the process, he had uncovered deep layers of his soil. It was the soil that stunned the hydrologists: Its deep red color was a sure sign of oxidation.

Why the surprise? On a typical farm with soil that's been depleted, eroded, and compacted, once you get below a certain level, there simply is no oxygen. Where there is no oxygen, there is no life.

Healthy soil is the foundation of a healthy farm. And as you'll learn, it also helps make the crops, and the farm as a whole, more resilient in the face of climate change. It's also the foundation for a climate-friendly farm, for healthy soil holds more carbon, keeping it out of the atmosphere. Globally, more than twice as much carbon is stored in our soil as in our living vegetation, and maintaining that soil—and getting more carbon sequestered in the land—is a key part of mitigating the crisis.[5]

The yellow sweet clover we pass on the way to the wind-turbine ditch may not seem like a part of solving the climate crisis, but it is, as are the trees covering the land. Both the trees and plants like that sweet clover foster vast, deep, and permanent networks growing down, at various levels, into the soil. When the rain comes, instead of eroding the topsoil and creating surface ruts that carry water and soil away to creeks and then rivers, the water is absorbed in tiny pathways created by the roots. The topsoil is left intact; soil carbon is maintained. And there's another benefit. Soil that holds water is a boon in droughts. As a result, the farm is better able to withstand, or even thrive in the face of, either extreme: flooding or drought.

The land we can see from Shepard's ridge, on the other hand, is releasing stored carbon into the atmosphere. These cornfields, like most annual fields on farms across the country, are tilled every year, speeding up the decomposition of organic matter in the soil. "You can't plant lettuce seeds on a parking lot," says Shepard. "It's not going to work." So industrial farmers take out the plow and dig into the soil to prep the earth for seeding. But the process is highly destructive, leading to soil carbon loss. Or, industrial farmers bypass tillage by using herbicides, instead of the plow, to kill the vegetation. Herbicides to fight weeds or tillage to loosen the soil are both expensive—not just for your wallet but also for our climate.

So instead, Shepard taps nature for help. On his farm, his crops do much of the work. For example, he plants daffodils, irises, and comfrey greens to loosen the soil instead of plowing it with heavy machinery.

He asks me to reach my hand into the earth and *feel* what he's talking about. The warm, crumbly soil is easy to dig my fingers into. The plants' rich root structures have aerated and loosened it. I can sense that it would be a welcoming patch for a newbie seedling. Plus, with only 4 percent of Shepard's farm planted in annuals, at any one time only 2 percent of the farm is being actively prepared for the current crop. The farm, as Shepard explains, has all the phases of soil, from bare black dirt to soil for annuals, grassy perennials, brushy perennials, and trees.

All this biodiversity benefits Shepard's pocketbook in another way, too. With a variety of crops that thrive at different levels of growth— some are root crops, others are low to the ground, still others are hip-height bushes, and others are towering trees—he is able to get multiple yields from one plot of land. With mixed cropping and plants maturing at different times, you've got cash inflow throughout the year. "We get three cash flows that all accomplish the same objective of loosening the soil underneath," he says.

It's not just healthy soil that helps climate-friendly farms like Shepard's heal the climate. The trees, and all the other perennials, are doing their fair share of the work, too. The upside? Every single year, this vegetation is sequestering more carbon.

Jump from Wisconsin to the whole country: The Pew Center on Global Climate Change estimates that if the nation's farmers adopted certain more-sustainable farm-management techniques, ones leading to more stored carbon and reduced greenhouse-gas emissions, total U.S. greenhouse-gas emissions could be reduced by 5 to 14 percent.[6]

Now cast your gaze around the world. Research suggests that sustainable agricultural practices like Shepard's have the potential to sequester so much carbon in our soils that we could make a significant dent in global emissions.[7] Based on its own long-term studies of carbon sequestration, the Pennsylvania-based Rodale Institute estimates that if we converted the globe's 3.5 billion tillable acres into organic production, we could sequester as much as 40 percent of our current carbon emissions. Okay, before you go rolling your eyes, I know the likelihood of transitioning the entire planet to organic production is slim, but the scale of this figure powerfully points to the potential here, potential we can't ignore if we know we need every sector to work overtime to avert this planetary catastrophe.

Ingredient 3: Regenerative—Mitigating Climate Change on the Farm

The more time I spend on Shepard's farm, the more I get how sustainable farms use so much less fossil fuel than industrial farms. There are no fossil-fuel-based chemicals here; no major irrigation systems powered by the same; no extra-large oil-hungry tractors and natural-gas-dependent synthetic fertilizers. Being on New Forest, I'm less puzzled by studies that are showing that organic farms can emit between one half and two thirds less carbon dioxide than industrial farms for every acre of production.[8]

"If we're using our tree crops as human food, and the grass between is livestock feed, we've got a perennial system that requires zero fossil fuel inputs and creates enough energy to sell as well," explains Shepard. Because perennials need only be planted once, they require less energy. Plus, weed control is only a concern when the crops are newly planted. Once they have good roots, they can hold their own against the weeds.

"Most mowing or fertilizer needs can be taken care of with animals," he adds.

The net energy gain for the system is huge, says Shepard. "Once you're in the ground and established, you don't have to do any planting again—just harvest the yields." And the yields are plentiful. Shepard farms at every step in the life cycle of plants, from the annuals, like squash and peppers, all the way through to the decomposition, when their shiitake mushrooms are finest.

I'm struck that this isn't a farm of sacrifice and limits; it's a farm of abundance. I see the abundance in the towering chestnuts, the lush berry patches, the thriving grapevines. At one point, as we're standing in a patch of shade under particularly tall trees, Shepard takes a piece of paper from the pad on which I've been busily scribbling.

"You see this sheet of paper?" he says. "Lying flat, it provides a certain amount of surface area exposed to the sun. Bend it, and all of a sudden you've got all this surface area." To demonstrate, he folds the paper, and then he points to the tree towering above us. "Now, when you've got plants that love the shade, you've also got all that area for them below the trees, too."

Research the world over confirms my anecdotal observation of abundance. In one of the largest studies of sustainable agriculture, covering 286 projects in fifty-seven countries and including 12.6 million farmers, researchers from the University of Essex found a yield increase of 79 percent when farmers shifted to sustainable farming practices across a wide variety of systems and crop types.[9] Harvests of some crops, such as maize, potatoes, and beans, increased by 100 percent.[10] A study author wrote, "Sustainable agriculture practices, such as conservation tillage and integrated pest control, also reduced pesticide use and increased carbon sequestration." The study also found that these sustainable farming practices require less water, especially important considering that developing countries will face increased water shortages.[11]

In a virtuous circle, these climate-friendly farming practices also enhance biodiversity. In one study comparing organic and conventional agriculture in Europe, Canada, New Zealand, and the United States, researchers found that organic farming increased biodiversity at "every level of the food chain," from birds and mammals to flora and all the way down to the bacteria in the soil.[12] Such biodiversity will be essential as we face a climate-unstable future.

New Forest's energy self-sufficiency is another aspect of the farm's regeneration. The self-sufficiency comes from tapping the energy of nature—of the sun and the wind. There's the wind turbine that will be used for the apple cider mill and the solar panels Shepard has already installed on his family's home, which help to heat the house during the cold Wisconsin winter. Then there are the crops he's growing especially for fuel, like his hazelnuts. "The hazelnut is the nutritional equivalent to soybeans with three times the oil per kernel weight. But you have to plant soy every year," Shepard explains. "While the hazelnut kernel yield may not be quite that of soybeans, you can use it for energy: Half the weight harvested is the shell, which can burn as hot as coal."

Ingredient 4: Resilient—Food for the Future, Too

Dodging the Deluge

I am visiting New Forest Farm just weeks after a flood devastated the Midwest, costing the state of Wisconsin millions of dollars in cleanup. On my way here, I passed fields that still looked like they'd be better for swimming than farming. The rain and wind were so strong on Shepard's farm, they upended a three-thousand-pound fuel tank. A cornfield across the valley still has a huge black gully where the earth was torn up by the torrent.

Curious, I ask how Shepard's crops withstood the downpour. "It's been brutal on the 4 percent of our land that's planted in annuals, but the rest couldn't care less. In fact, our hazelnuts have never looked better. They've gotten all the water they need," he answers.

No matter how quickly we ratchet down our emissions—and if citizens don't stand up now and demand it, "quickly" won't happen—we will still face the ramifications of our current (and recent) activities, whose emissions will have consequences for decades to come. Climate chaos—worse droughts, heavier flooding—is guaranteed. In short, we know we don't just need a regenerative food system; we need a resilient one as well. That's where farms like Shepard's come in.

How did New Forest evade the disaster that befell its neighbors' fields? Shepard's farm managed to absorb the year's record-breaking rainfall (and mind you, this was after the year before had broken all previous records). In one one-hour period, the land was deluged with twelve inches of rain. Despite the torrent, though, there is no evidence of overland water flow leaving the farm.

Shepard dodged the bullet with agroecological solutions.

First, the healthy soil he has been building since day one was critical. What's healthy soil? It means it's rich in microorganisms, fungi, bacteria, and worms that are all "breathing, pooping, and peeing," as Shepard says. It's alive.

Healthy soil doesn't go anywhere; it stays put, getting new carbon every year from roots and from leaves deposited on the surface, which then become food for all the soil life. The process is called "aggradation," and climate-friendly farmers strive to foster it. Over time, soil should get thicker, deeper, richer, and more diverse. What most of our farms across the country do is the opposite: It's called degradation.

Healthy soil benefits plant growth and plant resilience. Healthy soil is better able to absorb water, making the land more stable during floods, droughts, and extreme weather. In one example from Japan, rice farmers using chemicals were nearly wiped out by an unusually cold summer, while sustainable farmers in the same region still reached 60 to 80 percent of their typical production levels.[13] In a study by the Pennsylvania-based Rodale Institute, organic crops were shown to yield 35 to 100 percent more than conventional crops during drought years.[14]

Then there are the swales: the ditches Shepard has gouged every fifty feet across his land that together store as much as fifty acre-feet of water. (That's like covering one acre with water fifty feet deep.) They're dug in the shape of herringbones all along the hills. When the floodwater hits, it spreads out back across the land in these crafted channels.

In comparison, the industrial farm is a flood disaster waiting to happen. For eight months of the year, a typical corn farm is just bare soil, which gets washed away by the rain and blown away by the wind.

"Say you've got two thousand acres," Shepard tells me. "You're going to have to pull out the crop when you have to, whether it's wet out or not." And all that driving across wet soil essentially squeezes the air out of it, compressing it. The other reason these cornfields are so vulnerable is that when they're pounded by rain, the clay particles settle to the top. When the water washes away, this tiny clay layer is left. Then the sun comes out and bakes it.

"It becomes as hard as concrete," he says. "Now you have an almost impervious surface. The next time the rain comes, it just washes off."

In contrast, when the rain comes to his farm, the intensity of the downpour is diminished. At New Forest, the rain falls through trees, then bushes, then grass, slowing as it goes. By the time it reaches the soil, Shepard says, "it's just drip, drip, drip."

Then the healthy soil absorbs the precipitation and the swales fill, becoming pocket ponds crawling with amphibians. And another beneficial cycle begins: The bugs that love the water on his farm draw the American toads that love the bugs. The toads, it turns out, are the only creature known to eat plum curculio, a long-snouted beetle that's a major threat to apple trees—including those spread out across Shepard's farm. Beat the deluge; you beat the bugs, too.

There Are No Pests Here

Scientists worrying about the impact of global warming on agriculture are especially concerned about insects. Picture the tropics and what do you see—besides piña coladas and white sand beaches? Mosquitoes and other flying creatures that love the warm, damp weather. Climate scientists worry that as temperatures warm, these insect populations will migrate into temperate regions; some are already heading north as the climate becomes more hospitable.

So how does ecological farming protect us from pest infestations, especially when one of the core philosophies is to keep chemicals (including potent chemical pesticides) off of fields? It's about relationships.

"It is basic population ecology," Shepard tells me. He's talking bug populations, I realize, as his farm buzzes with bees and butterflies and is alive with predatory insects, like the soldier beetles and dung beetles that crawl at our feet. It might seem like a paradox, but it's about getting enough predator insects, the right kind, on your land and ensuring that they have enough pests at their disposal.

Take the cucumber beetle. "If you're a chemical farmer, as soon as you get an economically harmful threshold of cucumber beetles, you spray," he says. "And if you're a straight organic farmer, as soon as you get cucumber beetles, often you'll just use an organic spray." Either way, you're limiting the polyculture of insects.

"You've got to let the population run naturally," says Shepard. At first, this might mean you have some losses, but you can plan for that, plant more of different kinds of crops. What happens next might seem miraculous to the uninitiated, though it could just be called nature. Through a cycle of death and reproduction, you start getting new populations that arrive to eat, and thrive on, those beetles. "Eventually you find a certain stability," he says.

There is another operating principle here: a way of thinking holistically about your crops and creatively about your income. "Everyone says apples are so hard to grow organically because of the pest problem," says Shepard. "They're right, *if* you're trying to get 90 percent of your apples picture-perfect. Apple orchards around here are going out of business as fast as can be, because it's costing them more to produce table-quality fruit than the fruit sells for." But there's another way to approach growing apples.

Shepard says he does virtually zero pest control, zero fungus control, and zero weed control on his apple orchards—bringing his input costs down to nearly zero. He may get only 10 to 15 percent Grade A fruit at the end of each harvest, but he still makes a profit. How? By putting to good use the rest of the pockmarked fruit. He feeds some to the pigs. (Grass-fed and apple-finished hogs are selling on the market for four to six times more than feedlot pork, he tells me.) The rest of the cosmetically challenged fruit he presses into juice or hard cider. That's nearly 100 percent use, nearly zero input costs, and a guaranteed profit.

There is a deep trust in the rightness of the natural world underlying this process, a deep acceptance that we can't control everything (and shouldn't try). It's a trust, writes Fukuoka, that "the environment will move back toward the natural balance and even troublesome weeds can be brought under control."[15] The New Ager might call it "trusting the universe." The biologist, like "biomimicry" expert Janine Benyus and Bioneers founder Kenny Ausubel, might call it following "nature's operating instructions."[16] But uncertainty is hard to accept and trust is hard to come by when you're a farmer indebted to the bank for costly chemicals and machines, surrounded by others who have bought into the industrial dogma, and living on the margin, so that risk and experimentation seem foolhardy. Thankfully, there are more and more farmers like Shepard, who are showing us a path so that more and more of us can trust, letting nature lead us to a food system that will help cool the planet.

Down on the Farm

A climate-friendly farm's resilience is integrally tied to the quality of life of its farmers. How can a farm be resilient if the farmers are not being taken care of? I think about this the moment one of Shepard's two sons comes whizzing by on a muddy mountain bike.

"Hey, Dad," fourteen-year-old Erik says, "when are we headed to karate?"

After they discuss the details for the pickup of two of his friends, Erik bikes off, down through the pepper patch.

Shepard says, "Me and the kids, we're all one belt away from our black belts."

Quality of life may seem like a tangent, just an added perk on a farm that's performing all these wondrous ecological services, but it's an integral part of the story. As I read *The One-Straw Revolution* or listen to Shepard talk, this point is brought home. Writes Fukuoka, "I do not particularly like the word 'work.' Human beings are the only animals who have to work, and I think this is the most ridiculous thing in the world."[17]

Shepard was inspired by this sentiment. When we visit his four hogs, he offers this example of how he's created the farm with his and his family's leisure in mind: In the mornings, he comes out to visit the pigs, bringing them the kitchen scraps and checking up on them. He collects his eggs, maybe some shiitake mushrooms for an omelet and some greens and other produce for the day's meals.

"I've fed the pigs, taken out the garbage, gotten my food for the day, all in about fifteen minutes," he says. As he's telling me about his morning rounds, he sweeps his arms open, across to the thick patches of trees, shrubs, and flowers. "How much maintenance does this require? You're looking at it! We select our plants for 'sheer, utter, total neglect.' If a crop fails to thrive, we don't care. Anything that's here is here because it's highly productive and virtually pest free," he says.

As Shepard and I talk about his life here on the farm, I'm reminded of a comment from a corn farmer in Missouri. While he was vehemently opposed to genetically modified foods and the increasing consolidation of ownership in the food system, he felt he had made the only choice he could: to grow GM corn. He explained to me that he simply couldn't find any non-GM seeds in his area. When I asked why he chose to keep farming at all if it meant growing a crop he was so opposed to, he said, "I didn't have a choice; I didn't want to give up the farm. No one ever talks about this, but there is an emotional side of farming: This is the kind of life I want for my family." And though you may not be able to quantify this emotional side, or put a price tag on it, it's a core part of the story of a sustainable way of farming.

I got back in touch with Shepard while I was working on this chapter. I told him that when I described his farm to a friend she said it sounded almost too easy, too perfect. So I asked him about the challenges, too. Here's what he rattled off: Up at five in the morning, by two that afternoon he had already picked two football fields' worth of asparagus, cut it, bundled it, and delivered it to the warehouse to be shipped out to his produce buyers. Next, he turned to the peppers and got eighty-five hundred planted. A fourteen-hour day later, he was ready for dinner.

"Ever planted a tree? Ever planted a thousand trees? Ever planted a thousand trees a day, by hand, for years?" said Shepard. Too easy? Just because he's working with nature doesn't mean he's not working.

As for the farm seeming perfect, Shepard described to me this scene: The birds were singing in the trees; the rays of the last of the day's sun were catching the green of the leaves. He detailed the dinner that awaited him: Hard-cider-glazed pork chops made from his own grass-fed and hazelnut-finished pigs, cooked with cider-glazed onions, morel mushrooms, and gobs of butter. Fresh mixed-green salad with homemade apple-cider-vinaigrette dressing made with toasted-hazelnut oil. Steamed asparagus sprinkled with homemade Parmesan cheese. All washed down with ice-cold fresh milk. All certified organic, most of it from the land outside his kitchen door.

But is this all fantasy? Is Shepard's farm a quirky anomaly? New Forest may seem a novelty to those of us more familiar with the monochromatic fields that spread across the Midwest or with the factory livestock operations I chronicled earlier in the book. But there is growing consensus that this way of farming is no sideline act to "real" food production, but is actually thriving around the globe—and is a key to our salvation.

We're learning that natural farming systems can produce more abundant food, foster healthier soil, all while mitigating climate change by reducing emissions. In April 2008, an international initiative— cosponsored by the World Bank in partnership with the United Nations and representatives from the private sector, NGOs, and scientific institutions from around the world—released the International Assessment of Agricultural Knowledge, Science, and Technology for Development reports (pardon the mouthful). The IAASTD, as they're collectively known, is considered perhaps the world's most credible research-based assessment of global agriculture. It's the result of four years of collective work by more than four hundred authors and peer reviewers.

Among its conclusions, the IAASTD stresses the benefits of agroecology and small-scale farming and the importance of sustainable management of livestock, forests, and fisheries. Indeed, it urges a transition to "biological substitutes for agrochemicals" and "reducing the dependency of the agricultural sector on fossil fuels."[18] In effect, its conclusions represent a "significant departure from the destructive chemical-dependent, one-size-fits-all model of industrial agriculture," notes Greenpeace.[19] The international Pesticide Action Network summarizes the IAASTD's conclusions this way: "Reliance on resource extractive industrial agriculture is dangerous and unsustainable."[20] A statement by civil-society organizations timed with the release of the report declares that, overall, the IAASTD offers "a sobering account of the failure of industrial farming" and represents the beginning of a "new era of agriculture."[21]

Shepard's farm is just one glimpse of the kind of agriculture that is emblematic of this new era. But, of course, not all climate-friendly farms look like his. Indeed, a core principle of climate-friendly farming is that methods develop in concert with local climes and needs, with local cultures and tastes. The five ingredients are constant; the particularities are unique.

The Long View

At the top of one of the farm's ridges, Shepard shows me the Winnie-the-Pooh house. Well, it's not a house, really. At the moment, it's just a circle of saplings. But in thirty years, he swears, these saplings will have grown into tall, thick trees, wide enough, with a little grafting help, to form a house of sorts made of living trees.

"Then, when families come to the farm, the kids can play inside the house," he says. "There will be bunk beds and honey pots."

In the middle of this growing house, he has added two poplar trees. "Those will form the ladder," he explains. "So kids can climb up to the bunk beds."

Shepard's thirty-year time frame is foreign to most of us modern humans. Thirty years? We want to see results now. But he underscores that to farm as he does requires the long view. It is perhaps a paradox that the rapid regeneration Shepard has already seen on his land was borne of choices he made that took a long view of sustainability. With tree crops, you put them in the ground and can wait decades before you can harvest; you've got to believe in the transition.

Unfortunately, we live in a culture that's dominated by eight-minute abs and "five weeks to your best size now!" diets. A thirty-year return? That's anathema to our timescale. The typical corporation can barely think beyond the next quarterly returns (and with corporations driving so much of our food system, no wonder we're in such trouble).

However, the long view is a vital part of climate-friendly farming; it forms the heart of sustainability. One oft-repeated and, dare I say it, now-cliché sustainability sentiment, attributed to the Great Law of the Iroquois, puts it this way: "In every deliberation, we must consider the impact on the seventh generation."

A consciousness of the generations that come after us was brought home to me as soon as I became pregnant. All the abstractions about environmental sustainability and global warming, about toxins in our environment and our food, about the future of the planet and our species, are no longer abstractions. All of it is very real as I sense my daughter swimming inside me. At thirty-three weeks, she has already formed her fingers and toenails, her lungs and a four-chambered heart. And she has inside her all the eggs she will ever create. So that in me are the seeds of my grandchildren, just as inside my grandmother was born the seed of me. This is no metaphor; it's biology.

Ingredient 5: Community-Empowered—Promoting Sustainability in Economics

Taking It to Scale

Shepard's style of farming embraces the long view as a key ingredient of climate-friendly agriculture. But this perspective requires a different kind of business, too. You can't drop this philosophical approach into the instant-gratification culture of the profit-hungry, what's-the-next-quarter's-earnings business mind-set.

That's where Shepard's distribution network, Organic Valley farmers' cooperative, comes in. Since he started farming in 1995, Shepard has been working with Organic Valley to distribute his produce. The co-op was founded just a few miles away from New Forest Farm in 1988. Today, over a thousand farmers are members; two hundred grow produce.

For Shepard, Organic Valley provides the cash flow that keeps his operation afloat. The other big benefit of the Organic Valley relationship, though, is that it lets Shepard be Shepard.

"I could have partnered with other produce buyers, but I would have had to have a larger quantity of any one crop," he says. The magic of Organic Valley is that there are dozens of growers who pool their produce so that smaller-scale, diverse farmers can get access to big markets. The co-op helps farmers like Shepard make those big-time connections.

Organic Valley's new processing plant, opened in 2007, in Cashton, Wisconsin, is a part of furthering this goal. The co-op uses it as the main distribution center, where many products come before being taken to the stores. "That thing is the size of the Death Star," says Shepard.

The relationship with Organic Valley is notably different than if Shepard were simply selling to any distributor. The farmers themselves call the shots, and they deliberate as a group, deciding big questions like "Do we expand?" and "How much do we charge?" They also determine their own internal policies about quality standards.

"It's complicated," says Shepard. "But it's a democracy, and I guess that's how democracies are."

At the end of my visit, Shepard shares with me a tattered *National Geographic* from 1993. Sun-worn and weathered, the magazine includes a feature story about his hometown, the one with the multicolored river.

He flips the magazine open to two full-page color photos. In one, a bright red river bubbles past an old brick factory. The other was taken at precisely the same spot many years later. There is one significant difference: The river runs clear.

For Shepard, the lesson of these photos is the lesson his farm teaches him every day.

"We can turn it around, and we can turn it around so fast," he says. "Just yesterday, my wife and I noticed something in the pocket ponds we had never seen on our farm. The ducks are back."

As I pull out of Shepard's driveway a few minutes later, heading past the three-thousand-plus-acre chemical farms and back through the tiny 667-person town of Viola, Wisconsin, I keep thinking about rehabilitated rivers and resuscitated fields, about nature's gravitation toward health, abundance, and renewal. For this moment, I am buoyed by the clarity that we have nature on our side; if only we would remember that we're batting for the same team.

Comparing Climate-Intensive Farming and Climate-Friendly Farming

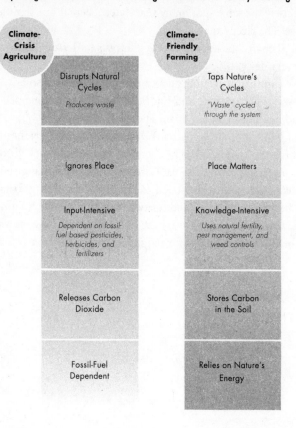

Climate-Crisis Agriculture

Disrupts Natural Cycles
Produces waste

Ignores Place

Input-Intensive
Dependent on fossil-fuel based pesticides, herbicides, and fertilizers

Releases Carbon Dioxide

Fossil-Fuel Dependent

Climate-Friendly Farming

Taps Nature's Cycles
"Waste" cycled through the system

Place Matters

Knowledge-Intensive
Uses natural fertility, pest management, and weed controls

Stores Carbon in the Soil

Relies on Nature's Energy

7
MYTH-INFORMED: ANSWERING THE CRITICS

Six Myths About the Future of Food

1: The inevitability myth
Isn't industrial agriculture the only realistic path?

2: The false-trade-off myth
Don't we have to choose between essential forests and sustainable farms?

3: The poverty myth
Won't climate-friendly farming curse people with unending poverty?

4: The prosperity-first myth
Don't people need to be prosperous before they can even think about the environment?

5: The hunger myth (see Chapter 8)
Can sustainable agriculture really feed the world?

6: The technology myth (see Chapter 9)
Don't we need biotechnology to save us from climate change?

1: THE INEVITABILITY MYTH

When you disembark at Mali's Bamako airport, a gust of thick, hot wind greets you. It carries the smell of burning wood, burnt rubber, and the sweat of workers who run across the tarmac, readying the airport for your arrival.

It was nine o'clock and dark when our flight from Paris landed on a warm night in February 2007. Among the passengers were the usual—Malians returning home, aid workers back from break—and dozens of the not-so-usual: small-scale food producers from Indonesia, Iran, Louisiana, Mozambique, and elsewhere. They were just a small sampling of the more than six hundred who were headed for a dusty outpost a few

dozen miles from the capital, a village, of sorts, built in the months leading up to a conference gathering far-flung members of the international
peasant and farmer movement La Via Campesina.

For me, these folks were, and are, a living response to an oft-heard refrain: Planet-friendly farming could help us mitigate and adapt to global
warming; too bad industrialization of agriculture is inevitable. As
Margaret Thatcher imprinted on our minds in the 1980s, "there is no
alternative"—her mantra referring to the march of corporate capitalism
disconnected from democracy. From this perspective, monocultures—
one crop covering vast expanses—dependent on ever more fossil fuels
and chemicals are the only way to feed a hungry planet, and because this
is perceived as the only realistic path for our food system, its logic is unstoppable. All the industrial food and farming trends I've described in
earlier chapters add up to make us feel that this food system is an inexorable force, as fated and inevitable as Kenny getting killed in every
episode of *South Park*.

But try explaining this inevitability mind-set to the hundreds of
people I met in Mali and all those who are a part of La Via Campesina,
which counts among its coalition organization an estimated two hundred million members worldwide.[1] These members believe in the power
of the peasant and in the role of small-scale agriculture to mitigate
and adapt to climate change—because they are living it. The movement's stance is neatly summed up in one of its simple, but profound,
mottoes: "Small-scale farmers can feed the planet and cool the
world."

After a few hours spent waiting for our visas to be processed by airport officials unaccustomed to handling such a flood, we packed into
buses that inched their way along bumpy roads to the staging ground
for the five-day conference. On the prolonged bus ride—we were
stopped for an hour and a half at a security roadblock—dozens of lan-
guages mixed in the stuffy air. And in the darkness, I heard about the
struggles, but also the resilience, of these food producers from around
the world. There was Margaret Curole, a shrimper from Louisiana who
had seen her local economy collapse with the introduction of industrialized jumbo shrimp from China's aquatic factory farms. There was
charismatic Mohammed Ikhwan, the translator for the Indonesian
delegation, who shared stories about how palm oil plantations were
expanding and devastating communities in his region. And M.O.

Arigbede of the Union of Small and Medium Scale Farmers of Nigeria, who would later tell me about the heavy-handed propaganda campaign that Monsanto surrogates are waging to push GM crops into his country.

We also hear that the industrialization of agriculture is inevitable, in part, because we're made to believe no one wants to farm anymore and there simply are no farmers left. Here in the United States, we've lost our farmers fast. In just one century, we went from 41.9 percent of our population working in agriculture in 1900 to 15.3 percent in 1950 to less than 2 percent by 2000.[2] But in many other countries, farmers still make up the bulk of the population. Globally, nearly half the world's economically active population, and six in ten workers in Asia and Africa, work in food production and agriculture.[3] According to Professor Louis Ferleger, China and India, with the two largest populations in the world, "together account for over fifty percent of the total agricultural workforce worldwide."[4] Even these figures, though, are only our best estimates of global agricultural populations, they inevitably undercount the multitudes in the developing world who are involved in small-scale food production, working in kitchen gardens and informal markets—food producers who don't, and won't, appear in official registries.

Ask the successful food producers I met in Mali if they are history. Ask the Iranian pastoralists, the women farmers from Mozambique, the cheese producers from the Basque region of Spain, whether they want to continue to farm and they won't even understand the question. It's not a choice; it's a way of life.

The Via Campesina members' comments on this subject resonated with what I'd learned from Marek Kryda, an advocate for small-scale farming in Poland, who stressed the resilience of Polish farmers. "Here in Poland, we have peasants. When I am a peasant, my son is a peasant, my grandson a peasant. For peasants, it's an identity. If we have a problem, then they say, you can just become a truck driver or something. But when it's your identity, it's different. It's who you are."

When I asked Kryda to explain how farmers in his country are able to fight the incursion of Smithfield, he responded, "My fellow food producers survived Stalin and Hitler . . . They'll survive Smithfield, too." (Keep in mind that we are trained to imagine, when we hear the word "peasant," some hardy soul in a sixteenth-century rural-landscape painting. Or we associate "peasant" with poverty. We might reimagine the word, picturing instead an innovative food producer with our interests—and the planet's—at heart.)

The sister argument for industrialized agriculture's inevitability is that sustainable farming—on the scale necessary to feed the globe and reduce the food sector's climate impact—is just not practical. I'll dive further into this hunger scaremongering, but in the meantime, let's stop to ask what's "practical."

Is it really practical to be reliant on a food system addicted to fossil fuel? Is it realistic to build a food system entirely dependent on energy from ancient sunlight—from the coal, oil, and natural gas reserves we are quickly depleting—when instead we could build a food system tapping current sunlight?

We can flip the argument on its head: What's naive—utterly impractical—is the belief that we can continue along the path of corporate-controlled, industrialized food and survive and thrive as a planet. Especially when even a short list of industrial farming's impacts should make us shudder: from losing topsoil in the United States seventeen times faster than we're replacing it to the more than three million people globally who are poisoned by pesticides and more than a quarter of a million who die from these poisonings every year to the 405 dead zones worldwide from agricultural-chemical runoff.[5] And when, as you're learning in this book, the industrial food system is a key contributor to climate change. In other words, the dominant food system is undermining the very abundance and health we've been told it provides us.

Okay, maybe you've been convinced—you buy it; this *isn't* inevitable—but we still must contend with the final drumbeat of the inevitability message: It's too late for another path; industrial agriculture is a fait accompli. It's a done deal. This is certainly what the biotech industry wants us to believe: Agricultural biotechnology has spread so far, so fast, that there's no turning back.

That would certainly be the impression you'd get reading the American Dietetic Association's biotech position paper. "Over half of the world's population lives in countries where biotechnologically modified crops have been officially approved by governmental agencies and grown," the paper states.[6] Wow. It certainly does sound like these crops are everywhere. But hold on. It turns out that 92 percent of biotech crops are grown in just five countries: the United States, Canada,

Argentina, Brazil, and India.[7] The United States alone represents half of the world's biotech-planted acreage.[8] (Only thirteen other countries have planted GMOs on more than 120,000 acres, which is about the size of the small island nation Palau.)[9] This is a great example of how even correct stats can mislead: Because both China and India have such large populations and˜have recently allowed the commercial planting of biotech crops, the statement is technically accurate. Yet what the association doesn't say is that only 3 percent of mainland China's farmland is planted with biotech crops.[10]

Yes, biotech crops are spreading, but the planet isn't blanketed yet. Yes, industrial agriculture and intensive livestock production are expanding, but we can change course before it's too late. In fact, there's widespread resistance and the emergence—even rebirth—of vibrant, sustainable farming communities worldwide. As I write this section, I reflect on the farmers I met in Mali and the thousands who attended the 2008 Organic World Congress of the International Federation of Organic Agricultural Movements (IFOAM); I reflect on the Department of Agriculture figures showing a spike in new organic farmers here in the industrialized-food capital of the world.[11]

Now, I'm no naïf. An economic logic driven by the interests of global corporations continues to push the anti-ecological industrialization of farming. And we citizens have let these huge companies use their political clout to garner subsidies and secure trade policies taking us further in this destructive direction. But does it mean the industrialization of food is inevitable? Actually, it means the opposite. Anti-ecological agriculture is driven not by its inherent superiority but by specific beliefs and corporate forces, neither of which are unchangeable.

Remember, too, that anti-ecological farming has emerged in a historical blink of the eye—primarily in just about half a century—which itself should bolster our sense that this path is not inevitable.

After I returned from Mali, I spoke for some time with Annette Desmarais, an associate professor in the Department of Justice Studies at the University of Regina, in Canada. She's been involved with La Via Campesina since it formed in 1993. When I asked her about the view that family-scale farming is doomed by the inevitable march of industrial agriculture, she said, "For over a hundred years, people who thought they knew what was happening in countrysides around the world predicted the disappearance of the peasant. If they were right, surely by now they'd all be gone."[12] But they're not. And their music and voices were heard loud and clear in the hot desert landscape of Mali.

THE FALSE-TRADE-OFF MYTH

The more than one thousand attendees of the 2008 IFOAM international conference were packed into rows under the sweltering white tent watching a presentation by a fellow from Mars Inc.

Mars? you might ask. Organic Mars bars? Well, no. Not exactly. We were all listening to Howard-Yana Shapiro, formerly with Seeds of Change and now director of plant science with the maker of familiar brands like Snickers and M&Ms. Mars, Inc. prides itself on being a leader "in the industry's global effort for cocoa sustainability."[13]

We have a tough choice, he told us. We can either protect vital forests *or* expand farming. We can't do both. As Shapiro talked, a slide popped up on the screen in front of us, showing an aerial image of a lush rainforest with a scar: a square carved out of it. The scar was a farm. The more productive the farm, he argued, the smaller the scar, and the fewer the forests that would need to be cleared to make way for it. While it's true that agriculture pressure on forests has been a significant factor in deforestation, hastening the release of carbon dioxide into the atmosphere, most of the other presenters at the conference had been making a different point, emphasizing the role agroecological farming could play in providing us food, all while protecting biodiversity and creating carbon sinks in healthy soils.

Instead Shapiro's message seemed to echo what I'd been hearing from industrial-agriculture and biotech advocates. Using the forest versus farm trade-off, industry bigwigs have been pushing biotechnology and chemical agriculture as an essential part of the climate change solution. The underlying assumption being that these industrial operations are more efficient than any agroecological alternative.

"The world will have to accept biotech crops, especially if we all agree that we cannot keep cutting trees to increase farm land," Jerome Peribere, chief executive of Dow AgroSciences, said earlier that summer.[14] Repeating this theme in remarks that spring, Syngenta's Chairman

Martin Taylor said, "The world has to choose between technology, deforestation and hunger. I can't see another way out."[15] Taylor even described organic farming, the kind practiced by many of the conference attendees, as a "mediaeval agriculture."[16]

This is not a new meme. Back in 1998, Hendrik Verfaillie, then the head of Monsanto's agricultural division, said that if we were to move the planet toward organic agriculture, "we would have to burn down the rain forest. We would have to eliminate all the wetlands and tax the environment in a way that would be totally unacceptable."[17]

Back at the conference much of the evidence displayed and presentations made belied the biotech industry's message: Sustainable food systems could provide enough food for us all and do so while protecting ecosystems and enhancing carbon sequestration. There was no zero-sum equation. Indeed, new research, highlighted in the next chapter, demonstrates that agroecological systems can secure abundant food supplies without taking unnecessary risks with our ecology.

There's a second powerful argument against the "chemical-intensive agriculture saves forests" falsehood we hear from the biotech industry. As industrial agriculture expands, it's expanding to provide not just food for humans but food for animals and now "food" for vehicles, too. Often, the pressure agricultural expansion puts on forests is totally unrelated to feeding people, in a world where hunger is worsening. The real way to remove pressure on forests? Assert real democratic control of our common resources, including giving voice to the communities most affected by agricultural expansion.

THE POVERTY MYTH

A few years ago, I was listening to economist Jeffrey Sachs in a second-floor Columbia Journalism School auditorium speak at a conference for journalists from around the world. In response to a question about the food system here in the United States, Sachs cheerily responded that we'd basically figured it out: You can walk into any grocery store and eat like a king (or queen). Plus, we grow more than enough food for us all, and for exports, with just 2 percent of our population producing that food. He neglected to mention the millions who are still necessary to bring us our food; the work just moved off the farm and into the meat-processing plants, the retailing outlets, the shipping industry, the chemical-manufacturing plants, and more. The actual percentage of workers in the food industry has remained relatively constant over the decades, USDA data show, with the workforce shifting from the field to the factory, where many face arguably worse conditions and less freedom.

But that day, Sachs was celebrating our industrialization, and industrialization of agriculture specifically, for helping to end poverty and address hunger here. This message is one he repeats in his book *The End of Poverty* when he describes the inexorable path of economic development "that moves from subsistence agriculture toward light manufacturing and urbanization, and on to high-tech services."[18] It's a ladder to success that everyone wants to get on, his theory implies.

The summer before the Sachs conference, I was at a swank reception in New York's tony West Village. Gripping my cosmo and feeling that I fit in about as well as a PETA activist at a rodeo, I politely answered when one of the investment bankers in attendance asked about my work. And so, one topic led to another, and we got to talking about farmers in the United States.

He had one question for me: "Why should Americans farm anymore, anyway? If other countries can produce food more cheaply than we do, we should let them, and specialize here in what we do best."

A gulp of the cosmo. A deep breath. I didn't launch into much of a response then. But listening to Sachs echo this sentiment, I was reminded of the pervasiveness of the myth that sustainable farming equals poverty. The not-so-subtle message is that to advocate for small-scale farming, for climate-friendly, chemical-free production by independent farmers not beholden to corporate giants, is to condemn the world to the dark ages, to lock billions into poverty.

Actually, the opposite can be true. Sustainable agriculture can help us mitigate climate change, adapt to it, and at the same time empower billions of people to feed themselves.

This win-win-win can be hard to see, I admit. Of the 1.2 billion people in the world suffering from extreme poverty, three quarters live and work in rural communities, and half of all the undernourished are farmers.[19] But this doesn't mean that family-scale farming has *caused* their poverty, nor does it mean that family-scale, sustainable farmers must suffer from hunger and poverty.

We could draw a very different lesson from these numbers: that the foreign-aid encouraged drive for industrialized, export-oriented agriculture has squeezed out family-scale farming, depriving so many around the world of their food self-reliance. We could also point to the dramatic dis-investment in agriculture over the past several decades. Between 1980 and 2004, spending on agriculture as a share of total public spending in developing countries fell by half. And what investment has been made has mainly targeted large-scale operations and export production. With decades of trade and economic reforms pushing exports, by 2004 forty-three developing countries had become dependent on just one commodity—like coffee or sugar—for one fifth of all their export revenue, according to The Oakland Institute, a policy think tank. As real prices for these agricultural exports tumbled over the past three decades, developing countries have further lost out. In addition, many governments and international development institutions sold farmers on costly chemicals and seeds, undermining financial well-being, independence, and community health.

We're told that corporate-friendly economic policies will decrease hunger, but what do the folks who are "being developed" say about this claim? I traveled to South Korea to find out. It may seem odd, I realize. The nation, after all, is held up as the poster child for what rapid industrialization can do: Only slightly larger than Indiana, it transformed itself from one of the world's poorest economies into the thirteenth largest in just under three decades. Since 1970, those laboring in the fields have dropped from half to just under 7 percent of the population.[20] Today, one quarter of the country's forty-nine million people call the city of Seoul home. A major exporter of electronics—think Samsung and LG—South Korea is also among the world's largest exporters of petrochemicals. But maybe if we can find inspiration for embracing small-scale farming in hyper-industrialized South Korea, we can find it anywhere.

Despite the country's urbanization, burgeoning farmer and consumer movements have emerged since the heady days of the pro-democracy activism of the 1980s. The people I met who are part of these movements—from the charismatic leaders of a consumer co-op whose membership tops 150,000 to farming activists with La Via Campesina who were organizing a regional summit for colleagues from Thailand, Malaysia, Japan, and beyond—offer an alternative view of development.

As we ate steaming bowls of traditional Korean soup, Byeong-Seon Yoon, a professor at Konkuk University, told me that corporate-friendly food policies have done little to address food independence or help end poverty in his country. These policies have mostly "increased people's dependence on agricultural imports and strengthened industrialization of agriculture, forcing hundreds of millions of farmers to give up traditional practices," he said, above the din of lunchtime diners from the bustling restaurant.

Like the pull of South Korea, I was drawn to Mexico because there, too, farmers have been working to retain their traditional farming practices, healing and restoring their land. I was also drawn to these countries because they are among the nations whose markets have been most flooded with our artificially cheap food—primarily corn in Mexico and beef in South Korea—and whose farmers have felt the pain of those imports. By 2004, ten years after the passage of the North American Free Trade Agreement (NAFTA), the 15 million Mexican farmers who depend on corn had seen the real prices for their crop drop more than 70 percent. An estimated 1.5 million corn farmers have been forced to leave their land post-NAFTA, devastated by cheap imports.[21]

In the heart of the dry and dusty Mixtec region of Oaxaca, where much of the topsoil had been scarred with deep gullies of water erosion, Abhaya Kaufman, a friend and colleague, met with the founders of the twenty-five-year-old CEDICAM, a rural education and development organization, to hear from farmers directly. Small-scale farming is thriving here in large part because farmers have been taught to look beyond the temptations of industrialization.

Kaufman joined in the CEDICAM farmer workshops, held next to a village basketball court, where farmers got to shoot a few hoops between workshops on seed saving and composting. In between one of the workshop sessions, Kaufman sat with Phil Dahl-Bredine, an American missionary who has become a part of the community and has a passionate respect for local knowledge. Dahl-Bredine explained that because of farmers' use of local sources of fertilizers, natural pest controls, native seeds, and inexpensive technologies, the community is well nourished. The very practices they've embraced that heal the planet go a long way toward explaining their community's abundance.

Jesús León Santos, the soft-spoken yet strong-willed founder of CEDICAM, described his work as a dual and parallel process. Detoxifying the land, getting it off chemical dependency, also means detoxifying the people, freeing their spirits from ideas "of the North": ideas that make them feel dependent, believing that their knowledge is somehow "less than." A large part of the organization's work focuses on promoting and improving on farming methods that many in the community already practice, but don't necessarily recognize as "technology." The workshops validate traditional techniques and identities; these identities are inscribed in the land and infused with traditional farming practices.

Communities like the one Kaufman visited in Mexico and the ones I saw in South Korea belie the poverty myth, which is based on a narrow idea about farming and its place on the planet. The "corporate-driven model," writes Annette Desmarais, sees agriculture "exclusively as a profit-making venture," with resources "increasingly concentrated into the hands of agro-industry."[22] It is a view of industrialized agriculture that ignores its human and climate cost while at the same time grossly underestimating the social and ecological benefits of sustainable farming.

Shedding this myth, the "detoxified person" holds a vision of farming shared by the people I met in South Korea, the farmers I saw in Mali, the organizers Kaufman shot hoops with in Mexico. They embrace a different path of social and economic development, one that values farmer-driven food production, celebrates food independence, and acknowledges the beneficial role that sustainable agriculture can play culturally, economically, and environmentally in addressing the crisis of the climate.

THE PROSPERITY-FIRST MYTH

There's a dangerous corollary to the poverty myth; it holds that we as nations will be able to address our environmental crises—particularly the biggest ones, like climate change—only after we lift people out of poverty. (When coupled with the myth that prosperity will only be achieved through the industrialization of agriculture, it sure makes the prospect of addressing climate change through sustainable farming that much more challenging.)

This myth presumes that people can only become environmentally aware once they're prosperous enough to think beyond their basic needs. It pops up throughout the popular press, but you know it's really pervasive when even so-called environmentalists echo it. Authors Ted Nordhaus and Michael Shellenberger insert the prosperity-first myth front and center in their 2008 book *Break Through: From the Death of Environmentalism to the Politics of Possibility*. They argue that the environmental and progressive movements of the 1960s "were born of the prosperity of the postwar era" and the "widespread emergence of higher-order postmaterialist needs."[23] The clunky term "postmaterialist" is intended to suggest that these needs "emerge only after individuals or societies have met their basic material needs."[24]

No prosperity, no environmental consciousness. Period. To bolster their theory, Nordhaus and Shellenberger trot out this evidence: "Ecological concern remains far weaker in Brazil, India, and China than in the United States, Japan, and Europe. And it explains why, when environmentalism does emerge in developing countries, such as Brazil, it does so in Rio de Janeiro's most affluent neighborhoods, where people have met their basic material needs, and not in its slums, where people live in fear of hunger and violence."[25]

You don't need to be a historian of social movements to have an inkling that these guys might not be telling us the whole story. Numerous examples of environmental campaigns and movements exist in each of the countries these two identified as ecologically unenlightened backwaters. And the last time I checked, it was the United States—not Brazil, India, or China—that refused to ratify the Kyoto Protocol.

Yes, the Chinese government may be pushing coal-fired power plants, with a new one going up every week, but let's not be misled.[26] The government may not broadcast the news, but "ecological concern" is alive and kicking in China. Even a top environmental official, Zhou Shengxian, estimated that the country was rocked by fifty-one thousand pollution-related protests in 2005.[27] That's nearly one thousand protests a week.

Or consider the environmental battle heating up in Ecuador, not exactly a high-income country. The fifteen-year clash is between indigenous tribes in the country's Amazon and energy giant Chevron over what may be the worst oil contamination in history.[28] In some ways, you can't get "poorer"—by Nordhaus and Shellenberger's narrow definition—than the Amazonian tribes waging this fight. According to the authors' logic, though, these communities should be preoccupied with meeting their "basic needs," not with taking on the Herculean challenge of standing up to one of the world's largest companies. Yet these communities are.

When Abhaya Kaufman visited Mexico, she was invited by Yolanda Giron, a local guide, educator, and community activist from Oaxaca's Etla Valley, to go "tree watering." Two decades earlier, Giron and several friends had come together to start addressing environmental concerns in their community by planting trees. In the twenty-five years since, they had planted forests across four hillsides and were expanding to more.

Perched in the bed of a pickup truck that wove through village streets collecting passengers, Kaufman met Sam, Soledar, and Adelpha, founding members of the group they called Yutnuu Cuii, Mixtec for "green tree." By the time the crew arrived at the grove, it had swelled to ten adults and twenty kids. As they neared the place, all could see the work they'd accomplished: Beside the riverbed, thick pine trees now grew, dropping a blanket of needles on the ground. The kids headed straight for the well they'd built the previous year to fill buckets to water the seedlings up the hill. Yes, they'd planted thousands of trees, but their biggest accomplishment, said Giron, as she surveyed the kids dashing about, was the change of consciousness.

"I know we will keep doing this work as long as we have to," she said. "I know the next generation will keep it up."

How can you explain Giron and her community's passion for the land? The indigenous Ecuadoreans' dedication to a decade-and-a-half-long struggle? Those environmental protests in China? In my own travels, interviewing organic-farmer activists from Kenya and land reform movement leaders in the heartland of Brazil, I've met the most courageous, visionary, and dedicated environmental stewards. These people are not prosperous by any material definition, but they have a much deeper appreciation for the environment, and greater savvy about how to protect it, than some of the wealthiest people I know. Yet their stories

simply don't make sense if you buy Nordhaus and Shellenberger's sentiment, if you've been snookered by the prosperity-first myth.

There's a grave danger in getting this wrong. For in doing so, we miss
seeing the potential of billions of the world's poorest people to be part
of creating compelling, urgent solutions, particularly to global warming.
We are made blind to the ways in which they already are. Free from this
myth's hold, we see real possibility, particularly in the hearts and minds
of small-scale farmers the world over. To perceive the radical environmental movements, including those addressing climate change, that are
emerging in indigenous farming communities, rising up among slum
dwellers, and spreading in economically forgotten neighborhoods is to
discover real hope where people like Nordhaus and Shellenberger see
none.

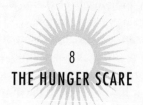

8
THE HUNGER SCARE

Catherine Badgley, an assistant professor in the Department of Ecology and Evolutionary Biology at the University of Michigan, likes to take the students in her graduate course Food, Land, and Society out of the classroom and onto the farm. On one of these visits, in late May 2004, Badgley traveled with her students to Rob MacKercher's organic farm on the outskirts of Ann Arbor.

MacKercher had been farming his 1.5 acres for four years but had been farming before that for more than fifteen. Now, an acre and a half is far from huge, yet every nook was being used to grow a profuse variety of produce, from kale to kohlrabi, from summer squash to sweet corn. Struck by the abundance on the relatively small farm, Badgley casually asked how much food MacKercher produced every year. When he replied, "Twenty-seven tons," Badgley did a quick calculation.

Her math told her that if a salad for a family of four included a pound of produce—radishes and spinach, onions and tomatoes—then this farm could produce a salad every day of the year for 150 families.

"I thought to myself, if you can grow that kind of quantity here, why *can't* organic agriculture feed the world?" said Badgley.

That chance encounter set Badgley and a team of six other researchers on a two-and-a-half-year odyssey to explore one of the more compelling, and common, concerns about organic agriculture: Can it sustain us all? As Badgley put it when we discussed her study, "a long-standing argument by proponents of chemical agriculture is that it's superior because of strong yield performance."

From the pages of *Time* to the halls of biotech-industry conferences, I've heard this critique of sustainable agriculture and claim for chemical agriculture lobbed at organic enthusiasts. It is a seemingly persuasive argument. For decades, it has been one of the most gripping defenses of biotech and industrial agriculture. After all, who among us would want to deprive the hungry of food? At a Biotechnology Industry Organization (BIO) workshop I attended in 2005, one participant went so far as to proclaim that pro-organic—and anti-biotech—activists should be "tried for crimes against humanity."[1] (As I slunk down in my seat, the audience of several hundred made no verbal protestations to the contrary.)

When the world faced the global food-price crisis of 2008, news reports that choosy consumers were now willing to stomach biotech foods hit the wires. Andrew Pollack of the *International Herald Tribune* wrote that in countries like Japan and South Korea manufacturers were turning to genetically engineered corn to make soft drinks and other foods. "Until now, to avoid consumer backlash . . . companies have paid extra to buy conventionally grown corn," wrote Pollack. "But . . . it has become too expensive to be so finicky."[2]

The businesses profiting from industrial agriculture—chemical and biotech companies among them—have certainly mastered this talking point. Chemical giant Syngenta has claimed that disregard for the company's technologies would limit "agriculture's efforts to meet future crop needs."[3] Speaking to the *Independent* in 2001, Michael Pragnell, CEO of Syngenta, one of the world's largest agricultural-chemical manufacturers, said, "We need to recognize that were agriculture to go organic again, we would have an enormous food deficit."[4] He continued, "I hesitate to say it, but I do tend to think of the organic movement as a western European luxury."[5]

Comments like Pragnell's pop up again and again. Consider this sentiment from Carlos Joly, then director of sustainability for Monsanto. Speaking at a 1998 conference in London, Joly argued that the company's biotech wheat would boost yields, while a shift to organic wheat would lead to a "35% to 44% drop."[6] To drive home his point, he continued, "If organic methods were widely adopted here in the UK you would have to import an extra 5 million tonnes of wheat a year or expand your wheat growing area . . . Organic farming is like all good things—when it is taken to extremes it becomes a poison."[7] Never mind that fifteen years on, biotech wheat has still not been commercialized *and* we still have plenty of production.[8]

Now such charges are being thrown at advocates for a climate-friendlier food system. Because, remember, when we speak up for climate-friendly farming, we're arguing for farming that embraces non-fossil-fuel sources of fertilizer and weed and pest control, farming that depends on nature, not chemicals made by multinationals, for innovation and greater yield performance. To speak up for this farming, we need to take seriously Pragnell's and Joly's arguments. What's the truth? Is there a trade-off between farming that is good for the climate and farming that can feed the world?

Badgley's study, among others, can help us dig into the answer.

WE'VE GOT THE WHOLE WORLD IN OUR HANDS

Egged on by the question that had popped into her head on MacKercher's fields, Badgley, along with her research team, crafted a study investigating how a shift toward organic production would affect the world's food supply. If the world went organic, would we be left starving? A big question, indeed, and to answer it, Badgley and her coauthors would spend years exploring the data.

Ultimately, they tracked down nearly three hundred studies of yield data from certified-organic, industrial, and low-input agriculture, from peer-reviewed articles and the gray literature.* From these studies, they

* "Gray literature" refers to studies that haven't been peer reviewed and published in academic journals. Some critics of the study have lashed out at the authors for using gray literature data, but just because these studies had not been peer reviewed doesn't mean the research was not solid. The research used was from leading academics, often from long-term studies that were still in process. "It is an appropriate caution," said Badgley, "but we look at where the data is coming from, and if it's coming from people, for instance, who may have had seven years of data and are waiting for ten to write their journal article, that data was still useful for us."

calculated average yield ratios for nonorganic versus organic production for a range of crops in developed countries (where high-input,
chemical agriculture reigns supreme) and in the developing world
(where low- or no-input agriculture has historically meant extremely
low yields).

In developed countries, they found that across nearly all food products, the exceptions being eggs and sweeteners, switching to organic
production either did not affect or slightly decreased average yields.
The average yield ratio ranged from .891 to 1.060. In other words, organic yields ranged from slightly less to the same as the conventional
yields. (And, when we're talking about yields here, we're only talking
about on-farm production, not about the other benefits or drawbacks
of these production systems, such as the climate impact of chemicals
used in industrial farming.)

When you look at what happened with yield ratios in developing
countries, the story gets even more interesting. The average yield ratio
in these countries jumped from 1.736 at the low end (for sugars) to as
much as 3.995 (for legumes and pulses). By adopting agroecological
approaches, farmers could grow "almost twice as much to four times as
much of the crop as with his/her previous practices," explained Badgley. Because most farming in these regions is currently low input and
low yielding, shifting toward more climate-friendly organic agriculture with the help of capacity building and research would result in relatively higher yields and improve local food security.

And, if we really care about the total food supply for the planet, we
should also look at what the data tell us about the world's overall food
supply if we shifted toward organic. And the researchers' conclusion?
The estimated food supply for the world, if we went organic, would be
greater for *every single food category they investigated*, which includes
all the major foods that contribute substantially to our caloric and nutritional needs. Since all food categories in the developing world would
experience yield increases, in some cases significant ones, the overall
estimated global food supply would go up, way up. In grain products
alone, a global transition to organic production would trigger a 45 percent jump in food supply.[9]

There's another interesting detail in the data, one that gives us even
more reason to shake off our worries about yield drag from shifting
toward organic production. We could more than make up for some of

those small yield declines that would occur in developed countries if we simply addressed one problem: food waste.

Industrialized countries waste food in every category, and in some, egregiously so. Grains? Less than half of all grains ends up in our food supply; the rest goes mainly to livestock feed, with some going to seed and postharvest waste. Even more startling, only 10 percent of sugars and sweeteners and a quarter of oil crops and vegetable oils are in the actual food supply, because so much is diverted to soft drinks, livestock feed, and industrial uses of vegetable oils, explained Badgley. We would only need to *slightly* reduce this waste, and we could more than make up for the small average yield decline in a shift to organic production in developed countries.

The study concludes that planetary caloric needs and yield data from around the globe indicate that "organic agriculture has the potential to contribute quite substantially to the global food supply, while reducing the detrimental environmental impacts of conventional agriculture."[10]

Now, as Badgley herself stressed, these figures are just estimates, but they certainly suggest a powerful potential in organic agriculture, one that the crime-against-humanity screecher at the BIO conference was seemingly unaware of—or intentionally ignoring. "The point of the study was never to show that organic production yields more than industrial agriculture," Badgley told me, "but to discover whether we could shift toward organic production and produce as many calories as industrial methods currently do and produce enough calories to feed the world." And the answer is a resounding yes.

What of the other big barrier that critics of organic pose, the limits of natural fertilizer? Industrial-agriculture proponents have long argued that we simply do not have enough organic sources of fertilizer to maintain high yields. So Badgley and crew also evaluated the amount of nitrogen potentially available from organic sources, such as nitrogen-fixing leguminous cover crops, manure, and compost, as well as the potential of organic techniques to reduce crop loss (the other side of the yield equation) through crop rotation, intercropping, and biological pest control. Here again, their research gives weight to the organic argument. "Data from temperate and tropical agroecosystems suggest that leguminous cover crops could fix enough nitrogen to replace the amount of synthetic fertilizer currently in use," they write.[11]

And Badgley's study is not the only one to make such claims. Other studies from around the world have come to similar conclusions. In Jules Pretty's University of Essex study of sustainable farming that I mentioned earlier, researchers found a 79 percent yield increase in the shift to organic production across a wide variety of crop types.[12]

MISREPRESENTING THE DATA

Despite the evidence from these studies and many others, the fearmongering about a starved organic planet is still being parroted in print. The week after the 2008 Slow Food Nation bonanza in San Francisco brought together fifty thousand organic enthusiasts, *Time* popped the question "Can Slow Food Feed the World?" and answered with this buzzkill: "Sure, slow food tastes better, but agribusiness has long argued that industrial farming is the only way to economically feed a global population nearing 7 billion."[13]

In the next sentence, journalist Bryan Walsh makes the real dig, stating, as if as fact, that "organic farming yields less per acre than standard farming, which means a worldwide Slow Food initiative might lead to turning more forests into farmland."[14] To nail the case, he references the Food and Agriculture Organization of the United Nations. "In a recent editorial," writes Walsh, "FAO director-general Jacques Diouf pointed out that the world will need to double food production by 2050 and that to suggest organics can solve the challenge is 'dangerously irresponsible.' "[15] (That quote was actually lifted from an early version of the director-general's op-ed, which was given to Walsh for background purposes, according to a media relations officer at FAO. While the final statement still raises doubt about organic agriculture, its wording is less extreme.)[16]

Eric Reguly over at the *Globe and Mail* sounds a lot like *Time*'s Walsh. In a column published a few days earlier in that Canadian paper, Reguly rebukes organic farming: "I've now concluded that it's a land-gobbling luxury," he writes.[17]

His reasoning? "Generally speaking, organic harvests per hectare fall short of conventional ones," says Reguly. He adds, "Growing a tonne of organic wheat—depending on where you do it—*might* [emphasis mine] require one-third more land than raising a tonne of conventional wheat, which has its yield pumped up by fertilizers, herbicides, and insecticides."

So if he bypassed Badgley—and the University of Essex study, among others—who does Reguly cite to back up this claim? The chairman of Nestlé, Peter Brabeck-Letmathe: "We cannot feed the world on organic products." Reguly also quotes Syngenta's head of business development, Robert Berendes, who says organic farming is "a waste of agricultural land in times when the world needs more crop output."[18]

Wouldn't you think Nestlé and Syngenta would have a stake in maintaining the myths about the benefits of chemical agriculture? Syngenta, as I mentioned earlier, is among the world's largest agricultural-chemical companies, and Nestlé is the world's largest publicly traded food company, pulling in nearly ten billion dollars in 2008 and manufacturing products chock-full of ingredients from the industrial-food pipeline.[19]

Reguly also relies on a study by Niels Halberg, head of the International Centre for Research in Organic Food Systems, in Denmark, to defend his down-with-organic diatribe. According to Reguly, the study found that in "some areas with intensive, high-input agriculture, conversion to organic farming will most often lead to a reduction in crop yields per hectare by 20% to 45%."[20] He follows that with a slight nod to organic production, acknowledging that "introducing organic farming methods—crop rotation, natural fertilizers and the like—to farms in developing countries . . . has boosted yields."[21] But then delivers this final hit: "But more modern fertilizers and pesticides *might* [emphasis mine] have boosted the yields even more."[22]

The Halberg study sounded familiar; I'd seen it quoted by an organic-farming advocate, not a Reguly-styled critic. So I fired Halberg off an e-mail. After reading the article, he wrote back, "Shrewdly enough the writer did not misquote me, but surely misinterpreted my conclusion."[23]

Halberg and colleagues have been exploring this question for years. In a paper they published in 2005, they estimated that conversion to organic agriculture in Europe and North America, where high-input, high-yield farming is the norm, could indeed reduce yields by as much as 35 percent.[24] But they also found that the indirect effect on food security where it matters most would be very small, because shifting farmland to organic production in sub-Saharan Africa, where hunger is so acute, would actually *increase* food self-sufficiency, decreasing dependency on food imports and thus reducing hunger.[25]

This is the key point of Halberg's study that Reguly missed: If we are truly worried about the hungry—now nearly a billion and counting—we have to look at *who the hungry are, where they live,* and *how they will be affected by changes in farming systems.* Looking only at absolute yields doesn't tell us enough. So what do we know about hunger? It's concentrated in rural areas in sub-Saharan Africa and south Asia, and three quarters of undernourished people on the planet live in poor agricultural regions.[26]

If we are really concerned about addressing climate change and ending hunger—or even just ensuring that hunger doesn't get worse—we need to be supporting sustainable and local food production precisely in these regions. With this in mind, FAO has a four-point commitment to food security, which includes food abundance, yes, but also food access, stability, and how food is used. Food abundance (that seemingly all-important yield factor) is only one aspect in addressing hunger. Indeed, millions of poor people will remain undernourished unless local food production is given higher priority and inequality of access to food is reduced. Halberg offered this example: "India has been a net food exporter the last five years, but still there are approximately two hundred million food-insecure people there."[27] From Badgley's study we know that organic farming can be a sure path toward increased yields—that come without the financial and ecological cost of pesticides and genetically modified seeds—in precisely those places where hunger is so pronounced.

EAT THESE WORDS

We need not let ourselves be silenced by foes of organic agriculture. I hope you see—from the Badgley, Pretty, and Halberg evidence and more—that we've got a strong defense if we're ever called out for being "callous elites" in claiming that organic agriculture can be part of the climate-change solution.

Here are a few more points to add to our rebuttal.

Let's take a moment to remind ourselves of the places and people we're talking about: the world's hungry, most of whom live in rural areas. Why does that matter for organic agriculture? Because in developing countries, where labor costs are low, organic agriculture can benefit communities in two ways: providing employment for the landless and reducing the burden of costly inputs, like pesticides and synthetic fertilizers. Agroecological farmers can substitute these expensive materials with a farm's own, or local, resources.[28]

As Badgley says, "Industrial agriculture may have high yields." "That's what these crops and chemicals were designed for. But advocates of industrial agriculture have failed to appreciate that alternative methods have strong yield potential as well but with fewer synthetic inputs and fewer purchased inputs, making alternative methods potentially more environmentally *and* economically sustainable."[29]

Plus, we've got to remember that current yield data don't provide a crystal ball for telling us the *future* of productivity as organic farmers develop agroecological methods. As this knowledge deepens and spreads, yields will only further improve. Current yield data also don't tell us how industrial agriculture will fare in the face of greater climate change.

The next time someone tells you that you're being narrow-minded by promoting climate-friendly farming when as many as a billion are going hungry every year, you can reply with confidence. You can share some of the specific arguments you've learned here, evidence from Badgley, for example, that we could convert all current cropland to organic production and still yield enough calories for all. Tell them about the family farmers who are choosing to reject emissions-intensive chemical farming in favor of ecological farming and how they and their communities are thriving.

You can explain that moving toward a food system that encourages low-input local production, with organic practices where viable, will not only help address the climate crisis but also help redress one of the most painful facts of the modern world: hunger amid plenty.

9

THE BIOTECH BALLYHOO

A DAY AT THE MUSEUM

Walk past the flashlight-wielding security guards peering into purses, through the grand atrium and up the wide stairs, sidestep the screaming kids and double-wide strollers, continue beyond the replicas of Galápagos turtles and the dioramas collecting dust, and, until it closed in August 2009, after a ten-month run, you found yourself at the American Museum of Natural History's climate-change exhibit.

Beyond the glass doors and a pile of fake coal, you first saw the neon red line that showed the spikes in the levels of carbon dioxide in the atmosphere over the past century, from 260 parts per million to 350 to 385 and beyond. Fork over the twenty-four dollars to tour the entire exhibit and you discovered dozens of panels about the crisis, explaining everything from nuclear energy to the impact of coal plants, and multimedia messages from "green jobs" superstar Van Jones and MacArthur genius and Bronx sustainability maestro Majora Carter, extolling the economics of sustainability and a renewable-energy infrastructure.

The exhibit's Take Action section offered inspiration in the form of simple things you could do. Tucked into one corner of the display you could find details about how to choose climate-friendly food: Cut down on packaging, eat more local foods, and eat more fruits and vegetables. But after all those planes, trains, and automobiles you saw towering above you in the opening mural, you probably walked away without realizing that our food system's climate impact trumps them all. Only if you were the type of museumgoer who reads the small print would you have seen the text in the Take Action section noting that livestock is responsible for 18 percent of the total global warming effect.

(Remember, that's 5 percent more than the total emissions of the transportation sector.)

Other than these small mentions, the exhibit was largely silent about the role of agriculture in both contributing to the crisis and offering solutions. It was completely silent on the importance of nonchemical approaches to farming.

But even more than what the exhibit *didn't* say, it was what it *did* say that struck me. Two panels about the future of food offered dire warnings about the threat of climate change to our food supply. But they claimed there was a solution: the brave and relatively new world of genetically modified foods. The panels focused on the threat to rice faced with increased flooding and corn devastated by droughts. The solution for vital corn crops in sub-Saharan Africa was apparently clear: the drought-resistant seeds being developed by the Water Efficient Maize for Africa (WEMA) project.

For nearly a decade, I've been tracking the biotech-industry hype about the heroic role it will play in saving us from famine, farmer bankruptcy, blindness, disease, and poverty, and even in preserving biodiversity. Now it seems the biotech promoters have a new PR twist: protecting us from climate change.

At first blush, these climate-change promises seem like just another version of those we've been hearing since the FDA approved the commercial sale of genetically modified foods in 1994. Back then Dan Verakis, a spokesman for Monsanto, one of the biggest producers of GMOs, was claiming that biotech crops would benefit biodiversity by reducing herbicide and pesticide use, in effect reversing "the *Silent Spring* scenario."[1] In 1999, we heard from Monsanto that it had developed a genetically engineered rice strain that would become a vital source of vitamin A, reducing blindness caused by its deficiency.[2] In a speech that same year, then–Monsanto CEO Robert Shapiro boasted that GM technology would reduce the use of insecticide, claiming that we had already seen an "80 percent reduction in insecticide use in cotton crops alone in the United States as a result of the introduction of insect-resistant plants."[3]

None of these promises, among many more, have borne fruit. Instead, the biotech crops that have been commercialized—and now grow on more than three hundred million acres worldwide—are largely just two types: herbicide tolerant and insecticide resistant.[4] And these crops, we're finding, have been fostering herbicide-resistant weeds and pesticide-resistant pests and reducing biodiversity, among other consequences.

After spending time at the museum, though, I realized that we have more than just PR fluff to challenge. The push for biotech crops as a climate-change solution is a multi-billion-dollar business and one that I believe—and I'll share with you why—is a tragic distraction from the powerful ways we can address our very real concerns about hunger and global warming without creating new ones.

BIOTECH AND THE PROMISED LAND

Back at the museum, the panel about GM drought-resistant varietals posed this ominous question: "Will they take root soon enough?" The panel promised that genetic engineering would create supercrops, able to handle the demands of the extreme floods and intense droughts that are inevitably part of our climate-unstable future.

It doesn't take an agronomist to know that stable and predictable sources of water are essential to food production. Farmers have always been concerned about inadequate and erratic rainfall, and for generations they have been selectively breeding varieties for resilience in times of drought.

With climate change, drought will no doubt become more common, and the need for resilient varietals will be even more paramount, especially in sub-Saharan Africa, where so many of the world's undernourished live and where drought is, and will remain, particularly prevalent.

According to the museum display, salvation rests with WEMA, a "public-private partnership" led by the African Agricultural Technology Foundation (AATF) that is developing bioengineered maize. Curious, I dug into what WEMA is and what we know about what biotech crops might—or might not—achieve, as well as what alternatives we could embrace.

WEMA is a five-year project to "develop new African drought-tolerant maize varieties" funded by the U.K. Department for International Development, the U.S. Agency for International Development, and the Rockefeller Foundation.[5]

Rockefeller rang a bell. I flipped back to the "Climate Change: The Threat to Life and a New Energy Future" exhibit brochure. And there, down in the right-hand corner, I read that major support for the exhibit had been provided by the Rockefeller Foundation, along with presenter Bank of America.[6]

Rockefeller, among the largest private-sector supporters of scientific research, has deep roots in biotechnology. As far back as 1932, Rockefeller's Warren Weaver, a mathematical physicist, birthed the foundation's work in biological sciences. By 1938, Weaver was steering the foundation's research toward what he liked to call the "ultimate littleness of things," or, put more scientifically, "molecular biology," on which modern-day biotechnology rests.[7]

The WEMA project also receives funding from other sources with a firm faith in biotechnology, including the Bill and Melinda Gates Foundation and the Howard G. Buffett Foundation, which together have contributed a total of forty-seven million dollars.[8] (Howard is the son of Warren Buffett and serves on the boards of mega food company ConAgra and the Lindsay Corporation, an irrigation-systems provider for industrial farms.)

The Gates Foundation is no stranger to the biotech industry. In October 2006 it brought on board Rob Horsch as a foundation senior program officer. Horsch's last job was head of International Development Partnerships at Monsanto, where he worked for twenty-five years.[9] And along with fifty million dollars from Rockefeller, Gates's Foundation has given an initial commitment of one hundred million dollars to the Alliance for a Green Revolution in Africa, which has been pushing biotechnology-based agricultural development on the continent.[10]

In 2008, the interim executive director of AATF, the foundation that houses the WEMA project, also had long-standing ties to the biotech community, including roles as a member of the South African Genetic Engineering Committee and a board member of the International Service for the Acquisition of Agri-Biotech Applications (ISAAA), which is helping to market and distribute biotech crops globally, particularly in the developing world.[11] Launched in 1991 with a million-dollar anonymous donation, the nonprofit ISAAA is funded by the major biotech companies, including Bayer CropScience, Monsanto, Syngenta, and Pioneer Hi-Bred, and has received grants from Rockefeller, among other foundations.[12]

The WEMA project itself is also receiving support from biotech industry giants, including behemoth Monsanto and German chemical group
BASF. Monsanto is providing proprietary germplasm and expertise
as well as allegedly drought-tolerant transgenes developed with BASF.[13]

At first glance, this might seem to be an odd pairing. BASF and Monsanto are rivals in the marketplace. BASF's genetically modified canola,
resistant to its Clearfield herbicide, is up against Monsanto's Roundup
Ready, which dominates the market. Dominates is putting it mildly.
Monsanto's genetically modified corn, cotton, soybeans, and canola grow
on more than 90 percent of the total global biotech acreage.[14] But partnerships like this one help expand the market—for both companies. And
BASF, the world's largest chemical company, is certainly interested in
expanding its agricultural division as it watches sales slump for its other
products.[15]

When I inquired about the timeline for WEMA's work, spokeswoman
Grace Wachoro told me that the foundation had made regulatory sub-
missions in the United States and expects the first drought-resistant
crops to be commercialized by 2013.[16]

But some industry execs are skeptical that agricultural biotech will
turn in real results anytime soon, and they acknowledge that varieties
developed so far would provide little help in a climate-unstable future.
In the summer of 2008, Syngenta chairman Martin Taylor said it would
take up to twenty years for useful biotech varieties to be developed and
tested. Existing biotech varieties, Taylor explained, which are "largely
designed for the climate, chemicals, and pests of the northern hemi-
sphere, would be unsuitable."[17]

The ten years predicted by those industry observers is a long way
off. Even five is a long time to wait. Many regions are already experienc-
ing record droughts—today. Smallholder farmers are already suffering.
Shouldn't we be celebrating solutions that we know will work, now, and
questioning these hollow promises?

Jack Heinemann, for one, is.

QUESTIONING BIOTECH

"All stress-tolerant GMOs—like drought-resistant and flood-resilient
varietals—remain only promises, not products, despite a dozen years of

commercial GM agriculture and over twenty-five years of research," said Heinemann, an expert on gene ecology and one of hundreds of researchers responsible for the IAASTD reports, which I mentioned earlier.

Heinemann is a professor of molecular biology and genetics at the University of Canterbury, in New Zealand, and was formerly with the U.S. National Institutes of Health. His research, in part, focuses on the transfer of genes from biotech crops to non-biotech plants and on the genetics of plant traits such as drought tolerance.

"A plant's resilience in drought conditions or to other stresses, like too much water or too much salt, are complex plant characteristics," he told me from his office in New Zealand. The biotech crops commercialized to date are engineered to express qualities that are, in comparison, relatively simple, like resistance to one herbicide or a single insecticidal protein.

Chemical farmers typically buy a "technology package," which includes the seeds and the associated herbicide. They sow the herbicide-resistant crop, and then as it matures, they spray with the herbicide, killing off the weeds while the crop remains unharmed. Sixty-three percent of biotech acreage in 2007 was growing herbicide-tolerant crops, while insecticide-resistant and "stacked"-trait (a combo of herbicide and insecticide resistance) crops split the rest.[18]

"Getting an organism to display a specific trait based on the inclusion of roughly a single gene is not the same as asking a plant to live in a fundamentally different physiological space, as is required for drought and salt tolerance," said Heinemann. Unlike herbicide or pesticide resistance, drought resistance involves a multitude of genes, each playing various subtle roles. Scientists don't even have a handle yet on how many, or which, genes serve these functions. And even when a plant has expressed this tolerance, it has only been achieved in the controlled environs of a lab.

"But traits like resilience are response networks, the plant adjusting to its environment," Heinemann stressed. It's a whole different ball game when you take that plant out into the real world. And the truth is, it's nearly impossible to predict how different real-world effects will ultimately affect the plant. Whether genetically engineered crops can produce reliable drought tolerance in the fields is still a serious question. "When we start to change the relationship of these traits in the real world, we get highly unpredictable behavior," he said.

And because of the complex genetic interactions, these interventions can lead to unintended consequences in the plant, consequences that are "undesirable and have nothing to do with drought tolerance," says the Union of Concerned Scientists' Doug Gurian-Sherman.

But Heinemann's skepticism is not just based on his concern about whether bioengineered crops can be engineered to handle being thirsty for a long time. It derives also from the nature of the business. "The change in intellectual property law that allowed someone to own a piece of DNA and therefore own the plant in which that DNA could be found, caused a shift in agricultural innovation from seed developers to people who develop herbicides and pesticides," he said. "The companies that make biotech plants are not plant-breeding companies; they are agrochemical companies. They're chemistry-based companies." As a result, agriculture is increasingly driven by chemical companies' desire to profit on their products, not by what's in the best interest of all of us.

His skepticism also comes, in part, from recognizing a fundamental flaw in biotechnology, a science that is based on a misconception about the nature of genes. And he's not alone in raising his eyebrows at both biotech's promises—and premises—and the dangerous timing of pushing this technology as climate change makes our ecosystems increasingly vulnerable.

Dogging the Dogma

Since the 1960s, our understanding of genes, and how information is transferred across genes, has been dominated by what is known as the "central dogma" of molecular biology. We have Nobel Prize–winner Francis Crick to thank for it.

In a 1958 paper, and in later publications, Crick articulated the concept, which argues that biological information in the DNA of an organism—whether we're talking about humans or hamsters or habañeros—is transferred, via RNA, to proteins. According to this take on molecular biology, the transfer of information is unidirectional.

"Particles—the genes—are decoded or expressed into proteins that are directly responsible for form and function. This is the dogma," University of California at Berkeley associate professor of microbial ecology and biotechnology expert Ignacio Chapela explains to me. From this assumption about how information transfers and how proteins work—they're the "cogs and motors" driving the functioning of cells (and ultimately organisms)—it's a short intellectual jump to assume that genes can be tidily identified, spliced, and diced. Agricultural biotechnology rests on faith in the Central Dogma; the science assumes that you can confidently take a gene from one species and neatly transfer it and the functions you're seeking will be replicated like carbon copies. No feedback loops, no unknowns—no worries. (If scientists admit unintended consequences, which some do, the line is that none are serious enough to make us lose any sleep or make the whole enterprise suspect.)

There's only one problem: Genes don't work this way.[19] Decades ago, scientists determined that genetic-information transfer isn't a one-way street; information is transferred not just *from* DNA but *from* proteins through RNA back to DNA, too.[20] And DNA, we're discovering, does more than just direct a single protein. Depending on the context, the same piece of DNA can have entirely different effects in an organism. That goes a long way toward explaining why human beings are such complex organisms when "we are only about as gene-rich as a mustardlike weed (which has 26,000 genes) and about twice as genetically endowed as a fruit fly or a primitive worm," as biologist Barry Commoner says.[21]

We also now know that RNA—what we learned in high school biology class was the postal servant, obediently delivering information from DNA to proteins—is actually highly complex. RNA can behave like a protein; it can behave like DNA. It can even affect how DNA is being expressed at different moments in life.

"There is a whole world of DNA and RNA that is playing by its own rules and has nothing to do with form and function in the way the Central Dogma articulated it in the 1960s," says Chapela.[22]

And if the Central Dogma is wrong, then one of the very foundations of agricultural genetic engineering is compromised. For this reason, skepticism about biotech crops goes deeper than whether biotech can reliably produce qualities like drought tolerance. It goes to the scientific underpinnings of the technology. Flaws in the foundation explain the world of unintended consequences we've already tracked as this technology has been released into the wild, onto farm fields, and into our food supply, and they explain why each discovery of the unintended impacts of transgenics is deepening concern within the scientific community.

Says Chapela, "Despite a third of a century and more than $350 billion invested . . . a hurricane remains more predictable and a wildfire remains more controllable than GM organisms."[23]

Contamination Damnation

Early one October morning in 1999, Chapela was jolted out of bed by the ringing of his phone. It was his graduate student David Quist calling from Mexico—and he had some unexpected news.

Quist was delivering a workshop that day in Sierra Norte, nestled in the state of Oaxaca, where Chapela had been working for more than a decade. A mycologist by training, Chapela had been approached to work there by a coalition of indigenous residents. This coalition, Unión Zapoteca-Chinanteca de Comunidades Forestales, had been contacted by Japanese businessmen interested in a specific mushroom that grew in the area's forests—very interested. These importers were willing to pay as much as five hundred dollars a pound for *matsutake*, Japanese for "pine mushroom."

"The community called me because they didn't want to be involved with drug dealers. They didn't understand why anybody else would pay such a price for just food!" Chapela explained. Convinced that these businessmen just wanted to sell the mushrooms for *eating* purposes, Chapela became a broker between the two groups.

After this initial project, Chapela continued to work with the community to help foster an appreciation of its common resources—and thus the need to protect, preserve, and benefit from them. Through working with Chapela, the community became aware of the unusual genetic diversity of its native plants and began to see that diversity as an asset, providing a vital supply of varied seeds.

Back in the late 1990s, the commercialization of genetically modified foods was still mainly a U.S. affair. In fact, in Mexico there was a government moratorium on the planting of GM corn. There were exceptions, though, for substantial experimental fields at the International Maize and Wheat Improvement Center, according to Chapela. And many Mexicans felt that someday (and possibly quite soon) commercialized GM corn would land on their soils—invited or not.

"The community became clear that if they didn't have the capacity themselves to look, they would never know when it had arrived," said Chapela. Along with graduate student Quist, he decided to offer a transgenic-detection workshop in the community of Xiacuí to teach residents how to spot GM contamination.

"We were sure there wouldn't be any contamination, yet. The propaganda was so strong that transgenics weren't moving into the environment, I guess I believed it," Chapela said.

The night before the scheduled workshop, Quist ran the detection process to be sure everything was set up for the next day. And thus the morning call to Chapela.

"I've got a problem," Quist said across the wires. "My negative controls are showing up positive."

The test had been designed to include one positive sample—a can of Del Monte corn, which was definitely GM—and samples from the region. Chapela and Quist had assumed that the latter corn, in the remote and pristine areas where they were working, would be among the purest sources they could find.

"We thought, let's just go there and take some samples from the field. Those will certainly be negative. That was our mistake, thinking that way," Chapela said. Because here was Quist's call, and those samples from the field that were supposed to be pure? Six out of nine had come up positive; they were contaminated.

These findings so stunned them both, and would, they knew, be so controversial, that they ran four months of additional tests to be 100 percent confident in their results. Once they were, they published their findings in *Nature*.[24] The revelations sent a shock wave through Mexico, across the border, and throughout the industry. If GM corn was *already* appearing in Mexico, what did this mean for the extent of potential contamination?

Their findings were so troubling, in fact, that they started a firestorm of attacks against the researchers. Investigative journalists would later uncover that an online smear campaign against Chapela and Quist had been driven by paid communications staff for the biotech industry, but not before these criticisms had succeeded in garnering a retraction from the magazine.[25]

But Chapela and Quist's discovery was not an anomaly, nor should it have been that unexpected. Cross-crop genetic contamination is well known, and of all crops, corn is particularly susceptible.[26] Explained Chapela, "There is a whole range of degrees of exchange of genetic material when a plant reproduces. Corn is on one extreme of the spectrum; there are a huge number of opportunities with every pollen grain for cross-contamination."

For the corn in Mexico, the most likely source of contamination was the wave of U.S. corn imports after the 1994 passage of NAFTA. Though the imported corn was marketed as a grain, not as seed, Chapela explained, people didn't make such clear distinctions. "People eat what they plant and plant what they eat," he said. So it wasn't odd that people would plant the imported corn, and that some of that seed would be GM and would contaminate the fields.

Why should we care about such contamination? Because it affects everything from biodiversity to plant yields. To underscore why this matters, it might help to take a detour to a cautionary parable from the land of Maker's Mark.

The Kudzu Factor

While my college classmates were learning to roll their *r*'s in Spain, gain a taste for smelly cheese in France, or perfect their capoeira in Brazil, I spent my junior year teaching at a small school in Harlan County, Kentucky. Set inside the deep V of a holler—Southern speak for "valley"— the Pine Mountain Settlement School offered weeklong immersions in rural life. We taught kids how to card wool, read a compass, and distinguish harmless black racers from the venomous copperheads that roamed those valleys.

After a day's work, I'd trudge across the narrow county road to my single-room cabin, surrounded by kudzu. The entire holler, in fact, was full of the stuff.

If you're from the South, you know kudzu well. As a California girl, I'd never heard of it. The green vine originated in Japan and China. Brought to the United States in the late 1800s, it was considered just an ornamental plant until some smart folks realized the hearty vine could be used for erosion control—and the kudzu crisis was born.

During and after the Great Depression, when the Works Progress Administration hired millions of Americans for massive public infrastructure projects, road-building campaigns took off and kudzu was king. The plant prevented erosion along miles and miles of carved-out roads throughout the South.

But there was a problem with kudzu. The plant loved—I mean really loved—the hot, humid, wet Southern clime, and it grew like crazy. By 1953, the USDA was having second thoughts about dear old kudzu, and that year it did an about-face. Overnight, kudzu went from patriotic plant to official pest weed. Decades later, those tenacious fronds were still invading Kentucky hollers.

Kudzu is a symbol of the unintended consequences of intervening in ecosystems when you don't focus on the "systems" part, when you have blind faith that by dissecting complex systems down to their minute parts, you can best address the crisis at hand. In ignoring the systems, we blind ourselves to the inherent interconnections.

As we scramble to confront one of the most complex challenges our species has ever faced—climate change—our "solve by dissection" tendencies tempt us toward new modern-day kudzus: biotech crops that, allegedly, can withstand the vagaries of climate change, like the drought-tolerant WEMA crop the Museum of Natural History exhibit celebrates.

Consider the promises from Gramina, an Australian and New Zealand joint venture. The company claims to be at work on a genetically engineered grass that can withstand global warming's soaring temperatures.[27] The grass, say the developers, might have another benefit for the cattle munching it: It is being designed to prevent the expression of a specific enzyme, and this, the company says, could lead to better digestibility and fewer nasty methane burps.[28] But some scientists are already raising red flags. The very changes to the grass that the company says might *decrease* methane could actually trigger a chain reaction that creates a more acidic stomach environment, which could lead to more (not less) methane emissions.[29]

The jury is still out. Meanwhile, the company recently announced it's taking its trials from lab to field. Which should get us asking, what if the new grass, with its built-in ability to withstand greater extremes in temperature, ends up displacing native grasses? What if the grass becomes a twenty-first-century kudzu? The company assures us that field trials will be contained, but talk to Oregonians about containment.

A field test of GM creeping bent grass in Oregon jumped the curb, and the genetically modified plant is now spreading across the state.[30]

If we learn anything from our prior missteps—like kudzu—it should be that while we must move fast to respond to climate change, we shouldn't leap without fully comprehending the systems implications of our actions. We can replace our "solve by dissection" approach with what Wendell Berry dubs "solve for pattern." Solving for pattern asks that we focus on the intersections, not ignore them. And solving for pattern is what we do when we see the interconnections of our food system and climate.

If I have a bias, it stems from a conviction that this solving for pattern is how we evolved and how sustainable agriculture works; it is also how we will best address our most entrenched social, environmental, and economic problems. We will not find technological silver bullets to solve the climate crisis, the promises of biofuels backers and biotech promoters notwithstanding. Yes, we can experiment, but as we do so, we would do well to remember the kudzu: There may be benefits, but there could also be unanticipated, disastrous results.

Biotech Blunders

Since biotech crops were first introduced commercially in the 1990s, scientists around the globe have raised a host of concerns about the interaction of these human-made crops with the environment.[31] These concerns have not registered with our regulators, in part because companies have hidden information behind trade secrets claims, which "hampers external review and transparency of the decision-making process," concluded a 2002 National Academy of Sciences report on USDA oversight of GM crops.[32] As corporations promote new GM varieties for vulnerable regions in Africa, these concerns about the technology are all the more relevant. Here are just a few.

Into the weeds: Since the earliest introductions of biotech crops, scientists have worried that the traits being bred could foster herbicide-resistant weeds that would be hard to control, crowding out native varieties and dominating ecosystems.

"In the past, farmers used a variety of chemical controls and manual labor, making it unlikely that any weed plant would evolve a resistance to all those different strategies simultaneously," says Jack Heinemann, "but as we oversimplify—as we industrialize—we make the agroecosystem more vulnerable to the next problem."

Already examples of herbicide resistance are popping up from canola fields in Canada to farms in Australia.[33] Perhaps we're seeing the problem most clearly with resistance to the herbicide glyphosate. In the pre-biotech era, glyphosate-resistant weeds were not a big concern, but because of the herbicide's widespread use on biotech crops, glyphosate resistance is emerging in every major environment where biotech crops are planted.[34] Today, multiple weeds in the United States are glyphosate resistant, covering as many as several million acres.[35] Weeds that are more naturally tolerant of the herbicide are also spreading. In response, farmers are spraying glyphosate more heavily, with more frequency, and on more acreage than ever before, making glyphosate the most widely used herbicide in the United States and exacerbating the problem.

Let's bring this back to Africa: Imagine that scientists are able to create a drought-resistant corn variety. But now imagine that this resistance transfers itself to an African grass. Suddenly, that grass, which was not previously a concern for corn, is adapted to the drought-prone ecosystem in which the new corn variety is growing. Sound far-fetched? It's not, considering that maize has been found to share viruses with African native grasses, viruses that can transfer between organisms.[36] At this point in the scenario, we're in trouble; we have, my friends, what could be called a "superweed." And, warns Heinemann, the very trait that we saw as answering our needs for tomorrow "may cause the loss of that technology the day after."

The rise of superpests: Then there are the pests. Part of the biotech promise has been reducing pesticide use, but researchers around the world, including here in the United States, are finding that pesticide use is going up—not down—in the era of biotech. In one survey of cotton growers in China, researchers found that seven years after GM crops had been introduced, farmers were using as much pesticide as they had before, mainly because secondary pests that had historically been contained by extra sprayings and had posed little or no threat to cotton had taken off.[37] Indeed, the crisis of these secondary pests emerging on GM-planted land has led to a "worldwide elevation of certain species from relatively innocuous to highly destructive," say the authors of a report on the crisis.[38]

The drag of yield drag: Among the biotech industry's top promises was the pledge of the almighty yield. In 1998, Monsanto president Hendrik Verfaillie said, "Biotechnology will help us produce more, and healthier, food."[39] Its boosters are still promising this in their latest round of advertisements, like this one from Monsanto: "Producing more. Conserving more. Improving farmers' lives. That's sustainable agriculture. And that's what Monsanto is all about." We're still waiting on the proof.[40]

In one of the most comprehensive studies of field trials of biotech soy, Dr. Charles Benbrook reviewed eighty-two hundred university-based soy-varietal trials in 1998 and found that Monsanto's Roundup Ready soy produced a yield drag, on average across all the trials, of about 5 percent, with a drag in some areas as high as 10 percent.[41] For those of us for whom that means little: "If not reversed by future breeding enhancements, this downward shift in soybean yield could emerge as the most significant decline in a major crop ever associated with a single genetic modification," explains Benbrook.[42]

Select studies have shown a relatively small jump in yields in the first years of planting biotech crops, but the yields soon drop and in some cases even fall below the initial level after a few years. Some are now wondering if the decline might not be the result of the Bt toxins produced by certain biotech crops, toxins that can accumulate and remain active in the soil. Researchers are exploring whether these toxins are disturbing the multitudes of microorganisms abundant in healthy soil and fundamental for fertility and that holy grail genetic engineers are striving for: productivity.[43]

There's another way to think about yields and biotech: Yield on the field matters; so does how much of that yield gets into our mouths. With multiple cases of unapproved genetically modified foods getting into the food supply and requiring massive recalls, that, too, should be considered "yield drag," for those are crops that ultimately go to waste. Consider the 2001 StarLink corn recall. This variety of Syngenta biotech corn had only been approved for animal feed, but it turned up in products throughout the human food supply. The recall included half a million cases of taco shells, one and a half million pounds of ConAgra corn products, 441,206 cases of veggie corn dogs, 180,798 pounds of chili mix, and much more.[44]

The loss of biodiversity: The other big concern is that the spread of genetically modified crops will dangerously impact biodiversity, first by reducing crop diversity. In 2007, just three biotech crops accounted for 95 percent of the total acres planted with GMOs: Biotech soybeans covered 51 percent of the total, corn covered another 31 percent, cotton another 13 percent, and canola 5 percent.[45]

The contamination of non-GM varieties with biotech traits also threatens diversity. Yet as we enter a time of critical and dramatic climate change, diversity will be at a premium.

"Climate change means unpredictability and a diversity of challenges," says Ignacio Chapela. "The only possible answer is to have as many and as varied possible answers as we can, since we do not know, by definition, the nature of the challenges ahead."

In addition, GM crops impact on-farm biodiversity, not just because of what the farmers are planting (or not planting), but also because of what they're killing. Though weeds get a bad rap, they can play an essential role on farms. Bees feast on their nectar and pollen; birds munch on weed seeds; worms and other soil invertebrates that help control pests live among them; the list goes on.[46] In one three-year farm trial in the United Kingdom, commissioned by the government, the use of herbicide-tolerant GM canola, beets, and maize meant indiscriminate spraying of weed killers. The study found, maybe not so surprisingly, that the spraying of herbicide on crop fields significantly reduced farmland biodiversity, creating a cascade effect: the herbicide affected the bee population, fewer pollinators meant less production of insect-pollinated plants, which meant even less biodiversity . . . and so on.[47]

"The world depends not just on the plants we harvest; it depends on the very many different kinds of plants, animals, microbes in ecosystems that we *do not* harvest that ensure the plants we *do* harvest have in them the things we need to eat," stresses Heinemann.

As GM crops are pushed into regions like sub-Saharan Africa, we could be shutting down options just where we need them most.

The biggest biotech players, particularly Monsanto, are also impacting biodiversity by buying up seed companies. In 2004, just four seed firms, DuPont/Pioneer, Monsanto, Syngenta, and Limagrain controlled 29 percent of the world market for commercial seeds.[48] Monsanto increased its share in 2005 with the purchase of Seminis, which controlled a significant segment of the U.S. vegetable-seed market: 55 percent of the lettuce on our supermarket shelves comes from Seminis seeds,

75 percent of our tomatoes, and 85 percent of our peppers.[49] With Monsanto's 2008 purchase of Dutch company De Ruiter Seeds, the industry giant further expanded its market share.[50] (Ironically, Monsanto is one of the major funders of Norway's Svalbard Global Seed Vault. Colloquially referred to as the "doomsday vault," the repository will eventually hold 2.25 billion seeds. That's a lot of seeds, yes, but still just a fraction of the planet's biodiversity that is quickly disappearing— thanks in part to the consolidation of the seed industry driven by companies like Monsanto.)[51]

What's worse, the focus on biotech crops is taking our eye off the ball. A majority of the agricultural research and development dollars in the past decade has been directed toward genetic engineering, not new conventional hybrids and certainly not organic production. But what furthers a company's bottom line is not necessarily what our ecosystem most needs. This missing eco-wisdom is felt on the farm, as biotech crops and the industrialization of production methods snuff out knowledge-intensive, climate-friendly farming. "Companies are defining what solutions to make available to humanity based on what solutions they can practically own. That's not a rational way to run an agroecosystem," says Heinemann.

In the face of the climate-change threat, now is not the time to undermine biodiversity; it's the time to protect it. And that diversity on which we so depend "may be very thin," cautions Heinemann. "There may be very few copies for a particular trait or a particular type of gene. We have to maintain this natural biodiversity as a real, evolving incubator of new genes, or old genes that we haven't seen before or that we never knew were relevant. We need this biodiversity as our reservoir. If we jeopardize this for the sake of a possible wonder trait for tomorrow, then we won't have any wonder traits for the day after tomorrow."

As I reread my notes from the Heinemann conversation, review the results from the Chinese cotton growers study, or hear Chapela talk about his Mexico bombshell, I keep thinking about kudzu. We already know biotech crops don't grow in a hermetically sealed box; they function in an environment, interacting with it in ways we can't predict. When I attended the Biotechnology Industry Organization's annual convention in Philadelphia a few years ago, the trade association was offering as a prize a glass "eco-orb" that contained a fully self-sufficient ecosystem. The eco-orb seemed to me to signify that this point—the beautiful complexity of the real world—is lost on the biotech industry. Yet we are lunging forward with this next big experiment, a genetically engineered food supply, blind to the most simple of lessons: that it takes hubris to believe we can control nature and know precisely the impact of our crude reengineering of it.

WHO SAYS?

Don't just take my word for it. These concerns aren't just the fears of the fringe; many scientists around the world have raised similar alarms.

That groundbreaking United Nations report, the IAASTD, for example, raises serious questions about the role of genetic engineering in the future of farming. Agricultural biotechnology, the IAASTD warns, "lags behind" in its development; "information is anecdotal and contradictory, and uncertainty about possible benefits and damage is unavoidable."[52]

Although signed by fifty-seven governments, the IAASTD's 2008 final conclusions didn't please everyone.[53] Chemical giants like Syngenta and industry trade association CropLife International refused to sign the document.[54] In a comment in *New Scientist* magazine, Deborah Keith, a crop-protection research manager for Syngenta, explained; "When it comes to the pressing issue of climate change . . . genetically modified crops . . . can help by developing traits such as drought resistance. This potential and the science supporting it were ignored in the report."[55] In an interview, Syngenta's head of biotech research and development Martin Clough told me; "When it became pretty evident that the breadth of technologies were not getting equal airtime, then I think the view was that there was no point in participating. It's important to represent the technological options, and it's equally important to say that they get fair play. That wasn't happening."[56]

THE UNSUNG HOPE

Let's rewind for a moment and return to that biotech corn being celebrated on the walls of the Museum of Natural History. Maybe, despite all the concerns I've just laid out, you're still thinking, But aren't we talking about the fate of millions of some of the hungriest people on the planet? By rejecting GMOs are we just exerting "an imperialism of rich tastes," as Wellesley political science professor Robert Paarlberg, author of *Starved for Science*, says?[57]

"This postmodern resistance to agricultural science," argues Paarlberg, "becomes dangerous, however, when exported to countries in Africa where farmers remain trapped in poverty because they are starved for science."[58] This is Paarlberg's, and other biotech proponents', preferred mantra: Biotech is science-based; agroecology is not. "But Paarlberg doesn't seem to realize, or doesn't acknowledge, that agroecology *is* science," Dong Gurian-Sherman tells me. In many ways, it's more complex science than biotech. "Paarlberg also equates agriculture of resource-poor farmers in Africa with organic, apparently because they don't use much synthetic fertilizer or pesticides, but modern organic practices are much more than just the *absence* of synthetic chemicals and can often produce yields in sub-Saharan Africa even higher than industrial agriculture," he stresses. There's a certain "imperialism of the lab": Science is only that which is abstracted from nature and relies on microscopes and petri dishes. Studying the intricate relationships of microorganisms, plants, insects, and animals in the field it is not.

So is biotech worth the risks I've detailed? Yes, would seem to be the museum display's answer. The unspoken assumption is that we should embrace risk, because we don't have any choice.

Beneath a photograph of a tractor in a field, the display reads, "As climate change affects rainfall, farmers are looking to hi-technology answers such as genetically modified seeds for food security. Many farmers in southern African countries hope genetically modified maize will help them grow crops despite projected increases in drought."

Are farmers in southern African countries really waiting for biotech to save them? Is there really no alternative? Standing there in the museum, I knew I had to ask Sue Edwards. A botanist by training, the Ethiopian-based, British-by-birth Edwards is the director of the Institute for Sustainable Development's Tigray Project, in Addis Ababa, where she works with farmers on increasing productivity through ecological agriculture.

"No," she answered frankly, "farmers we work with don't hold much hope for GM maize." (Maybe this disconnect is not so surprising. According to an Oakland Institute review of Gates Foundation internal documents, "not one of those consulted for the foundation's agricultural strategy—not the reviewers or the external advisory board members—is a farmer from Africa."[59])

Edwards already has hope at her fingertips; she's seen hope in her fields. It's not coming from an unproven technology developed in laboratories halfway around the world; it's coming from the farmers themselves.

I first met Edwards and her husband, Dr. Tewolde Egziabher, in Modena, Italy, at the 2008 International Federation of Organic Agricultural Movements convention, which brought together more than a thousand farmers and scientists, consumer advocates and government officials, from nations ranging from Azerbaijan to Zimbabwe. One night, we strolled down ridiculously cute cobblestone streets in the center of town, through an evening farmers' market where we tasted Modena's famed balsamic, past a town square where lilting classical music was being performed, before dining on homemade ravioli and salads doused with the syrupy-sweet vinegar. Over that dinner, I heard about Edwards's home garden in Addis Ababa—her "forest," as she called it—and about a remarkable project that was showing the power of farmer-led, agroecological projects to transform lives in one of the most drought-stricken regions of Ethiopia. Call it the anti-biotech.

Beginning in 1996, Edwards and her colleagues set out to work with smallholder farmers to investigate whether resilient food systems can be fostered by tapping natural systems like ecological agriculture and building the skill base of the farmers themselves. More than ten years later, they've got some pretty impressive results.

For the project, Edwards and her team wanted to focus on a particularly drought-prone region with especially income-poor farmers to see whether an ecological approach could help restore soil fertility and raise crop yields.[60] Tigray, Ethiopia, was the perfect place. Home to an estimated four million people, 85 percent of whom live in rural areas, Tigray gets only five hundred to seven hundred millimeters of rainfall every year. To put that in perspective, that's less on average than falls in San Antonio, Texas. But in Tigray, even this precipitation is concentrated in a short rainy season, often falling as intense storms. The rest of the year is dry, very dry.

The homes of the Tigray farmers with whom Edwards works typically have no sanitation, no running water, and no electricity. It's not unusual for the women to walk two or three hours a day, or longer, to fetch five to seven gallons of water for their daily cooking and cleaning. Their houses are made of thick stone roofs and mud floors, and their incomes average just three hundred to four hundred Ethiopian birrs a year, roughly equivalent to twenty to fifty cents a day. The poorest farmers only manage to store food reserves for four to five months. "They harvest on empty stomachs," said Edwards.

Working at first with four farming communities and eventually expanding to fifty-seven in one quarter of the districts in the region, Edwards and her colleagues began their farmer trainings in 1996. They enlisted the farmers to do field trials, comparing crops grown using ecological methods like composting, crops raised with chemical fertilizer, and others grown without any inputs at all. Using sampling systems accepted by the United Nations' agricultural agency, the FAO, they were able to get rigorous data on all three.

The results were resounding and exciting. By 2006, researchers were finding significantly higher yields in the ecological test sites of *every single crop* compared with the chemical-fertilizer plots and even more dramatic yield benefits compared with the plots using no inputs.

And corn? Maize produced using ecological methods on average had a 129 percent higher yield than that in the plots that used chemical methods and a 213 percent higher yield than that in the no-input fields.[61] Other meta-studies have shown similarly dramatic results. In a 2008 study from the U.N. Conference on Trade and Development, an analysis of 114 projects in twenty-four African countries showed consistently that yields more than doubled when ecological practices were used, compared with chemical agriculture and no-input agriculture.[62]

And there were other benefits as well: The compost used in the ecological systems helped maintain soil fertility from year to year, so farmers could rotate compost applications, meaning they didn't have to produce enough compost for all their land every year. Farmers also discovered that they faced fewer challenging weeds, such as the Ethiopian wild oat *Avena vaviloviana*, and that their plants were more resistant to pests, such as the teff shoot fly.[63]

Plus, the program was much more than a one-dimensional intervention; it was also about building relationships. Many communities found, too, that this program helped them discover solutions for managing animal grazing, which before had been a big barrier to crop development.[64]

Edwards's work, and numerous similar initiatives, shows that there are already under way, in semiarid regions in Africa, strategies that greatly increase yields without depending on costly and climate-costly inputs. Right now. Not in five years. Not in ten. Right now. Right when we need them. Better yet, these techniques can be developed and embraced by farmers themselves, without their becoming beholden to corporate execs a world away, or burdened with the high costs of GM seeds or chemical inputs, or subject to the mercy of an international market where fertilizer prices, for example, jumped more than 200 percent in 2007.[65]

The improvements in crop productivity have meant that families for whom food insecurity—and real hunger—was a constant threat have been able to produce enough food to have a full year's reserve. Some are now even producing a surplus that they sell, nearly doubling their annual incomes to seven hundred dollars a year.

"These farmers, they're getting out of grinding poverty," said Edwards.

As I talked with her, she also stressed a bigger point: why the focus on GM corn itself is so misguided. Biotech firms focus on corn, Edwards emphasized, not because of any particular human-health benefit of the yellow stuff, or an inherent potential for drought resistance, but because of the way the crop pollinates. Its design makes it easy to breed and to genetically alter. "As a result, it's the most fiddled-with crop," she said.

WEMA argues that it is focused on corn because the crop is the continent's key staple, claiming that "more than 300 million Africans depend on it as their main food source."[66] But Edwards and other ecological-agriculture proponents argue that corn is only so widely grown because it's been pushed onto populations. Before colonization, populations throughout the continent survived on more nutritious and varied food sources; some of the most widely consumed crops, like sorghum, were particularly health supportive and well adapted to drought-prone regions of Africa.

Said Edwards, "It is true now that corn is a staple, but even pre–Second World War, Africa was dominated by sorghum, pearl millet, and many of the other indigenous crops." Indeed, corn itself is not native to Africa, but was brought to the continent via slave-trading ships. For Portuguese slave traders' long voyage, corn was the preferred food because of its caloric density and its tough outer shell that prevented spoiling. It continued to be popular for the colonial industrialists as a food for workers in the growing numbers of mines and plantations.[67]

A myopic focus on corn simply reinforces the problem. Edwards would argue that we should be looking not just at different corn-growing methods but also at revaluing indigenous crops that are so nutritious and naturally suited to difficult climate conditions, including drought.[68]

Her critique also stems not just from skepticism about the specific technology but from skepticism about the entire approach. "The best way of trapping your farmer, getting him on the treadmill, is to start to undermine the confidence, then take away the seed, and he or she is trapped," she pointed out.

Like Heinemann and others, Edwards is dubious that biotech crops can deliver on their promise and concerned about their unintended effects. Plus, she has seen the alternative, seen where real hope lies. After more than two decades of working in the fields with farmers themselves, she's seen an impressive jump in yields, without the costs—financial or ecological or human—of biotech. In these ways, what Edwards—and Ignacio Chapela and Jack Heinemann—is really suggesting is a shift in paradigm, to addressing a system problem with a system solution.

THE POWER OF METAPHOR

How is it that despite what we know about the complexity of genetics and of ecological systems we continue to embrace the Central Dogma's simplistic notions and remain blind to the unintended consequences of tinkering with genes?

Maybe one answer is the power of metaphor. Chapela and I discussed the way we talk about genetic engineering: Scientists and journalists translating for laypeople describe DNA as our "code," "blueprint," or "instruction book." Computer metaphors seem apt, so we hear of switching a gene on or off, like the 0s and 1s of the digital age. "The computer-world metaphors are beautifully adapted for this view of the technology," said Chapela. Precise, controllable, and neat, though—in the real world—this technology is anything but.

Those tens of thousands who passed through the halls of the American Museum of Natural History may never get to weigh the warnings from the fields of biotech crops against the possibility of environmentally sound climate-resilient crops that Sue Edwards's research represents. Those of us who know, and learn about, this ecological path, though, can challenge the dogma—even if sometimes doing so doesn't feel that comfortable. Just ask Chapela.

IV
ACTION

10
EAT THE SKY: SEVEN PRINCIPLES OF A CLIMATE-FRIENDLY DIET

At some point, we've all been scolded about food: Finish your spinach, cut your calories, stop snacking. Or experienced global warming finger-wagging: Turn off those lights, give up your car, cut back on your flights. I'm not going to do either. We need all hands on deck to address the climate crisis, and guilt-tripping is never an effective way to inspire us to hoist the sails.

It's time to drop the "you should" rhetoric and go for the "we can" chorus—with a tip o' the hat to our president, of course. These seven principles are delivered in that spirit. Consider them a road map for eating with the sky in mind—more inspiration than commandments.

Seven Principles of a Climate-Friendly Diet

Principle 1: Reach for real food
Principle 2: Put plants on your plate
Principle 3: Don't panic, go organic
Principle 4: Lean toward local
Principle 5: Finish your peas . . . the ice caps are melting
Principle 6: Send packaging packing
Principle 7: DIY food

Some of you may already embrace these principles; you just might not have thought of them as climate-friendly ones. Others might find these novel notions. But for all of us, following them is not always easy. We live in a world where most of our food options are a far cry from the morsels I suggest you munch. These barriers to healthy eating—for ourselves and our planet—are very real. As you come up against them, consider them as signs, signals of just how much change is needed—and where it's needed most. Get reinforcement. Hook up with a food campaign in your community. Be active beyond your fork. And have fun. Food is pleasure, after all, and these principles will guide you into a world of food that delivers the goods—without the guilt.

PRINCIPLE 1: REACH FOR REAL FOOD

For years, Hellmann's mayonnaise has been calling itself "real." Now a movement named the Real Food Challenge is spilling onto campuses across the country, and a bestselling book called *Real Food* has recently hit bookshelves. But what does "real" really mean? The concept is relatively simple. I would say that "real foods" are "whole foods," but ever since Whole Foods supermarkets swept the nation, I've found myself having to either qualify the term (er, not the grocery chain) or not use it at all. So, real foods it is: They're foods that are as close to their natural state as possible, that haven't undergone energy-intensive processing and don't contain chemically laden ingredients. Strawberries freshly picked = real. Strawberry-flavored Pop-Tarts = not so real.

Real foods are grown by farmers who tap their knowledge about natural systems to raise their crops, not their wallets to purchase synthetic fertilizer and fossil-fuel-based chemicals. Real food comes from land that is being nurtured so that it retains more water, stores more carbon, and is more resilient in the face of climate instability. Real food comes from land that becomes healthier as the farmer does his or her work. Think Mark Shepard's farm versus the destroyed peatlands of Malaysian palm plantations. And real meat and dairy come from animals raised humanely, on pasture or on organically grown feed, with care taken for their well-being, not those poor CAFO-trapped animals.

Finally, it may be a bit of a cliché by now, but if you've ever tasted a tomato from the farmers' market, you know that real food has real flavor. It's the kind of flavor you find in plants that have been raised in healthy soil, bred for taste, not for shipping.

Finding Real Food

Unfortunately, finding real food isn't always easy, especially where most of us now shop. By 2005, one in four of our food dollars was spent at a Walmart.[1] When seeking real foods in processed-foods-laden box stores, take the advice of New York University professor Marion Nestle, author of *Food Politics* and *What to Eat*: Stay to the periphery. There, in those aisles, you'll find the healthy fruits and vegetables, the least-processed options.[2] I also like to use the "rule of thumb." If the ingredients list is longer than the width of your thumb—retreat.

Or, bypass the supermarket altogether and try out these sources for real food:

Farmers' markets: Farmers' markets are one of our best sources for real food. With more than 4,685 markets in the United States, nearly double the number that existed a decade ago, many more of us have the option of purchasing our food directly from the source, from the farmer who grew it.[3]

Community-supported agriculture (CSA): First launched in the United States in 1986, CSAs are farms supported by eaters who make an investment at the beginning of the harvest season and are then rewarded with weekly deliveries of fresh produce, and sometimes even cut flowers, honey, coffee, meat and dairy, and more. The relationship means that farmers know their customers and we eaters know where our food comes from. Today, tens of thousands of people are members of CSA farms across the country, and new ones are starting all the time.

Community-owned stores and food coops: You can also seek out real food at community-owned stores and food cooperatives in your community. Many have buying codes-of-ethics and food buyers who do the hard work of finding foods grown with the most ecological principles possible.

Avoiding Genetically Modified Foods

Real food also means produce and grains that have not been genetically modified and meat and dairy that have not been raised on GM ingredients. Eschewing these products makes a difference for the climate and for a host of other reasons, including many I shared earlier in the book. But how to avoid GM foods in the United States? I've got good news and bad.

First, the bad: To date, we are one of the few countries that have commercialized genetically modified foods, yet our government still refuses to require that products containing them be labeled. Even undemocratic China requires GM labeling.

Now for the good news: Despite our lack of labeling, you can still avoid GM ingredients by following some of these tips:

Choose organic: USDA-certified organic foods cannot be genetically modified or raised with genetically modified feed. While organic farmers are increasingly concerned about GM contamination, the organic seal is still one of the best ways to try to avoid GM foods.

Avoid processed foods: Most processed foods contain derivatives of corn or soy, so you're likely to be consuming GM ingredients unless the label explicitly says otherwise.

Go for fruits and veggies: Only a handful of GM produce has been commercialized—papaya from Hawaii and possibly small amounts of sweet corn and summer squash—so you can chow your carrots sans worry.[4]

Resources for Principle 1: Reach for Real Food

- *Learn more about real foods and why they matter:* Check out Web sites devoted to the ethics and politics of eating. Two of my favorites: www.grist.org and www.ethicurean.com.

- *Speak up for real foods:* Let your store buyers know you care. For those of you who might not be the bold, can-I-speak-with-the-manager? type, you don't have to go it alone. Connect with groups like Sustainable Table to find tips and real-foods comrades-in-arms: www.sustainabletable.org.

- *Find real foods:* At home and when you're on the road. Check out www.eatwellguide.org, which includes listings of real-foods-friendly restaurants, farmers' markets, and CSAs across the country. Or visit www.csacenter.org to find CSAs near you. Local Harvest also has great resources for finding farmers, stores, and other sources of real: www.localharvest.org.

- *Support real foods:* Help bring real food into your community or find groups that already are by seeking out members of the Community Food Security Coalition: www.foodsecurity.org.

PRINCIPLE 2: PUT PLANTS ON YOUR PLATE

We've long known the ecological, social, and animal-welfare costs of industrial meat and dairy production, but if that wasn't enough to get you salivating for your salad, we now have the climate to consider. I've already pummeled you with the facts about the impact of livestock on global warming—remember those shocking figures indicating that livestock production is responsible for nearly one fifth of the world's greenhouse-gas emissions? Here's a Cliffs Notes recap:

- Livestock production is responsible for more than one third of the world's methane emissions and two thirds of its nitrous oxide emissions.[5]

- Livestock production uses 70 percent of all agricultural land.[6]

- Half of all corn and 90 percent of all soy are diverted to feed animals on factory farms.[7]

- Half of all fossil-fuel-intensive synthetic fertilizer in the United States is used on feed crops.[8]

- Industrial poultry and swine consume almost half the world's fish oil and fish meal.[9]

- Fossil fuel use can be 2.5 to 50 times higher to produce meat protein than vegetable-based protein.[10]

- A Cornell study found that meeting the annual dietary needs of a typical meat eater requires as much as 2.1 acres of farmland, compared with just half an acre for a plant-centered eater.[11]

- A study of the environmental impact of different diets—omnivorous, vegetarian, and vegan—and farm production methods found that beef was the "single food with the greatest impact on the environment" and that across the board "greater consumption of animal products translates to a greater impact on the environment."[12]

This is just some of the evidence pointing to why the livestock sector is such a factor in the climate crisis and why rethinking our relationship to meat and dairy, especially from industrial farms, is such a key principle.

Kicking the Habit

Farro and fennel, quinoa and kale, persimmons and parsnips. The plant kingdom is bursting with flavors, nutrients—and some very odd names. Thankfully, putting more plants on our plate doesn't mean sacrificing flavor or variety; it means discovering it. Plus, for most of us in the United States, and in industrialized countries in general, reaching for the rutabaga wouldn't be such a bad idea for our health, either.[13] Americans today consume 222 pounds of red meat and poultry annually for every man, woman, and child. That's more than three times the global average and roughly equivalent to an order of Chicken McNuggets, a Quarter Pounder, and a side of bacon every day of the year for every single one of us.[14] Cutting back on meat also means that for those of us who do choose to consume the stuff, we can be more selective: going for the real meat and dairy of organic, sustainable, and humane origins.

This eat-less-meat message is certainly not what you heard from the meat industry at the 2008 American Meat Institute conference. Speaking to a packed room of fifty executives, Mary Young, the VP of nutrition for the National Cattlemen's Beef Association, had a different yarn to spin.[15] Part scold, part cheerleader, Young gushed about the "powerful nutrition story" these guys had: Eating meat helps build muscle, boost immunity, provide energy, aid satiety, manage weight, and prevent disease, she claimed. "Everyone is trying to own protein," said Young, "but the meat case can and should uniquely own protein!"

Here in the United States, maybe we've heard too much Young-esque boasting, for the typical American now consumes *twice* as much protein as the body can actually use.[16] The nitrogen from the extra protein we eat, but don't need, ends up in our urine. And, if we don't burn the calories from the extra protein, we simply store them as fat.

We also know that overconsumption of industrially raised meat and dairy, particularly processed meats, has serious health implications. In its recent dietary recommendations, the World Cancer Research Fund puts it clearly, suggesting that we "limit intake of red meat and avoid processed meats" and "eat mostly foods of plant origin."[17] Red meat and processed meat, the organization states, are a "convincing or probable cause" of certain forms of cancer, particularly colorectal, lung, esophageal, pancreatic, and endometrial.[18] A just-released National Institutes of Health study of nearly half a million people found that men and women who consumed diets with the highest levels of red and processed meat were more likely to die younger—especially from cancer and heart disease.[19]

The take-home message, with apologies to Young, is that we can follow this climate-friendly principle without trading in our health, and indeed, some of us even stand a chance of improving it.

Resources for Principle 2: Put Plants on Your Plate

- *Viva veggies:* Check out the resources at www.meatlessmonday.com or page through these enticing cookbooks that abound with inspiration.

  - *Grub: Ideas for an Urban Organic Kitchen*, my second book, includes more plant-centered recipe ideas, shopping lists, and other culinary tips.

  - Any cookbook by Mollie Katzen (of *Moosewood Cookbook* fame). Katzen also has great books for cooking meals with kids.

  - *The Modern Vegetarian Kitchen*, by Peter Berley. I am obsessed— I mean really obsessed—with the vegan skillet corn bread. Just writing this, I start craving the jalapeño- and maple-syrup-infused delight.

  - *Vegan Soul Kitchen*, by Bryant Terry (my friend and the coauthor of *Grub*). Terry offers up a twenty-first-century twist on soul food. The black-eyed pea fritters are to die for.

  - *Lucid Food*, by Louisa Shafia. The beautiful photographs in this cookbook will seduce you, if the recipes don't first.

- *Support real meat and dairy farmers:* Visit www.eatwellguide.org and discover local meat and dairy producers at your nearest farmers' market.

- *Go for grass fed:* If you choose to eat beef, look for grass fed. (Check out the next section for more on grass-fed meat and dairy.)

PRINCIPLE 3: DON'T PANIC, GO ORGANIC

It was lunchtime at a meat-industry conference, and I was sitting at a table with a gaggle of guys. (That seems to be who shows up at these events.) The corporate executive next to me was in the business of food coloring; thanks to his company, your Hot Pockets look brown when you bake them. When I mentioned organic foods, he looked a little perplexed. "Organic," he said. "Is that like what your grandmother used to eat?"

Not exactly. Certified Organic foods in the United States are those grown following specific USDA requirements in place since October 2002.[20] While these standards are not explicitly framed as strategies to address the climate crisis, organic farming methods, as I've discussed, can help reduce food-related emissions in a multiplicity of ways.

To be certified organic, farmers and processors are prohibited from using most synthetic and petroleum-based pesticides and fertilizers. (Some synthetic materials are allowed, but they must be approved by the National Organic Program.) By reducing farmers' dependency on these chemicals, the guidelines directly diminish on-farm carbon dioxide emissions. Organic corn, for example, has been found to require as much as one-third less energy inputs per acre. By one estimate, this translates into sixty-four gallons of fossil fuel saved per acre of organic corn.[21]

Whether you call it "sewage sludge" or use its more euphemistic name—"biosolids"—certified-organic farmers are prohibited from using municipal waste as fertilizer. You might not have thought much about what happens to our waste after you kiss it good-bye, and your last guess might be that it ends up on farmland across the country. But it's not uncommon for municipalities to dispose of their waste (processed, of course) on agricultural fields. Critics of sewage sludge on farmland contend that it contaminates groundwater with pathogens, an oversupply of nutrients, and heavy metals. Organic advocates argue that natural fertilizer sources, such as compost, livestock manure, and legume cover crops, not only save us from these negative consequences but also increase soil fertility, helping to do that all-important work of building soil carbon and pulling carbon out of the atmosphere. Organic fertilizer can also be an effective way of reusing what would otherwise be considered waste on a farm, another net benefit for reducing emissions.

There are two other key prohibitions regarding organic production: no irradiation or genetic modification. Irradiation, exposing foods to a high dose of ionizing radiation, cannot be used on organic products. While the process has been promoted for decades as an allegedly effective way to kill bacteria linked to food-borne illnesses, public health advocates are concerned that it reduces a food's nutrient content and leaves behind potentially hazardous chemical by-products.[22] Irradiation is another energy-intensive step in the industrial food chain that organic production bypasses.

Genetically modified foods cannot carry the organic seal either. Given the concerns I've raised about biotech crops, this provision scores another point for the organic team in the fight against global warming.

Certified-organic meat and dairy producers must follow additional guidelines. To get the organic label, for instance, meat and dairy producers must use only organic feed—another climate plus. Below are more details about the difference between the production methods.

"Organic" vs. "natural": Slapped on green-looking foods, the word "natural" can be confused with "organic," but the terms are quite different. In the United States, to be certified organic, your farming practices must be verified by a third party and follow the standards encoded in the federal organic legislation. Willfully violate these rules and you could face a fine of up to eleven thousand dollars per incident. Although there have been frustrations among organic consumer advocates about companies stepping over the line and bending the regs, most organic farmers play by the rules.

"Natural," on the other hand, is a vague term, placed on products that are grown and processed under a wide range of production systems, some that may reduce on-farm emissions, some that may have no better climate impact than chemical farming.

"Organic" vs. "grass-fed": You may find the "grass-fed" label on products from those ruminants I've told you about, animals—like cattle, goats, and sheep—that can digest grass and other fibrous plant materials. Advocates argue that choosing grass-fed meat and dairy is one way to lower your carbon foodprint. One study found that grain-fed beef required twice as many energy inputs as grass-fed beef.[23] Another found that raising cattle on pasture led to at least a 20 percent reduction in greenhouse gases.[24] Grass-fed advocates contend that while the cow grazing in the field will still be naturally emitting methane

Organic versus Non-Organically Grown Produce

Organic Foods	Non-Organically Grown Foods
• Farmers use natural fertilizers, such as manure, cover crops, and compost, to build healthy soil.	• Synthetic or chemical fertilizers and sewage sludge bolster soil fertility.
• Crop rotation, hand weeding, mechanical cultivation, and mulching control weeds naturally.	• Chemical herbicides control weeds.
• Natural methods, including birds and beneficial insects and non-chemical traps, help to manage pests.	• Chemical pesticides, including insecticides and fungicides, are used to control pests and disease.
• Irradiation is not allowed.	• Irradiation approved to kill pathogens in select foods.
• Genetically modified crops are prohibited.	• Genetically modified seeds approved.

through digestion, it's merely playing its natural role in the carbon cycle, and it's certainly not contributing to the environmental costs of animal waste and other pollution of CAFOs.

These claims aren't going uncontested. Leafing through a recent *Wired* magazine, I stumbled on an article titled "Surprise! Conventional Agriculture Can Be Easier on the Planet." According to contributor Joanna Pearlstein, grass-fed cattle are not the better climate bet. A grass-fed dairy cow, she claims, actually emits 16 percent *more* greenhouse gases than her industrial counterpart.[25] And because grass-fed dairy cows live longer, they'll be producing more emissions over more time, making "organic dairies a cog in the global warming machine." As for grass-fed beef, Pearlstein quotes the United Nations' Food and Agriculture Organization, which estimates that pasture-raised cattle burp up twice as much methane as do grain-fed cattle.

But don't let the conclusiveness fool you, says Meredith Niles, cocoordinator of the Cool Foods Campaign at the Center for Food Safety

Organic Meat and Dairy versus Non-Organic Meat and Dairy

Organic Meat and Dairy	Non-Organic Meat and Dairy
• Livestock must be raised on 100 percent organically grown feed. • Antibiotics and synthetic growth hormones are prohibited. • Livestock must have access to outdoors and ruminants must have access to pasture. • Disease is prevented with a variety of natural methods including a healthy diet, humane conditions, and rotational grazing.	• No stipulations about feed. Feed can contain animal by-products. • Antibiotics and synthetic hormones can be used to speed growth. • Disease is prevented or treated with a host of pharmaceutical drugs. • Livestock may or may not have access to outdoors. Typically, livestock are raised in confinement.

and now a doctoral student at the University of California at Davis. These estimates don't incorporate the full picture; they ignore the benefit of carbon sequestration in grass-fed systems, for example. Plus, on the other side of the ledger, they don't factor in the "emissions associated with the pesticides and fertilizers needed to produce feedlot grain, or the transportation necessary to support such a system," Niles continues. In addition, when ruminants are raised on well-managed pasture, farmers are not tilling the soil and releasing carbon.

While we certainly need a lot more research to better understand the impacts of these different systems, for now meat and dairy eaters concerned about the climate can cut back as well as reach for grass-fed products. They now have new labels to help find these products in the marketplace.

In October 2007, the USDA refined its voluntary grass-fed standards, which require that cattle consume only grass or forage (plants eaten by grazing livestock)—except at birth, when they can consume milk or milk replacements. The standard also stipulates that animals have access to pasture during the growing season, which varies depending on where livestock is raised.

If you're choosing USDA grass-fed beef, be sure to look for the

Comparing Meat and Dairy Labels

	USDA Organic	Certified Humane§	American Grassfed Association (for ruminants only)
	USDA ORGANIC	CERTIFIED HUMANE RAISED & HANDLED	American Grassfed
Verification	Requires third-party certification.	Requires third-party certification.	For ruminants only. Requires third-party certification.
Feed is USDA-certified organic?	YES	NO	N/A livestock not raised on feed
Feed is not grown with pesticides, herbicides, fungicides, or synthetic fertilizers?	YES	NO	N/A
Feed is free of GMOs?	YES	NO	N/A
Feed is free of animal by-products?‡	YES	YES	N/A
Livestock is raised hormone-free?	YES	YES	YES
Livestock is raised without antibiotics?	YES	YES**	YES
Animals have access to outdoors and pasture?	LIKELY††	DEFINITELY	DEFINITELY
Waste is managed sustainably?	YES	YES	YES

Naturally Raised*	Conventional
No label	No label
No verification.	No verification.
NO	NO
NO	NO
NO	NO
LIKELY	NO
LIKELY	NO
NO	NO
NO	NO
NO	NO

Adapted with assistance from Consumers Union, Greener Choices. For more information, check out www.greenerchoices.org

* Meat and poultry with the "natural" claim should not contain artificial flavoring, color ingredients, chemical preservatives, or artificial or synthetic ingredients. Should be only "minimally processed." The claim does allow some antibiotic use and does not address how the animals were raised or treated.

‡ Animal by-products are any parts of slaughtered animals not consumed by humans, including bonemeal and blood. Since 1997, the United States banned "the use of nearly all tissues from ruminants—animals such as cows, sheep, and goats—in feed intended for ruminants" because of concerns about Mad Cow disease, though consumer advocates have raised concern that loopholes still allow this questionable feed into ruminant diets.

** Antibiotics can be used to treat sick animals

†† Pending final ruling for specific requirements.

§ Certified Humane has clear stipulations for animal care, which include nutritious diet without antibiotics or hormones, and animals must be raised with shelter, resting areas, sufficient space, and the ability to engage in natural behaviors.

"process-verified" seal. This is your indication that the farmer has had their farming practices verified by a third party. If you find this seal, you'll also know that the farmer is meeting the tougher, more recent guidelines from the USDA's Agricultural Marketing Service, says Consumer Union's Dr. Urvashi Rangan.

You can also seek out meat that's verified by the American Grassfed Association (AGA), whose farmers tend to have a more holistic vision of grass-feeding as part of a sustainable system, rather than just a discrete practice. The AGA strictly prohibits livestock from being confined to pens, except during weaning and sorting, and requires 100 percent pasture. Plus, you're guaranteed that the farmers are following the rules by the association's licensed third-party certifiers.

With all this complexity, the best way to ensure that your meat and dairy has the lowest carbon foodprint is to know your producer. I know for most of us this simply isn't possible, so that's why learning what labels tell you—and don't—can still be key to guiding your shopping choices.

Local-O

If you're with me so far, you've noticed that these organic and grass-fed guidelines make no claims about place. Indeed, processed organic foods may include ingredients that have traveled just as far as their nonorganic counterparts. Organic meat and dairy may be raised on feed shipped from thousands of miles away. Indeed, as demand for organic foods has sometimes surpassed supply, or as companies have looked for cheaper ingredients, the industry has searched far and wide for its ingredients. By one estimate, as much as half of the organic soy consumed in the United States is now imported from China.[26] So when you're seeking out the O, keep in mind two other principles in this chapter: Look for real and local, too.

How to Know Organic When You See It

Organic at farmers' markets: You may notice that not every farmer at the farmers' market plasters his or her stand with USDA-certified-organic stickers. For many small-scale farmers, the process of getting

Identifying Organic Produce

What Is It?		What the Label Will Say
Organic		**5 digits beginning with "9"** Grown under the production guidelines of the USDA National Organic Program.
Non-Organic		**4 digits beginning with "4"** Raised with pesticides, herbicides, fungicides.

the organic certification just costs too much. Plus, these farmers know they can explain their practices directly to their consumers. If you're wondering about the practices of farmers at your local market, just ask them, or talk with the market manager. For family farmers, not having a USDA-certified operation doesn't mean their practices aren't in line with ecological principles. Indeed, supporting these farmers may be among your best climate choices: You're guaranteed the food is fresh and harvested close to home. The choice is right up there with going for the climate-friendly and tasty food you grow yourself!

Organic produce: You might not pay much attention to those PLU stickers gumming up your Granny Smiths, but they provide an easy divining tool for finding organic. You'll find the stickers on individual fruits and veggies, on bunches of produce like kale, and on bags of goodies, like potatoes and onions.

Organic processed foods: When you're choosing organic processed foods, you've got to pay a little closer attention. See the chart on the next page to understand what the different "levels" of organic labeling mean.

Resources for Principle 3: Don't Panic, Go Organic

- *Learn more about organics:* You can find out more about the U.S. organic regulations at www.ams.usda.gov/nop. For an international perspective on organic food and farming, visit the International Federation of Organic Agriculture Movements at www.ifoam.org

Identifying Organic Processed Foods

	100% Organic	Organic	Made With Organic Ingredients	Ingredient Panel Only
Must be certified by a USDA-accredited certifying agent?	YES	YES	YES	NO
What it means	All ingredients and processing aids must be USDA-certified organic.*	Must contain at least 95% organic ingredients. May contain non-organically produced agricultural ingredients that aren't available in organic form and are approved by the National Organic Program.	Must contain at least 70% organic ingredients. May contain up to 30% non-organically produced ingredients as long as they're not genetically modified, have not been irradiated, and were grown without sewage sludge.	Contains less than 70% organic ingredients.
What you'll see	USDA ORGANIC	USDA ORGANIC Percent of organic ingredients and/or "organic" in the ingredients list.	Can't use the seal. Can list up to three organic ingredients on the front packaging.	Can't use the seal. Can only list organic ingredients in the panel.

* Percentage of organic ingredients measured by weight.
Water and salt are not included, since there is no certification for either of them.
Source: National Organic Program USDA

or the United Kingdom's Soil Association: www.soilassociation
.org. The Organic Center is also a great starting place for research
about the organic sector: www.organic-center.org. The USDA's
Cooperative Extension Service has recently gotten into the act, too,
with extensive information about organic agriculture, including
an organic YouTube channel: www.eorganic.info.

• *Speak up for organics:* We're starting to see more support for organic agriculture from the highest levels of government. For the
first time ever, in 2009, the USDA granted fifty million dollars to
organic farmers and to farmers interested in transitioning from
chemical production to organic, for implementing conservation
practices on their farms. In addition, organic farmers and processors are now eligible for an organic certification cost-share rebate
of 75 percent of their certification fees. Advocate for more support
through groups like www.fooddemocracynow.org. Join the Organic
Consumers Association to support organic farmers and speak up
for policies that promote organic food: www.organicconsumers
.org. Discover more resources at Consumers Union's www.notinmy
food.org.

• *Get the facts on organic integrity:* Concerned about the labeling
issues I've discussed here? Want to learn more? Visit www.greener
choices.org. Also check out the resources at the Cornucopia Institute, which is working to protect organic integrity. The institute has
great "scorecards" that rate the best organic milk and soy companies:
www.cornucopia.org.

• *Seek out farmers who go "beyond organic":* Meet them at your local farmers' market; support them with your championing of policies favoring small-scale, sustainable farmers. See the suggestions
in Principle 1 for more resources.

PRINCIPLE 4: LEAN TOWARD LOCAL

When the term "locavore" became a *New Oxford American Dictionary*
word of the year in 2007, it was a sure sign that the eat-food-close-to-
home movement had taken off. You can now find eat-local initiatives

popping up everywhere from Google's swank California headquarters to hamlets off the coast of British Columbia.

As more of us connect climate change with the food on our plate, the locavore message is getting another boost—but it's also getting some bruising. The boost? Most of our food travels vast distances before it reaches our plate and choosing local foods is one way to reduce those associated emissions.*

The bruising? As we learn about food and climate change, we learn that the bulk of food-system emissions don't come from "food miles." Indeed, reducing our carbon food print means considering more than just this distance from farm to plate.

But despite the "local" implied in their name, locavores get this complexity. Yes, food miles are important, but just as important is how your food was produced and by whom. For locavores, it matters that food has been raised sustainably and comes from people you know, or at least have the possibility of knowing, a sharp contrast to an industrialized food system whose practices and whose workers' faces, hands, and labors are hidden to us. For the locavore, "local" chicken is not the stuff coming out of the CAFO down the road. In this way, the "local" in locavore is really code for sustainability and connectivity. As one of the original locavores, Jessica Prentice, explained to me, "Eating local is about addressing the anonymity of our food system. More than anything, I want to eat in a way that is interconnected."

But this nuance of locavorism is often sidelined in coverage of the movement, coverage that tends to myopically focus on food miles, above all else. In one such media moment, author James McWilliams

---

* A note on food miles: I don't like putting a specific number on the average distance our food has traveled in the United States, though you might have noticed the fifteen hundred miles figure. That estimate comes from research headed by Rich Pirog at Iowa State University's Leopold Center for Sustainable Agriculture. But his study was an estimate of the average not for all food, but for just thirty-three U.S.-grown fruits and vegetables and the distance they traveled to the Chicago Terminal Market. The study didn't include the 18 percent of imported foods or any meat and dairy products. But the media have taken up the fifteen-hundred-mile figure, often presenting it as *the* definitive average. Pirog never meant the number to be used this way. "We hoped our study would be a consciousness-raising tool," he says. Considering what this figure doesn't include, the average food miles for *typical* food consumed in the United States is most likely significantly higher.

seemed to give a fatal blow to local-food advocates. In an August 2007 *New York Times* op-ed, McWilliams cited a study comparing New Zealand and U.K. foods and concluded that it was "four times more energy-efficient for Londoners to buy lamb imported from the other side of the world than to buy it from a producer in their backyard."[27] It was enough to leave the lamb-loving environmentalist pondering, to eat local or not to eat local?

His controversial conclusion had legs. It was echoed in a November 2007 *Forbes* piece, in a 2008 Slate.com article, even on a Web page devoted to the climate benefits of trade on the World Trade Organization's Web site.[28]

But dig into the study and the findings don't necessarily mean we should leap for that New Zealand lamb. The main reason British lamb loses the draw has less to do with the lamb's mileage and more to do with national energy policy and farming methods. It turns out New Zealand farms use significantly less fossil fuel energy; that's largely because of the Kiwi context. In 2008, New Zealand was getting nearly 30 percent of its energy from renewable sources.[29] Compare that to the United Kingdom's 2 percent.[30] The Kiwi lamb was also pasture raised, while the British meat was raised on feed grown with emissions-intensive fertilizer. As a result, lamb raised in New Zealand used seven times less nitrogen and came away with a lower emissions price tag.

One lesson is not that we should reach for far-flung meat, but that transport is just one consideration to be weighed within the larger story about how our food is produced. The other? Brits should push their country to get with the program and shift—now—to renewable energy and press the lamb industry to rethink raising animals on chemically grown crops. And in the meantime, maybe Brits should reach for the rhubarb instead.

Learning What Locavore Means

Though food miles are rarely the most significant source of a food's global warming impact, this doesn't mean we should toss the argument out the Prius window. Miles still matter. (And will only matter more. The United Nations suggests that transport emissions could grow by more than 70 percent by 2020, as global trade expands.)[31]

To take just one example, a study of key foods imported into California and also produced in and exported from the state—table grapes, navel oranges, wine, garlic, rice, and fresh tomatoes—found that greenhouse-gas emissions from transport were as much as forty-five times greater for the imported foods as for the local ones. Global warming pollution was five hundred times greater for foods imported by airfreight.[32]

Plus, to really weigh the emissions from transport, we've got to account for the full story, including emissions from the mileage of our food's inputs, too—not just the distance from field to plate. For conventional food, this could include inputs like ammonia from Morocco or feed from Brazil. This full story would also include the emissions from constructing the infrastructure our food system relies on—the highways and roads, trucks and trains—and from repairing it. Wear and tear is so severe that some states are even considering truck-only toll lanes on the interstates and major highways to bear the cost.

The full food-miles story would also include the emissions from getting us to the store. Sure, big-box stores, with their one-stop shopping, may seem more climate friendly than the farmers'-market-hopping of locavores, but most of these stores are now located outside of population centers, on the outskirts of towns and the edges of cities, where it takes us miles to get to them.[33]

Finally, when we consider food miles, we should count the impact on communities, too. That study from California also found that the state's poorest residents bore a disproportionate burden of the pollution, since transport hubs—airports, ports, rail yards—are typically located in low-income neighborhoods.[34] Soot, sulfur oxides, and nitrogen oxides emissions from the ships in Southern California alone have been linked to as many as seven hundred deaths in these communities and an untold number of illnesses.[35]

Building the climate-change argument for local also means stressing why farms are so essential. In the United States, two acres of agricultural land disappear to development every minute, every single day.[36] Loss of farmland to strip malls and condos means we also lose the potential to store carbon in healthy soils. Plus, as prime farmland is developed, farms are pushed onto less desirable land, leading to higher rates of erosion and greater reliance on energy-intensive irrigation.[37]

When I first wrote this section, I added bleakly, "I don't know about you, but I have yet to hear about a strip mall built on farmland that reverted back to a farm." I had to eat my words—and delete that line.

While I was working on the final edit, I came across news about a mall going under and a community garden going up. When a Glendale, California, shopping center declared bankruptcy, a group of activists decided to open the community's first garden within blocks of the closed mall. Though not exactly strip mall begets organic farm, maybe this is a sign of a trend of gardens popping up where we least expect them and where you and I can access local to our hearts' desire.

Resources for Principle 4: Lean Toward Local

- *Seek out local:* Check out the resources in Principle 1 for finding real, local food. (Remember, the more ingredients in a product, the more likely the more elaborate the food-miles story.) Visit www .foodroutes.org for Buy Fresh Buy Local efforts in your community. Some stores now label the distance that produce has traveled to get there. If your store doesn't, prompt the produce manager to consider doing so.

- *Support local food:* Your region might already have a local-foods organization or food-policy council helping to spearhead local-food initiatives, so poke around. Check out resources at the Community Alliance with Family Farmers: www.caff.org. To find out if your state has a food policy council and to get involved, visit www .statefoodpolicy.org.

- *Take part in an "Eat Local" challenge:* Roll up your sleeves, grab your fork, and take part in an "eat local" challenge or launch one of your own: www.eatlocalchallenge.com.

- *Speak up for farmers:* Join an advocacy group speaking up on behalf of our small-scale farmers, building a national case for local. Some groups to learn from: National Family Farm Coalition, www .nffc.net and National Sustainable Agriculture Coalition, sustain-ableagriculture.net.

PRINCIPLE 5: FINISH YOUR PEAS . . . THE ICE CAPS ARE MELTING

Down where the Brooklyn-Queens Expressway meets the East River, a postindustrial, potholed avenue is lined with warehouses. Behind the doors of one of these nondescript buildings lies the home of a unique monthly dinner party. The evening I attended, I dined on fresh zucchini salad, Mexican lasagna, garlicky kale, mashed broccoli and cauliflower, blue corn churro with nutty mole dipping sauce, and some sweet concoction named Cookie Mash, among other desserts. The ample food fed nearly fifty. But unlike the food found at my dinner parties, all the ingredients were free—carefully procured from the streets and curbsides of New York City.

Sometimes dubbed freegans, the folks at this dinner would argue that, whatever you call them, they're simply taking advantage of, and highlighting, a flaw in our food system: the waste embedded in it. Much of the food that's thrown out in our nation's restaurants, bakeries, and supermarkets is perfectly good to eat. "Stores can't keep it on their shelves, but it's fine for us," says Jeff Stark, one of the dinner party founders. Today, people across the country are staving off waste in the food system by intervening in this, and other, creative ways.

But you don't have to go diving in Dumpsters to help reduce food waste. You could join the gleaners.

I met Asiya Wadud a few years ago in the San Francisco Bay Area. By night, Wadud works at Alice Waters's tony Chez Panisse restaurant in Berkeley. By day, she pursues her "real passion": capturing the backyard fruit bounty of the Bay Area. When she first moved there, she was amazed by the plenitude and just as quickly by the fact that families were obviously overwhelmed.

"I watched fruit fill gutters and rot in backyards," said Wadud. Inspired by the wasted abundance, she launched Forage Oakland in early 2008.

It's a simple concept: People with fruit sign up to have her help harvest what they've got and share, or trade, with others.

"It's free, and anyone can join," said Wadud. In one year, two hundred families did. Now, her tweets read, "Making 51st Street grapefruit marmalade" and "Just returned from a middle of the night olive harvest."

Wadud's work helps bring the most local of local food to people's doorsteps. While her efforts may seem marginal—tinkering on the edges of a global food system gone haywire—they're not insignificant. She's connecting neighbor to neighbor and delivering a serious quantity of fresh food in the process. Plus, Wadud is not alone. Beyond Oakland, there is Fallen Fruit in Los Angeles, which maps public fruit trees across the city and holds jam-making workshops, and Tour du Citron in Davis, which canvasses neighborhood trees by bike and donates the harvest to a local food bank. The tree owners are rewarded with delectable edibles like homemade jams. The trend is catching on even outside of citrus heaven California: There's the Portland Fruit Tree Project in Portland, Oregon; the Philly Orchard Project in Philadelphia; and Not Far from the Tree in Toronto.

When I asked Wadud about the roots of the foraging enthusiasm, she answered without skipping a beat: "People are more and more aware of the impact of their food choices and how these choices are contributing to climate disruption—and they are seeking creative solutions." And what about *her* foraged food's greenhouse-gas emissions? Virtually zero. "I don't even have a driver's license!" she confessed. All of her food "shipments" are made via one very sturdy bicycle.

Not quite ready to ask your neighbor about the lemons poking out above the fence line?

You can support the movement among the nation's food banks to glean from farms across the country. The California Association of Food Banks, for example, launched its Farm to Family initiative in 2006 to collect "excess" and "secondary" produce from growers and packers. Within a year, the program was already distributing more than thirty-eight million pounds of thirty-eight fruits and vegetables across the state.

Or you could work with your city to reduce food waste ending up in your local landfill. Check out the Compostable Organics out of Landfills by 2012 (COOL 2012) campaign, which is working with state and local governments to keep food, and other stuff that could be composted, out of our methane-emitting landfills.

The campaign estimates that U.S. landfills' emissions are equivalent to those from 20 percent of all U.S. coal-fired power plants. Cutting the waste headed to our landfills by half would be equivalent to shutting down more than sixty coal plants. And since organic waste, largely food scraps and yard trimmings, as well as recyclable paper and other materials, makes up nearly half of the waste of many cities, attacking food waste would make a huge difference. Plus, there would be the added benefit of putting our organic waste to work, as compost to restore health to our nation's small farms and community gardens. As Linda Christopher from COOL 2012 stresses, "once organic waste ends up in a landfill or incinerator, its potential to feed our soil, our crops, and ourselves is lost forever." To date, more than a dozen large municipalities and dozens of other towns and small cities have adopted programs to reroute food waste.

Ensuring that food from our fields (and backyards) makes it to our mouths (or *someone's* mouth) is the first step in reducing our waste. Making sure that food waste from our homes and institutions finds its way into compost bins is another. And supporting policies that enable us to do both is the final one.

Resources for Principle 5: Finish Your Peas . . . the Ice Caps Are Melting

- *Do your own personal-waste inventory:* Take this next week to note what food gets wasted in your home—what could Dumpster divers find in *your* trash bin? Once you've done your own inventory, you'll have some ideas about how you can trim your food purchases to cut back on waste—and save money. Get inspired across the pond with tips and ideas from www.lovefoodhatewaste.com.

- *Compost from home:* Got a garden? Creating your own compost is an easy way to reduce your food waste and put it to good use. You can also create compost even if you don't have your own green space. Farmers' markets often have a setup allowing farmers to happily take home compost, or you can connect with local community gardens. (Just remember, most food scraps are okay—but no meat, fish, or animal fat.) Check out www.howtocompost.org.

- *Advocate at work:* Most of the waste in our food system is institutional waste; it's not what happens behind closed doors in our homes. Do you work at a school? Restaurant? Grocery store? Find out what happens to your institutional waste and look into ways to reduce and repurpose it through municipal compost programs.

• *Join the Compostable Organics out of Landfills by 2012 campaign:* Learn more about COOL 2012 at www.cool2012.com.

• *Find the foragers:* Find Asiya Wadud at her blog: http://forageoakland .blogspot.com where you can also discover other groups in Wadud's network.

PRINCIPLE 6: SEND PACKAGING PACKING

Every year, we in the United States toss out as many as forty billion plastic water bottles.[38] That's roughly 130 bottles for every single man, woman, and babe in the country. Each year in just one city, San Francisco, 180 million petroleum-based plastic bags find their way into shoppers' hands and then to the dump.[39] And McDonald's alone is responsible for as many as 550 million Big Mac wrappers and boxes ending up in U.S. garbage dumps annually.[40]

The paper and plastic, cardboard and bottles, cans and Styrofoam, that contain our food and our drinks play a big role in our food system's global warming impact, from the emissions related to producing the packaging to the emissions from those landfills clogged with the waste. (Those San Francisco bags? It took 774,000 gallons of oil to produce 'em.)[41]

We can reduce our ecological foodprint by thinking twice when we reach for that plastic bag, cup, fork, and plate and we can also get behind measures in our own communities to curb excess packaging and encourage reuse and recycling.

Take inspiration from the Board of Supervisors in San Francisco, which voted in early 2007 to ban plastic checkout bags at large supermarkets. Instead, customers would be encouraged to bring their own and offered compostable bags made of cornstarch or bags made of recyclable paper. (This groundbreaking ordinance wouldn't go unchallenged. The California Grocers Association protested, claiming it would increase costs to consumers and retailers; the ban eventually passed.)

Other countries have placed a tax on plastic bags, also helping to reduce their use. Ireland added a tax on plastic shopping bags in 2002 and quickly reduced their use by 90 percent.[42] Rumor has it Los Angeles is exploring a plastic-bag ban and Washington, D.C., is looking at an

Ireland-style levy on the bags, too. And why not think big—why stop at cities? On June 8, 2009, the executive director of the U.N. Environment Programme called for a global ban on plastic bags, much like the one in place in San Francisco.[43]

Communities are also looking to ban other products that clog up our waste streams. Santa Monica, California, passed an ordinance to ban to-go food and beverage containers made from nonrecyclable plastic.[44]

Find out if your city or state is exploring a ban like this one or a tax that could help cut down on packaging, or consider launching your own campaign.

Resources for Principle 6: Send Packaging Packing

- *Advocate for climate-friendly policies:* Connect with environmental groups in your community, or progressive elected officials, to push for package-reducing policies. Learn more and take action at www. storyofstuff.org

- *Reduce your own packaging:* Be conscientious about how much your own diet's packaging is contributing to our nation's landfills and do what you can to cut back. Use reusable mugs, water bottles, and napkins when you travel. Check out the new wave of high-design, reusable to-go containers and utensils from companies like To-Go Ware.

PRINCIPLE 7: DIY FOOD

Each one of these climate-friendly diet principles requires us to do one thing that's becoming increasingly foreign to modern *Homo sapiens* living in industrialized countries: spend time cooking our own food. Luckily, a slew of cookbooks and other resources have come out recently to help us make this move with ease. Unlike some of the other prescriptions for addressing global warming, choosing a climate-friendly diet can be fun, feel good, and taste scrumptious, too. And resources abound to get us back into the kitchen.

Climate-friendly farming is also going to require that people—real flesh and blood people—get their hands in the dirt. Unfortunately, after more than half a century of government subsidies that encouraged large-scale farms, thousands of small-scale farmers tossed in the spade. Thankfully, new farmers are picking up their hoes and digging in. Today, in nooks and crannies throughout the countryside and in cities across the nation, they're creating agricultural oases.

Now, we're not all going to become farmers and we can't all get down and dirty in our backyards. But for those of us who can, growing our own food is one of the best ways to take a bite out of climate change. And even if you don't have backyard space, maybe you've got roof space. A 2009 survey by Green Roofs for Healthy Cities found that the number of green roofs in the country had blossomed by 35 percent in just the previous year. The survey found gardens now spread across six to ten million square feet of roof space.

Don't have access to either? Consider joining a community garden or supporting edible gardens in your kids' school.

Resources for Principle 7: DIY Food

- *Reclaim your kitchen:* Pick up some of the cookbooks I recommended earlier in this chapter and get back into your kitchen.

- *Reclaim your hands:* If you're interested in studying organic farming, check out the University of California at Santa Cruz's Center for Agroecology and Sustainable Food Systems' Farm & Garden Apprenticeship program: http://casfs.ucsc.edu/training/index.html. Find out about farming opportunities at www.growfood.org. Learn about *The Greenhorns*, a documentary about young farmers in the United States, and find great resources for new farmers at www.thegreenhorns.net.

- *Community gardens:* Check out your local community-gardening organizations or visit the American Community Gardening Association Web site for more info: www.communitygarden.org.

- *School gardens:* Get inspired by the California School Garden Network at www.csgn.org, or find out about connecting your kid's school with local farmers through the national Farm to School network: www.farmtoschool.org.

The Seven Principles of a Climate-Friendly Diet

Embracing a climate-friendly diet is not rocket science;
it just takes a heightened awareness about the food you
choose for yourself and your family.

1. *Reach for real food:* Use the "rule of thumb" trick to limit the additives in your food and Marion Nestle's strategy to stick to the outer supermarket aisles to avoid processed foods when you can.

2. *Put plants on your plate:* Move plants to the middle of your plate. If you choose animal products, go for those raised humanely and sustainably, looking for the organic seal or grass-fed certifications.

3. *Don't panic, go organic:* Look for foods that have been produced without industrial chemicals and other high-energy inputs. Hunt for the USDA organic seal or talk to your food producer directly to find out about their practices.

4. *Lean toward local:* Support your local-food economy: Visit your locally stocked supermarkets, check out your nearest farmers' market, or join a CSA. Supporting our networks of small-scale farmers and local businesses is a key way to ensure that we have climate-friendly food today *and* tomorrow.

5. *Finish your peas . . . the ice caps are melting:* Pay attention to your food waste. In school? Push for institutional composting. Work at a restaurant or a catering outfit? Inquire about recycling and reuse programs. Connect with others in your community to uncover innovative ways to waste less and enjoy more local food.

6. *Send packaging packing:* Think creatively, from bringing your own bag to the store to buying reusable containers for your leftovers and coming up with tasty ways to make them into new meals. Perhaps the simplest of all the steps, this is also among the most difficult. We inhabit a throwaway world; trying to change our throwaway habits can be a challenge.

7. *DIY food:* One of the best ways to bring climate-friendly food into your life is to reclaim your own power to cook, grow, and create your own food.

For more inspiration, check out these resources:

Center for Food Safety's Cool Foods Campaign

Learn more about the choices we can make in the grocery store
to support a climate-friendly food system.
www.coolfoodscampaign.org

Rainforest Action Network's Agribusiness Campaign

Take action to ensure that food companies are protecting
our vital ecosystems.
www.ran.org

Bon Appétit Management Company Foundation's Eat Low-Carbon Diet Calculator

What's your ecological foodprint? Find out here.
www.eatlowcarbon.org

Institute for Agriculture and Trade Policy's Climate and Agriculture Research

Dig into the science. Learn from IATP's astute researchers.
www.iatp.org/climate

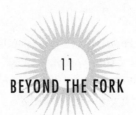

11
BEYOND THE FORK

In early November 2003, I gave a lecture at Arizona's Prescott College, the kind of school where you could easily stumble on Hacky Sack–playing students comparing notes on compost heaps. That evening, I stayed up late drinking tea with the professor hosting my visit. The conversation roamed into big-picture territory, and we found ourselves musing about our era's profound environmental challenges—global climate chaos perhaps the most obvious.

She confessed that though she'd been a die-hard environmentalist most of her life, she'd become disillusioned of late. For decades, she had been one of those greens who did "all the right things"—bringing her reusable mug to the coffee shop, composting and carpooling, diligently turning off her lights. You get the idea.

Then she went to New York City.

"I emerged from the subway into the heart of Times Square, and my heart just sank," she said. "In one minute of standing there with my jaw dropped, more energy was used up than I had personally saved in my entire lifetime."

I couldn't reassure her then by telling her she was wrong; she probably wasn't. And to be honest, I don't know what I said to her that night to make her feel better—if anything. But now that I think back to that conversation, I have some ideas about what I could have said.

I could have reassured her by reminding her that our actions, however small they may seem—like those she had been taking all those years and the ones I suggested in the previous chapter—do have global ripples. I've seen them with my own eyes. It's not hyperbole to say that every single organic farmer I've met simply would not be digging in the soil were there not eaters like you and me stepping up to choose their products.

And I could have reassured her by telling her about people like those in Güssing, Austria. I'm sure many residents there probably felt that same sense of disillusionment living in a community that had been dubbed a "dead-end town" and a "forgotten outpost" on the edge of the Iron Curtain. But in just one decade, the community of Güssing has transformed itself with green initiatives, creating a burgeoning renewable-energy industry of dozens of companies employing more than one thousand people.[1]

Or, I could have told her about Costa Rica, the small Central American country that had watched as most of its forest cover disappeared to deforestation and development. Residents there must have been disillusioned, too. Yet consider that thanks to progressive environmental policies and citizen pressure, the country has revalued the forests and replanted the trees, and today there is twice as much forested land as there was twenty years ago.

And I could have shared with her that night a sentiment that's clear to me now: As we make choices to align our daily decisions with our environmental values, like all those actions she was committed to and all those climate-friendly diet principles I've shared, we shift our sense of self. As we make these choices, we are no longer passive consumers; we are active citizens shaping the marketplace.

When it comes to our food, this means realizing the power of our fork to shape what gets sold (and what does not); which companies thrive (and which don't); and what policies are in place to incentivize the kinds of foods and methods of farming that are healthiest for the climate. And it means seeing ourselves as partners with food producers.

Consider this the eighth principle of the climate-friendly diet. It is also a reminder that the other principles aren't just tips for shopping differently; they're suggestions for modifying our mind-set to see ourselves not as isolated consumers but as members of a movement. Through an environmental lens, the lens of ecology, we see, as German physicist Hans-Peter Dürr reminds us, that in reality "there are no parts, there are only participants." And we are participants in a movement that ties us to a long history of effective social change, of ordinary citizens using the market to make their voices heard, dating back to the first boycott and beyond, to the very beginnings of market economies.

Turn back the clock to the 1880s, on Ireland's cold and wet west coast, and you'll uncover the origins of one of these strategies of flexing collective power: the modern-day boycott. For decades, the Irish Land League, working on behalf of the region's peasants, had been fighting against landowner exploitation. In 1880, the fight came to a head. British-born Captain Charles Cunningham Boycott threatened once again to increase rents for the poorest peasants. The league fought back. It called on the region's peasants to march on Boycott's house and persuade "all his employees inside and out, to quit."[2] They did. The organizers then went to all the community's shopkeepers, urging them to stop doing business with the family. The postman refused to deliver mail. The blacksmith stopped his smithing; the laundress ended her laundering; the harvesters refused to harvest. His family ostracized, Boycott backed down, and the concept of the "boycott" was immortalized.

Over the many decades since, we've seen a growing sophistication in how citizens have used collective power to influence the market. We are certainly seeing that sophistication play out in climate-change activism. And in just the time it's taken me to write this book, we've seen that same creativity emerge in collective actions linking the food system with global warming, from the cafeterias of community colleges to the candy aisles of Kroger, from city council offices in the Big Apple to the negotiating rooms where international climate-change treaties are forged. Though these efforts vary in size, scope, and strategy, they have much in common. They're each about getting us to think differently about the power of our fork, to see ourselves not as recipients of what we find on our supermarket shelves, but as participants in shaping the future of food.

SHAPING WHAT'S SOLD: REAL FOOD ON COOL CAMPUSES

It was a little after midnight, long after the official conference had ended and the five-hundred-plus attendees at the 2007 Food and Society annual get-together had hunkered down for the night. Tim Galarneau of the California Student Sustainability Coalition; Anim Steel from the Food Project, a Boston-based food and farming nonprofit; David Schwartz from Brown University; and a few other young people were still talking. Hunched over a table in an empty meeting room at the Grand Traverse Resort in Traverse City, Michigan, the group had already been together for hours, continuing a conversation that had been going on for more than a year.

What was keeping them up so late?

They were comparing notes. Each was witnessing a burgeoning student movement on college campuses to bring sustainably and fairly raised food into dining halls. From coast to coast, a similar energy and enthusiasm seemed to be bubbling up. Galarneau was seeing it in the massive effort to transform university food across California's esteemed public university system. Schwartz was seeing it back in Providence at Brown, where students were getting increasingly vocal about sourcing sustainable food. And Steel, a leader in the food-justice movement, had a frontline view from the Food Project's youth-run farm in Boston. From their unique perspectives, each sensed that students were hankering to speak up more loudly about sustainability and food; they just needed an effective way to do so. Out of this ongoing conversation, the group would launch the Real Food Challenge.

The concept is simple, really. Students, some who pay as much as one hundred thousand dollars, or more, for four years of private-college tuition, should have a say in what grub their schools serve—and that food should reflect shared values of fairness and sustainability. The Real Food Challenge provides an organizing tool to empower students to persuade their schools to make the move. Schools that join the challenge pledge to shift at least 20 percent of school food to real food—sustainably raised, grown with fairness, and from local and regional farms—by 2020.

In addition to this concrete goal, the challenge also offers schools and student organizers a support network, resources for sourcing real food, organizer trainings, and a "real food calculator." The calculator provides campuses with a mechanism for quantifying real food, for determining the percentage of real food they currently serve and measuring improvement over time.

Part of the excitement about the Real Food Challenge, Galarneau said, is that it taps into students' energy to address the global warming impact of their own campuses. A key strategy of student environmental activists has been to focus on persuading their schools to reduce their global warming impact through rethinking institutional energy use and turning to renewable-energy sources. One of the most successful campus-based efforts to date is the Campus Climate Challenge. The initiative has helped young people in colleges and high schools across the United States and Canada organize to campaign for—and win—100-percent-clean-energy policies at their schools. The Campus Climate Challenge served as inspiration for the Real Food Challenge founders interested in channeling student excitement in a new direction. "There was a lot of momentum around climate change on campuses. Al Gore had swept onto the scene," said Galarneau. "But the activism lacked a connection with the food system."

"Many young people are realizing that the food system is a key contributor to global warming. They know that we've got to talk about food if we're going to advance a broader sustainability agenda," he noted.

It would take another year and a half of conversations like the one back in that meeting room before the Real Food Challenge was officially launched in September 2008. But within a month, the original crew had hard proof that their hunch had been right.

The challenge launched with eleven pilot schools. Organizers hoped several hundred more would soon join. "During one of our conference calls that first month, we checked to see how many campuses had come on board. We had hoped for maybe 200," said Galarneau. "We already had 230; that's when we knew we hit a nerve. People were biting."

By the end of that first year, 329 campuses had joined the network from Brown University to City College of New York to DeAnza Community College in San Mateo, California. The determined young people who lead the challenge expect that in another year that number could grow to 1,000, about a quarter of all the two- and four-year colleges and universities in the country.

To put the potential impact in context, U.S. colleges and universities currently spend more than four billion dollars annually on school food. (Roughly half of school food is contracted out to food-service companies; the rest is managed by the schools themselves.) If it's successful, and the projected participating schools shift 20 percent of their purchases, the Real Food Challenge will have helped to move nearly one billion dollars of food purchases toward sustainability by 2020. "We're talking about shaking up the system," said Galarneau, "and young people like that."

Connecting the overarching mission of the Real Food Challenge—increasing the amount of fairly and sustainably raised local foods on campuses—to the effort to combat climate change is a complex challenge. First and foremost, there's the problem of quantifying the impact. Unlike getting data on campus energy use—emissions are relatively easy to measure and are usually the direct result of action (or inaction)—getting data on food is difficult. Campuses rarely know the full story of the food they purchase. In part that's because food-related emissions mostly occur during production, processing, and distribution—long before the food shows up in the cafeteria. Plus, even for the "direct" emissions—energy used in dining halls, food waste ending up in landfills—schools often don't have systems yet in place for accurate measurement.

But a data gap doesn't have to mean an action gap. Instead, the Real Food Challenge stresses the guiding principles for planet-friendly choices schools can make, including many I highlighted in the previous chapter. Real Food Challenge campuses can reduce meat purchases, re-think food-waste systems, cut back on packaging, and source more food locally—and they are, in fact, taking these steps.

Students are energized; campuses are paying attention. It was not long before the Real Food Challenge piqued the interest of food-service companies. In that initial launch month, said Galarneau, their phone was ringing off the hook with calls from Aramark, Sodexo, Bon Appétit—among the biggest players in college food service. "They were calling to say they wanted to be part of the challenge," he said.

But Galarneau and the other organizers were wary of official corporate partnerships, concerned that companies would just be latching on to the initiative without actually changing their practices. They'd already seen food-service companies pay lip service to sustainability in their contracts without embracing broad change in the dining halls. As we talked, Galarneau described a 135-page food-service contract he was reviewing, hunting for language that would provide the company loopholes to skirt sustainability. "The devil is in the details," he said.

In its own right, Bon Appétit, which serves 80 million meals a year at campus and corporate facilities, has launched a low-carbon diet initiative, reducing food waste, promoting composting, educating guests about their food choices and cutting back on beef purchases by 33 percent system-wide just from 2007 to 2009.

Organizers of the Real Food Challenge say their primary focus is on building student engagement. Because food-service directors typically don't have time to make the needed changes, schools rely on students to help make it happen. Plus, as Steel says, "no matter how committed many of these companies say they are, they can only go as far as students push them."

The challenge, while popular among students on participating campuses, still faces hurdles, including getting the ear of administrators facing one of the worst economic downturns in generations. But as the organizers like to point out, many of the climate-friendly principles actually help schools save money. Students at Stanford, for example, borrowed the Love Food, Hate Waste campaign from the United Kingdom to develop a way for people on campus to easily compost their waste. Erin Gaines, the sustainable foods coordinator at Stanford Dining and Hospitality, and an active member of the Real Food Challenge, told me about their success. In 2008, thanks to the campaign, the school composted 1.2 million pounds of food from campus dining halls and cafés. That's 1.2 million pounds that would have gone into a landfill. Instead, the scraps were taken to a local composting facility, and half of the compost was returned to the school to be used on its gardens and grounds.

Galarneau offered an example from the University of California system. In response to campaigning, the University of California at Santa Cruz decided to go "trayless" to address the pile-on phenomenon: students grabbing more food than their stomachs can hold. No trays also means less washing. The school has already calculated a savings of more than one million gallons of water a year. And no trays means less food waste. Since the policy's introduction, the campus has seen food waste decline by one third, and it has committed to diverting the remaining waste to compost. "The mantra is 'up-cycling,'" said Galarneau, "reducing waste before it becomes waste and then reintegrating waste, through composting, so that it never becomes waste." This one step has helped reduce energy consumption (less dishwater to heat) *and* emissions (all that food kept out of landfills), saving the school money, which in turn leaves more resources to invest in sustainable food choices.

Galarneau cited an observation economists have made about shifting markets: Once a consumer trend occupies 20 percent of a market, it can become an unstoppable force. "The young people in the challenge are testing that theory with a push toward purchases that value justice and sustainability," he said. When I talked with Katrina Norbom, a Real Food Challenge member at the University of North Florida, she said, "No matter what, it comes down to the students: If we can create enough support, we can make it happen."

This determination—embodied by people like Galarneau and Steel, Norbom and Gaines—is pushing the market to change by amplifying their voices. Call me cynical, but I don't think a multi-million-dollar food company, like those in the business of university food service, would listen to one lone student demanding a shift in waste policy or more organic kale in their dining hall. Multiply and magnify those voices, though, as the challenge does, and it seems corporate, and collegiate, ears perk up.

And this determination is making an impact well beyond the campus. Alumni of the Real Food Challenge are heading into communities where they're using their passion and organizing skills to expand the market for real food across the country. When I asked Galarneau and Steel for examples, they rattled off a bunch: Sue Dublieck from Iowa State University is running a farm-to-school project in Maine; Sam Lipschultz, a 2009 Sarah Lawrence graduate, is starting a youth-run farmers' market in one of Brooklyn's poorest neighborhoods; and University of California at Irvine's Hai Vo, who had been consulting with other youth-empowerment projects after college, just sent in his applications for apprenticeships in organic farming.

The organizers know that shifting 20 percent of school food to real, more climate friendly food, by 2020 is ambitious; but their vision is even bolder—and broader—than that. Currently less than 2 percent of food on most campuses is "real." Nationwide, the figure isn't much higher. As Steel said, "If we can't make this shift happen on a campus, how can we expect it to happen elsewhere? And if we can do it on campuses, then we can start asking, why can't we do it everywhere?"

CHANGING CORPORATE PRACTICE: THE PROBLEM WITH PALM OIL

To celebrate Easter this year, Chicago Art Institute senior April Noga headed to her local Dominick's. Not to buy Peeps or a PAAS egg-dyeing kit, but to "sticker" holiday candy made with palm oil—clandestinely.

And Noga was not alone. Across the country, from Fullerton, California, to Minneapolis and Chicago, and in cities throughout Canada, hundreds were slapping stickers on Hershey's Kisses, Reese's Peanut Butter Cups, Cadbury chocolates, and other palm-oil-filled candies, warning prospective buyers that their purchase "may contain rainforest destruction."

The Easter stickering was one of several actions that Rainforest Action Network (RAN) has coordinated as part of its Problem with Palm Oil campaign. The campaign was launched to raise public awareness about the connection between palm oil and global warming and to transform oil palm production practices to protect rainforests, communities, and the climate.

RAN was founded in 1985 to protect rainforests and the human rights of communities who call them home. Fifteen years later, as the connection between agribusiness and the destruction of precious rainforests was becoming clearer, RAN decided to create a campaign focused on those companies and practices most responsible for the damage. All roads led to palm oil, to the companies draining peatland and plowing down forests in Malaysia and Indonesia, where 80 percent of palm oil is produced.

The Problem with Palm Oil campaign was born in the beginning of 2008. For months, RAN dug into research, investigating the industry: where companies sourced their palm, which were the biggest buyers, what were the most destructive practices, and what could make the industry more socially and environmentally responsible. The group also explored approaches to getting palm oil buyers to put pressure on suppliers to improve their practices. As RAN did more research, it learned that public awareness about palm oil—let alone its impact on global warming—was virtually nil, despite the prevalence of the oil in so many of our products, from snack foods and cosmetics to detergents and biofuels.

After more plotting, the folks at RAN decided to kick off a three-pronged campaign: elevate awareness about this key climate-destructive ingredient, encourage companies to cut back on palm oil use, and give companies that wanted to source sustainably grown palm oil a way to make their demands known to suppliers.

In the summer of 2008, the group sent out citizen sleuths to unearth where palm oil pops up on our supermarket shelves. Spread out from Los Angeles to Washington, D.C., checking stock everywhere from food cooperatives like San Francisco's Rainbow Grocery to markets like Jewel in Chicago, the sleuths uncovered palm oil in the ingredient lists of more than five hundred products, made by more than 350 companies.

With the names and UPC codes for the palm-oil-implicated products, RAN launched its first stickering action to alert consumers about palm oil and rainforest destruction. That first day, more than two thousand volunteers participated across the United States, Canada, and Australia. Sabrina Lammé was one. A fifty-year-old Southern Californian who works at a medical-imaging company, Lammé got involved after discovering the issue surfing the Web. "Rainforest destruction and palm oil wasn't something I was aware of before," she says. Inspired by the seriousness of the campaign, she signed on for the action. By her estimate, she used up a couple hundred stickers tagging bags of candy, like Rolos and bright red Twizzlers, at her local Food 4 Less and Smart & Final.

While Lammé and other volunteers flooded stores with the yellow warning stickers, RAN sent letters to the 350 companies it had ID'd and asked its network of online activists to send e-mails, too.

"We wanted to put the companies on notice that they need to know what's in their products, where it comes from, and what impact their ingredients have on the environment," says the group's Leila Salazar-Lopez.

Collectively, the RAN-inspired activists sent out over one million e-mails expressing concern about palm oil, flooding the in-boxes of corporate e-mail accounts. From small soap companies to big palm oil suppliers, the reaction was instantaneous. Their calls tied up RAN's phone lines. "Companies wanted to know what they could do to get all these messages to stop," says Salazar-Lopez. Noticeably, the largest palm oil buyers—like Kraft, Procter & Gamble, and Unilever—were silent. "We had to reach out to them."

RAN was asking companies, from the biggest to the smallest, to sign a pledge, a simple statement committing to sourcing sustainable palm oil and to working with RAN to pressure the biggest suppliers, including Archer Daniels Midland and Cargill, to make good on their promises of sustainability.

In the first few days after that initial action, ten companies signed the pledge. By the end of September, twenty-five had. Still, the largest buyers—or at least RAN's best guess at the biggest—were absent.

Since there is no public data on palm oil purchasing, RAN hired its own researchers to head to the Midwest to follow train cars to find out where the palm oil was headed. "We're finding out this answer on our own," says Salazar-Lopez.

Based on its best researched guesses, RAN designated a "Dirty Twenty," major retailers and companies with recognizable brands that have palm oil in their products, yet who didn't respond to multiple attempts at contact by the group. By the next stickering action a few months later, on Halloween, volunteers were zeroing in on these companies, including Unilever and Whole Foods.

Many of the companies challenge RAN, asking why the campaign is necessary when the industry has the Roundtable on Sustainable Palm Oil (RSPO), which holds principles of sustainability and has established working groups exploring greenhouse-gas-emission reduction strategies.

RAN responds by pointing out that only about 40 percent of companies in the global palm oil industry are members of the RSPO. The rest aren't even at the table, and some of them are among the most egregious producers.

And, RAN stresses, the roundtable is a step in the right direction, but its membership guidelines and certification program aren't enough. It's made up of retailers and banks and investors, processors and buyers, and membership is open to anyone. Being a member doesn't mean your company is necessarily sourcing sustainably raised palm oil; it just means you allegedly agree with the principles and criteria and paid your membership dues.

Cargill, the largest importer of palm oil into the United States, did respond to RAN, but its reply was curt: "We're a member of the RSPO and our plantation just got certified." But that certified plantation? "It's just one of five of Cargill's plantations. The company needs to be a leader and get all their plantations certified and demand the same of all their suppliers," says Salazar-Lopez.

"We want the RSPO to improve," she says. "We don't want it to just be seen as an elaborate greenwash machine." Public and industry pressure on the roundtable to strengthen its enforcement and improve transparency is one strategy for changing that.

So RAN's campaign is asking companies to join it in forming a coalition, including companies that want to go further than the roundtable's standards and put pressure on the biggest suppliers, like Cargill, to exceed those standards and clean up their act.

"We have forty-five companies, including Whole Foods and Seventh Generation, as part of our coalition so far; twenty more are considering joining. These companies want to lead the industry, not be complicit in rainforest destruction," says Salazar-Lopez.

As stickerer Noga and I were getting off the phone, she had one last thought.

One of her "recruits" had been her sister. "She is one of those people who cares about the environment, but felt powerless," Noga said. "My sister would always say, 'I'm just one person. What difference can I make?'" After some cajoling, Noga convinced her to join in the action. Together, they ducked into the Dominick's in their northern Chicago suburb and left several dozen stickers lighter.

As they drove home, the sisters reflected on the shoppers who had picked up their bags of candy, silently read the added-on stickers, and quietly put the multicolored products back on the shelves. Noga's sister shared the feeling that maybe, just maybe, her small act did have a larger significance, educating consumers in their neck of the woods about rainforest destruction half a world away. She said she imagined multiplying that moment by the thousands of other people stickering, the who-knows-how-many other shoppers reading those labels, and the dozens of companies receiving their missives.

For the first time in her life, Noga's sister sensed, could really feel, that she was a part of a chain of events beyond anything she had imagined possible. She said to Noga that maybe, just maybe, one person *could* make a difference, "especially if enough 'one persons' take part."

FOSTERING CLIMATE-FRIENDLY FOOD: INSPIRATION FROM SOUTH KOREA

Around the world from the big-box stores on Chicago's urban edge, I traveled to South Korea to learn about other strategies for bringing to life a more climate-friendly food system. My research assistant and I arrived in Seoul at the end of a summer of protests that had erupted across the country. Tens of thousands had marched in the streets. With many protesters arrested and dozens still in jail, eight protestors still remained in refuge at Jogyesa, a Buddhist temple near the city's university district. What had ostensibly sparked the outrage was a presidential decree reversing a U.S. beef ban that had been introduced in 2003 because of fears of mad cow disease in our nation's meat. The ban was a major blow to the U.S. beef industry; South Korea was one of our biggest export markets.

But the real reasons for the South Korean fury were far more complex, originating in part in a collective belief in food self-determination: the right of the people themselves to choose what's on their supermarket shelves—not their president, the World Trade Organization, or lobbyists from the United States. (One Korean activist I met described his frustration in spotting the telltale cowboy hat of a rep from the U.S. National Cattlemen's Beef Association at President Lee Myung-Bak's inauguration.)

From the media reports and my own interviews with Korean food activists, it was also clear to me that the demonstrations showed just how many people in the country get it: Food is political. To change the food system requires organizing, whether one is speaking out against U.S. beef or speaking up for climate-friendly fare. The conversations I had in South Korea and beyond reminded me, too, that this activism isn't one-size-fits-all. Its spirit is alive in the students at Stanford as well as in those stickerers fanning out to supermarkets in Chicago. And we sensed that spirit even more deeply as we met members of South Korea's thriving food co-op movement.

My colleague Jessica Walker Beaumont, our interpreter, JiEun Choi, and I were offered the corner booth in a brightly lit bakery set off from a thoroughfare in a residential neighborhood of Seoul, South Korea's sprawling capital. As soon as we sat down in the cheery shop, with its green walls and hot pink trim, we found ourselves face-to-face with a traditional Korean decadence: a huge bowl piled high with vanilla ice cream and red bean candy, topped with diced fruit and crushed ice. Only once we were digging in to the delicacy did our hosts let us launch into our questions, accompanied by the dings of the glass doors as the day's shoppers came and went, picking up bread, dessert, and other treats.

We were talking with four leaders of iCoop, one of the country's largest consumer cooperatives and the "owner" of the sunny bakery. As a then-member of the Park Slope Food Coop in Brooklyn, I thought I had some perspective on co-ops. Park Slope, I like to note, with its more than fourteen thousand members, is the largest food co-op in the United States. So, sitting down with folks from iCoop, I was humbled when the region's director piped up to answer my first question.

The co-op was founded just a decade ago, we learned, and already has 50,000 member households, a staff of six hundred, one thousand volunteer educators, sixty-eight regional offices, a vibrant online store, and thirty-four brick-and-mortar grocery stores, all supporting three thousand farm families. And iCoop isn't even the biggest in the country. The next day, I would meet a leader of *that* co-op—Hansalim—whose ranks top 150,000 member families.

With memberships of this size, these co-ops are big business—and creative ones at that. The bustling bakery itself is an example of their human-focused business model. It was built with financing from sixty-two members who get repaid from the store's profits. At heart, the model and motivation of a co-op are a far cry from those of a for-profit enterprise: Co-ops are owned and democratically controlled by their members, not by the dictates of quarterly returns or shareholder whims.

The iCoop leaders talked about their philosophy as much as their business model. Like the furor in the streets that summer, these co-ops trace their origins to the decades-old pro-democracy movement here. The co-op leaders stressed that among their goals is to use their weight in the marketplace, and in society, to push for more "green food" policies and educate consumers about the environmental and social costs of the import-based, industrial food system their government has long been pushing. (We see an educational poster on display in the store: A graphic depicts how virtually all the country's wheat is imported. Just 0.3 percent of bread products are made from wheat grown by domestic farmers. In this bakery, everything is.)

Lee Jeong Joo, a mother of two and one of the co-op's volunteer activists—and, we would discover later, a cover model for the co-op's product catalog—explained that she first came to the co-op "concerned about food as a personal issue. Now I see it as a political issue, an environmental issue."

iCoop and the other co-ops we looked at are also helping their members understand the co-ops' efforts—for local foods, for chemical-free farming, for small-scale production—as elements of a climate-friendly food system. When I met Seong Hee Kim, one of the leaders of Hansalim, he stressed this point. Founded in 1985 by a Catholic priest, Hansalim grew out of an environmental philosophy that runs throughout all its work, especially its educational programs. The co-op runs a "life education" program for members' kids, taking five hundred children to visit member farmers for four days and five nights each summer. The immersion in sustainable-farming life is an eye-opener for urbanite South Koreans.

Kim gave me another example: Hansalim's no-waste policy. "We try to consume 100 percent of our production," he said. "When there's an overproduction of onions, for example, we let people know online that we have a surplus." And members step up to buy the extra.

iCoop, Hansalim, and the other food co-ops in South Korea seem a sophisticated far cry from our co-ops in the States, but they're not an anomaly globally. Worldwide, co-ops of all shapes and sizes number 750,000 and serve 730 million members, according to the National Cooperative Business Association.

As we work to build climate-friendly food systems, co-ops like these show us the leverage that can be found in building new systems—new linkages between consumers and food producers. These connections are all but impossible when our consumer food choices are so distantly removed from their sources. For an increasing number of us, our food is mediated by some of the largest corporations in the world: ADM, Bunge, and Cargill, Tyson and Smithfield, Monsanto and Syngenta, Unilever and Kraft, Coca-Cola and PepsiCo.

I don't presume that co-ops will emerge overnight across our food and farming landscapes; on the other hand, we shouldn't have the hubris to assume they can't or won't, either. When Organic Valley started in 1988 in La Farge, Wisconsin, the farmer-founders didn't know their co-op would grow into a $530 million company, helping keep more than thirteen hundred small-scale, climate-friendly farmers in their homes, on their land, and producing food for us consumers.

We also are only beginning to understand the radical shifts in identity, and self-interest, that occur when consumers and producers come together, as they do with co-ops like Hansalim. Unexpected conversations ensue.

Kim shared with us a running joke at Hansalim. Every year, without fail, when the farmer reps and consumer reps get together to determine the price of the co-op's basic basket of goods, it ends with a friendly fight. Rice is always the most contentious. See, each year, the consumers insist they should pay more to the farmers to match the market price for the commodity. But the farmers insist that their cost of production is less than the market price and therefore they should get *less*. "They get into a big argument," said Kim, laughing. "Our producers know our consumers; they see themselves as responsible for their lives. And the consumers, they know these farmers; they realize that they're responsible for the producers' well-being."

CRAFTING CLIMATE-FRIENDLY FOOD POLICY: FOODPRINT ALLIANCE

On an unseasonably cool and rainy summer day, half a dozen New Yorkers gathered in the cramped second-floor offices of the local-foods organization Just Food to discuss press conference plans for announcing city council resolution No. 2049 to reduce New York City's climate "foodprint."

Nearly a year before, a group of us had come together to share the frustration that New York City, like cities around the world, had launched initiatives to address its global warming impact, but had left the food system missing from the story.

Our fledgling group, the NYC Foodprint Alliance, representing organizations whose focuses ranged from animal welfare to local foods, had come together to do something about it. We decided to craft a city council resolution that would call on the city to incorporate sustainable- and local-food policy, programs, and public education into its climate initiatives, including PlaNYC, the city's blueprint for reducing greenhouse-gas emissions by 30 percent by 2030.

A few people from the group, including Mia MacDonald from the action-oriented think tank Brighter Green, and Jasmin Singer from Farm Sanctuary, took on the task of drafting the resolution. And from that day's report by the lead organizer, Just Food's Nadia Johnson, it sounded like we were one step closer to having the largest city in the country publicly connect climate change with food.

After learning about the resolution from MacDonald, city councilman Bill de Blasio and Manhattan borough president Scott Stringer had thrown their weight behind it. We had a sense from their enthusiasm it would be supported by the council.

Interested to see if other cities had crafted similar policies, we did some digging in the United States and overseas. We realized we were not completely alone.

When London passed its Climate Change Action Plan in 2007, it didn't mention food or farming, either, but thanks to pressure from local advocates, the city commissioned a study to make visible the story of food.

Annie Austin and two other researchers from Brook Lyndhurst rolled up their sleeves. "This report would be the necessary first step," Austin explained, "for the city to explore where the leverage points would be for reducing food-related climate impacts."

The researchers studied the emissions related to all eight billion meals served every year in the city.[3] They looked at the whole life cycle, from agricultural production and manufacturing to transportation and home use and concluded that food-related emissions make "a significant contribution to the capital's greenhouse gas emissions."[4] Probing into the sources of these emissions, they found that more than half came from food production, which indicated the relative significance of choices about agricultural practices. Transportation accounted for about one fifth, and one tenth of emissions came from storage and cooking food at home.

"Putting ourselves in the shoes of city hall, we looked at where are real opportunities and 'quick wins,'" said Austin. Identifying where the city was spending the most on food, the group noted that the public sector—schools, hospitals, and prisons—served around 110 million meals annually and could be one of those leverage points.[5]

From London to Manhattan's city hall and in cities around the world, folks like our eclectic group are inserting food into policy on climate change. In California, a new coalition is forming to introduce and advocate for food-and-farming-related climate policy at the state level. In Seattle, the city council recently passed a food-policy measure that will promote climate-friendly food for all the city's residents, from teaching more people how to grow their own food to strengthening the connection between urban consumers and farmers, from reducing food waste to protecting farmland in the region.[6]

At the federal level, advocates are pushing for policies that would incentivize farmers to increase soil carbon and reduce, or at least efficiently use, fertilizers, pesticides, and irrigation. They're also pushing for more funds for the research we need to measure and assess best practices for reducing greenhouse-gas emissions from our farms.

As I write, farmers and concerned citizens worldwide are gearing up for the climate negotiations in Copenhagen in December 2009, preparing to let the world's leaders know that sustainable food and farming, protecting rainforests from agribusiness destruction, and defending the livelihoods of smallholder food producers should be front and center in any discussion about how best to mitigate climate change—and adapt to our inevitable climate-unstable future.

A few weeks after that meeting in the Just Food offices, members of the NYC Foodprint Alliance, de Blasio, Stringer, and select members of the media stood on the steps of city hall for the announcement of the landmark resolution, among the first in the United States to connect the dots between local climate policy and food. (I was there, too, teetering on swollen ankles at thirty-nine weeks pregnant.) In his snappy remarks, Stringer said, simply, "This is a resolution to start a revolution." May his words come true.

I don't know if that Prescott professor would have gotten out of her funk if she'd heard these four examples of citizen power, but I certainly know they help me dispel mine. Embracing this eighth principle of climate-friendly food—going beyond our fork—tends to do that. Seeing our connection to broader efforts to shift our food system toward sustainability is downright energizing. Breaking out of the individual mind-set, we see ourselves (and food) differently; food can be that integrating lens that helps us absorb the otherwise abstract ideas of ecology and interconnectedness.

And food can help us see possibility where we might not have seen it before. Awakening to food and farming as part of the climate crisis, we see food choices and food activism as part of the climate solution. Awakening to food, we see the billions on the planet who are food producers as climate heroes, and we see ourselves, whether we have our hands in the dirt or just eat what comes out of it, as cocreators of the food system, too.

Perhaps, best of all, throwing your weight behind this climate-friendly food system will also deliver you hope. For, I've become convinced, hope isn't something we have to passively wait for until the news gets better;

hope is something we can choose, right here, right now; it's what we *become* when we take action.

It's pretty clear what human beings love. We love to feel challenged, to feel called to something historic. Really big. We love knowing we're shoulder to shoulder with buddies and brethren tackling projects that matter, from the big to the small. The barn raising, the sandbags at the levee . . . the fight to save our planet from climate chaos. Now that we see how our food can be part of the solution, how inspiring (and tasty) is that?

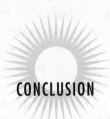

CONCLUSION

As I work on the final edits, I feel like the student at the final exam. My words have already spilled onto the inside cover of the Blue Book, and the proctor is calling time. I still have more to say, partly because so much is changing even as the ink dries.

When I began this book, the world was being rocked by a food-price crisis that had sent the cost of rice for billions doubling and pushed as many as one hundred million more people into hunger. As I am reviewing the final semicolons, the *Economist's* "food, feedstuffs, and beverage index" is expected to plummet another 25 percent.

When I began this book, my colleagues and I were lamenting that few people, anywhere, were talking about the connection between food and climate change. Dr. Roni Neff over at Johns Hopkins had the data to prove it, with that study showing a minuscule number of news articles on climate change even mentioned the food system. As I'm finalizing the endnotes, the media landscape feels flooded with food-and-climate-change news: Paul McCartney has just announced a campaign to go meatless on Mondays to help address global warming, and even Oprah's magazine mentions curbing meat as one way we can reduce our personal climate impact.

When I started this book, the meat industry was still giving global warming the silent treatment. As I finish, the American Meat Institute releases its latest briefing paper—with its entire focus on climate change.

When I began my research, George W. Bush was president, and climate-change deniers had a voice in Washington. Even NASA, at the White House's request, was censoring communications by government scientists about the crisis.[1] As I complete it, President Barack Obama has appointed as Energy secretary Nobel-winning Steven Chu, who has been warning for years about the urgent need to reduce emissions.

And over at the USDA the new head of the department just took a jack-hammer to a strip of asphalt in front of the administration building to plant a People's Garden—an *organic* People's Garden, mind you. And the recently anointed deputy secretary of agriculture, Kathleen Merrigan, is pushing for organic food and farming to be integrated throughout the entire department.[2]

Around the globe we're seeing similar tectonic shifts: Germany's Federal Environmental Agency is urging consumers to sideline their sausages to help fight global warming,[3] and the *Guardian* reports that British hospitals plan to promote meat-free menus as a way to cut emissions.

When I began this book, elected officials in the United States and globally were mostly turning a blind eye to connecting climate-change policy with food and agriculture. As I approve the final edits, at least a handful of cities across the country are now considering incorporating food systems into their initiatives to reduce municipal greenhouse-gas emissions. And in Denmark, voters just elected to Parliament a rep from the Party for the Animals, among whose main platforms is educating the public about the connection between livestock and climate change.

Every day brings new developments, new successes, but also new setbacks. Today, I received news that the indigenous peoples in Peru who had been peacefully protesting the government's decision to open up vast tracts of the Amazon rainforest to large-scale farming were attacked by government-sponsored special forces. The latest death toll stands at three dozen.[4]

Yes, history marches on.

I hope what I've written helps you realize we are not bystanders. Each of us is a player in one of the biggest stories ever. Global warming isn't just happening on the grand scale—to icebergs somewhere out there or in deliberations in capitals of far-off cities. Global warming is happening to us, right here, right now, in very real ways every day. And we, in turn, can be a part of transforming the climate-change story from one of hopelessness to one of renewal, regeneration, and resilience. There are powerful ways to be part of this historic shift: among them, aligning ourselves with a sane food system in our own communities, supporting the work globally to shift toward food sustainability, and honoring those farmers who are—we now can see—among the planet's real climate heroes.

In doing so, we never know the impact our actions may have. We never know who is watching. We never know, as April Noga's sister might say, how many "one persons" we may affect. Yet be assured, our choices will ripple.

Bill McKibben, who graciously wrote the opening words to this book, has set his sights on helping to mobilize the global community to stabilize the climate by pushing for a reduction of the concentration of carbon dioxide in the atmosphere to 350 parts per million; that's nearly 40 parts per million less than where levels stand now, and a major decrease from where we're headed. Doing so will require gutsy political leaders, savvy consumers, and empowered citizens. It will require that all sectors—including the food system—do their part, and that all of us citizens do, too.

I hope you can now see how we can help move the food system in a direction that would thrill Bill.

But even as I finalize these words, close my files, box up my notes, I can't help feeling . . . wait, there's more. Thankfully, I've got a built-in timekeeper. She'll be born any day now. It's time to put my pen down.

AFTERWORD

Biting into a Gloom and Hope Sandwich

On December 7th, 2009, hundreds of representatives in stiff ties and smart pantsuits from 192 countries gathered in Copenhagen to hash out global commitments to reduce greenhouse-gas emissions. Alongside the official meetings, more than thirty thousand activists gathered for hundreds of "side" events. Much of the world was hoping for real action and serious commitments—not just bluster. Eleven sleepless nights later, as delegates were packing up their bags to head home, we had a stalemate.

But communities around the world are not waiting idly for binding agreements. They're rolling up their sleeves and getting to work in every sector, especially when it comes to food and agriculture. They're also celebrating big wins.

Remember that Rainforest Action Network (RAN) campaign to expose the climate connection between palm oil and your Pop-Tart? For three years, RAN campaigners had been raising awareness among consumers and companies about the unsustainable practices of palm oil producers, especially those in the supply chain of Cargill, the largest U.S. importer. RAN found that once companies learned about the connection between their products and our climate, many were eager to jump on board and put pressure on suppliers to clean up their acts, though the biggest buyers of Cargill's palm oil—like Walmart, Kraft, and General Mills—were dragging their feet. Then, on September 22, 2010, the global food giant General Mills released one of the most forward-looking commitments to source sustainable palm oil. Said General Mills: "We are concerned about the role of palm oil expansion in the deforestation of the world's rainforests." Its policy puts the company "at the front of the pack" when it comes to addressing the problems with palm oil, said RAN organizers.

And remember those upstart students who launched the Real Food

Challenge in 2008? Today, seventeen universities have officially signed on to the Challenge. Collectively, these schools are committed to purchasing more than thirty million dollars' worth of "real food" annually; many more are imminently joining those ranks. In February 2011, campus organizers plan to host 600 students in Boston, 400 in Santa Cruz, 200 in Georgia, 150 in the Midwest, 75 in Arizona—altogether more than 1,500 student food activists will gather to hash out strategy for bringing real, climate-friendly food into university cafeterias.

And while food co-ops in the United States still fail to come close to the political prowess and consumer power of those I saw in South Korea, the National Cooperative Grocers Association's store sales have grown 58 percent in five years, surpassing $1.2 billion in 2010. These consumer co-ops are at the front line of bringing climate-friendly food—and public education—to millions. At the Association's annual meeting, I heard about their members' creative efforts to support climate-friendly farming, from Albany, New York, to Davis, California; from Ames, Iowa, to Ypsilanti, Michigan. There's the Bellingham, Washington, co-op that created "Food to Bank On," a program that supports new farmers by connecting them with experienced growers and area food banks. And the Albuquerque, New Mexico, co-op that distributes sustainable food not just to co-op shelves but to other area retailers, too, reducing food transport costs and increasing the diversity and availability of local foods.

Meanwhile, Bill McKibben's international network, 350.org, has exploded. On October 10, 2010, the movement launched arguably the largest global social action event in human history, staging a planetary "work party" in 188 countries. More than seven thousand communities got together to raise awareness about the climate crisis and engage in positive action, and many focused on the food, farming, and climate connection. In Dehradun, India, several dozen visitors to the Navdanya agricultural training center learned about the role of sustainable farming as a solution to climate change and etched a giant "350.org" in the soil. In Sagay City, Philippines, students gathered to plant hundreds of mangrove seedlings. In Flatbush, Brooklyn, neighbors came together to clean up a community garden and discuss the importance of urban farming for climate stability while dining on a potluck feast.

On a personal level, inspired by the research for this book, I've renewed my own commitment to climate-friendly food and farming. We rejoined our community-supported agriculture (CSA) farm and along with 222 other families have been getting food fresh from Green Thumb Farm, and our farmer, Bill Halsey, for months. My daughter tasted her first raspberries, pears, green beans, blackberries, basil, plums, peaches, summer squash, and more, thanks to Bill.

A friend described reading this book like dining on a hope-and-gloom sandwich: There are some pretty big slabs of gloom in these pages and in our current political setbacks, but there's hope, too. Yes, those international climate negotiations stalled, domestic climate policy with teeth is a pipe dream, and climate change denial is alive and well. (Of the thirty-seven Republicans vying for Senate seats in the 2010 mid-term elections, all except one disputes the global scientific consensus on climate science.) But hopefully you've been lifted up by the hope as well, and by these latest reports of committed action. I know I have. I also know, more than ever, that making the choice for climate friendly doesn't just feel good, it tastes good, too. My daughter agrees.

November 2010
Brooklyn, New York

ACKNOWLEDGMENTS

I would not have written this book, or believed in it, were it not for those around the globe who work doggedly every day for the radical and urgent transformation our planet so needs. For all these people, my profound appreciation.

I am also indebted to the dozens of scientists, researchers, and advocates whose work informed and inspired this project, as well as to the many people who gave generously of their time, offering their expertise and wisdom.

I'm especially appreciative of the individuals who gave insightful feedback on specific sections in this book. In particular, I would like to offer thanks to colleagues whose vision, research, and support are a source of inspiration: Peter Barnes at the Tomales Bay Institute, Mia MacDonald at Brighter Green, Dr. Roni Neff at the Center for a Livable Future, Danielle Nierenberg at the Humane Society of the United States, Meredith Niles, formerly of the Center for Food Safety, and Dr. Urvashi Rangan at Consumers Union. In addition, a big thank-you to my "dream team" readers who offered helpful comments on an early draft: Tim Galarneau, Dr. Roni Neff, Danielle Nierenberg, and Liam O'Donoghue.

I was also blessed with fantastic help from people who pitched in with research help at different stages of the project, including Zach Aaron, Jessica Bruce, Carolyn Daly, Deepa Ranganathan, Aaron Reser, Jill Richardson, Petra Tanos, and Laura Zaks. Special thanks to Jeanne Hodesh and Deepa Philips.

Abhaya Kaufman contributed reporting from Mexico. Anna Witowska offered assistance from Poland. JiEun Choi provided excellent guidance in South Korea, and Jessica Walker Beaumont made the South Korea research trip that much richer—and lots of fun.

I also want to express my gratitude to the online communities and listservs of the Food Climate Research Network, Community Food

Security Coalition, GENET, Food Crisis Working Group, Real Food Federation, and the Association for the Study of Food and Society. These are special virtual resources, and it's a pleasure to be a part of them.

Thanks also to the supporters of the Take a Bite out of Climate Change project, whose contributions helped launch the book's campaign Web site, including the Wild Rose Fund and several anonymous donors.

Special thanks to Dr. Ellen Berrey, my go-to gal, who for more than fifteen years has made time to offer moral and editorial support. I'm also grateful to longtime collaborator, coconspirator, and inspirer Bryant Terry.

In the turbulent world of publishing, I am blessed with a wonderful agent, Sam Stoloff, at Frances Goldin Literary Agency, who has been a tireless supporter and who is, by his very nature, a total gem. I have also been delighted with the stellar team at Bloomsbury USA, including Jeremy Wang-Iverson, Rachel Mannheimer, and my wonderful editor Kathy Belden, who was a joy to work with.

Birthing a baby and a book at the same time is not easy, but I am fortunate to have a wonderfully supportive family and circle of friends. In particular, I offer a couldn't-do-this-without-you thanks to my mother, whose wisdom and great sense of humor (not to mention editing skill) continue to astound me.

My penultimate appreciation goes to the magnificent man I have the privilege of calling my husband, John Marshall. I wouldn't have been able to pull this off without you, and it certainly wouldn't have been nearly as much fun. My appreciation for your patience and support—and for doing more than your fair share of the dishes.

My final, and most tender, thanks goes to the newest member of my family, Ida, who had all my love from day one.

ACRONYMS USED IN *DIET FOR A HOT PLANET*

AATF	African Agricultural Technology Foundation
AMI	American Meat Institute
BIO	Biotechnology Industry Organization
CGFI	Center for Global Food Issues (a project of the industry-funded Hudson Institute)
EPA	Environmental Protection Agency
FAO	Food and Agriculture Organization of the United Nations
FMI	Food Marketing Institute
FTC	Federal Trade Commission
GMA	Grocery Manufacturers Association
HSUS	Humane Society of the United States
IAASTD	International Assessment of Agricultural Knowledge, Science, and Technology for Development (a project of the World Bank and the United Nations)
IATP	Institute for Agriculture and Trade Policy
IFOAM	International Federation of Organic Agricultural Movements
IPCC	United Nations Intergovernmental Panel on Climate Change
NCBA	National Cattlemen's Beef Association
PETA	People for the Ethical Treatment of Animals
RAN	Rainforest Action Network
RSPO	Roundtable on Sustainable Palm Oil
SEC	Securities and Exchange Commission
USDA	United States Department of Agriculture
WEMA	Water Efficient Maize for Africa (a project of the African Agricultural Technology Foundation)
WTO	World Trade Organization

NOTES

INTRODUCTION: WHY THIS BOOK?

1. David Chandler, "Climate Change Odds Much Worse than Thought," Massachusetts Institute of Technology News Office, May 19, 2009. Study published in *Journal of Climate*, http://web.mit.edu/newsoffice/2009/roulette-0519.html.
2. David S. Battisti and Rosamond L. Naylor, "Historical Warnings of Future Food Insecurity with Unprecedented Seasonal Heat," *Science* 323, no. 5911 (2009).
3. Brian Halweil, *Vital Signs*, November 28, 2007, http://www.worldwatch.org/node/5440.
4. Henning Steinfeld et al., *Livestock's Long Shadow: Environmental Issues and Options* (Rome: FAO, 2006).
5. Ibid.
6. R. A. Neff, I. L. Chan, and K. A. Smith, "Yesterday's Dinner, Tomorrow's Weather, Today's News? US Newspaper Coverage of Food System Contributions to Climate Change," *Public Health Nutrition*, v. 12 issue 7, pp. 1006–1014.
7. Rajendra Pachauri, "Global Warning: The Impact of Meat Production and Consumption on Climate Change" (paper, Compassion in World Farming, London, September 8, 2008).
8. Tim F. Flannery, *The Weather Makers: How Man Is Changing the Climate and What It Means for Life on Earth* (New York: Atlantic Monthly Press, 2005), 256.

1. THE CLIMATE CRISIS AT THE END OF OUR FORK

1. IPCC, *Climate Change 2007: Fourth Assessment Report of the Intergovernmental Panel on Climate Change* (New York: Cambridge University Press, 2007), graphic 13.5.
2. Henning Steinfeld et. al., *Livestock's Long Shadow*.
3. IPCC, Climate Change 2001: Working Group I: The Scientific Basis, See "Chapter 6: Radiative Forcing and Climate Change." (Cambridge, UK: IPCC, 2007).
4. Kirk Smith, "Methane Controls Before Risky Geoengineering, Please," *New Scientist*, June 25, 2009, http://www.newscientist.com/article/mg20227146.000-methane-controls-before-risky-geoengineering-please.html.
5. K. Paustian et. al., "Agriculture's Role in Greenhouse Gas Mitigation," (Arlington, VA: Pew Center on Global Climate Change, 2006), 3.
6. Statement from Nobel Committee, http://nobelprize.org/nobel_prizes/peace/laureates/2007.
7. Spencer R. Weart, *The Discovery of Global Warming*, revised and expanded ed. (Cambridge, MA: Harvard University Press, 2008), 205.

8. Howard T. Odum, *Environment, Power, and Society* (New York: Wiley-Interscience, 1970), 115–16.

9. Diarmuid Jeffreys, *Hell's Cartel: IG Farben and the Making of Hitler's War Machine*, 1st. ed. (New York: Metropolitan Books, 2008), 56.

10. Ibid., 57.

11. Personal communication, Professor Jonathan Lynch, University of Pennsylvania. See also CNN, "All About: Food and Fossil Fuels," March 17, 2008, http://edition.cnn.com/2008/WORLD/asiapcf/03/16/eco.food.miles.

12. Datamonitor Premium Research Reports, "Fertilizer: Global Industry Guide," June 30, 2009, http://www.alacrastore.com/research/datamonitor-premium.

13. EPA, "U.S. Emissions Inventory 2006: Inventory of U.S. Greenhouse Gas Emissions and Sinks: 1990–2006," (Washington D.C., USEPA: 2008).

14. Danielle Nierenberg and Gowri Koneswaran, "Global Farm Animal Production and Global Warming," *Environmental Health Perspectives* 116, no. 9 (2008).

15. USDA Economic Research Service, "U.S. Fertilizer Imports/Exports: Summary of the Data Findings," http://www.ers.usda.gov/Data/FertilizerTrade/Summary.htm.

16. Ibid.

17. See, for instance, California Air Resource Board, "Research on GHG Emissions from Nitrogen Fertilizers," http://www.arb.ca.gov/ag/fertilizer/fertilizer.htm.

18. Personal communication, Dennis Keeney, Iowa State University, April 13, 2009.

19. USDA ERS, "Economic Information Bulletin No. EIB-48," April 8 2009, http://www.ers.usda.gov/Publications/EIB48.

20. Quoted in Jeffreys, *Hell's Cartel*, 68–69.

21. Office of Global Analysis, *Livestock and Poultry: World Markets and Trade* (USDA, Foreign Agricultural Service, Circular Series, 2008).

22. Steinfeld et al., *Livestock's Long Shadow*, xxi. See also P. Smith et al., "Agriculture," in O. R. Davidson et al., eds., *Climate Change 2007: Mitigation. Contribution of Working Group III to the Fourth Assessment Report of the Intergovernmental Panel on Climate Change* (Cambridge and New York: Cambridge University Press, 2007), 510.

23. Steinfeld et al., *Livestock's Long Shadow*, xxi.

24. See, for example, Carbon Farmers of Australia, http://www.carbonfarmersofaustralia.com.au.

25. Jacqueline Switzer, *Environmental Activism: A Reference Handbook* (Santa Barbara, CA: ABC-CLIO, 2003).

26. Lance A. Compa, *Unfair Advantage: Workers' Freedom of Association in the United States Under International Human Rights Standards* (Ithaca, NY: ILR Press, 2004), 94. According to Rodney Barker's account in *And the Waters Turned to Blood*, the state "courted the swine industry with tax breaks, protection from local zoning, and exemptions from tough environmental regulations." The constellation of benefits to the industry included laws that extended the preferential tax treatment that family farmers received to factory hog operations, which bore little resemblance to those traditional farms. Barker, *Waters Turned to Blood*, 234.

27. Smil, *Transforming the Twentieth Century*, 152.

28. Mary Hendrickson and William Heffernan, "Concentration of Agricultural Markets," University of Missouri, Columbia, Missouri, April 2007, 3.

29. Code of Federal Regulations 40 CFR 122.23 (4), http://cfr.vlex.com/vid/19812671.

30. X. P. C. Verge, C. De Kimpe, and R. L. Desjardins, "Agricultural Production, Greenhouse Gas Emissions and Mitigation Potential," *Agricultural and Forest Meteorology* 142 (2007), 255–269.

31. *World Agriculture: Towards 2015/2030, Summary Report* (Rome: FAO, 2002). Also quoted in Verge, De Kimpe, and Desjardins, "Agricultural Production."

32. Pachauri, "Global Warning" (see introduction, n. 7).

33. *World Agricultural Supply and Demand Estimates* (Washington, DC: USDA, 2009), 12. ERS, *Feed Grains Database: Yearbook Tables* (Washington, DC: USDA, 2008).

34. Steinfeld et al, *Livestock's Long Shadow*, xxi.

35. FAO, Fisheries and Aquaculture Department, "Fish Utilization," July 7, 2009, http://www.fao.org/fishery/topic/2888/en.

36. N. H. Stern, *The Economics of Climate Change: The Stern Review* (Cambridge: Cambridge University Press, 2007).

37. Greenpeace International, "Eating up the Amazon," (London: Greenpeace International, 2006), 5.

38. Cargill, "Cargill's View on the Greenpeace Report: 'Eating Up the Amazon' " May 2006, http://www.cargill.com/wcm/groups/public/@ccom/documents/document/doc-amazon-response.pdf.

39. Mary Hendrickson and William Heffernan, "Concentration of Agricultural Markets," University of Missouri, Columbia, MI (April 2007). Information on company activity from ADM, Bunge, and Cargill corporate Web sites.

40. H. Steinfeld and T. Wassenaar, "The Role of Livestock Production in Carbon Cycles," *The Annual Review of Environment and Resources* 32 (2007): 274.

41. Steinfeld et al., *Livestock's Long Shadow*, 87.

42. Ibid.

43. Nierenberg and Koneswaran, "Global Farm Animal Production." See also Steinfeld et al., *Livestock's Long Shadow*.

44. Rosamond L. Naylor et al., "Effect of Aquaculture on World Fish Supplies," *Nature* 405 (2000).

45. Explanation of conversion ratio: Frances Moore Lappé, *Diet for a Small Planet*, 20th anniversary ed. (New York: Ballantine Books, 1991), 445. For further discussion, see Paul Roberts, *The End of Food* (Boston: Houghton Mifflin Company, 2008), 293.

46. Quoted in Barker, *Waters Turned to Blood*, 234.

47. Smith et al., "Agriculture," 511.

48. Frank Spellman and Nancy Whiting, *Environmental Management of Concentrated Animal Feeding Operations* (Boca Raton, FL: CRC).

49. EPA, "U. S. Emissions Inventory 2006," Agriculture 6–7, http://www.epa.gov/climatechange/emissions/download09/Agriculture.pdf

50. Steinfeld et al., *Livestock's Long Shadow*, 99.

51. Mia MacDonald, *Skillful Means: The Challenges of China's Encounter with Factory Farming* (New York: Brighter Green, 2008), 3.

52. Andy Thorpe, "Enteric Fermentation and Ruminant Eructation: The Role (and Control?) of Methane in the Climate Change Debate," *Climatic Change* 93, no. 3–4 (2009): 408.

53. J. McMichael et al., "Food, Livestock Production, Energy, Climate Change, and Health," *Lancet* 370, no. 9594 (2007): 1253–63.

54. Figures from the U.S. Emissions Inventory 2009: Inventory of U.S. Greenhouse Gas Emissions and Sinks: 1990–2007, http://epa.gov/methane/sources.html.

55. Thorpe, "Enteric Fermentation," 411.

56. Based on calculations by Andy Thorpe of the emissions from the average New Zealand dairy cow.

57. Steinfeld et al., *Livestock's Long Shadow*, xx.

58. Ibid.

59. Ibid., xxi.

60. *Livestock and Soil Fertility: Exploiting the Natural Balance* (Nairobi, Kenya: International Livestock Research Institute, 1997).

61. Steinfeld et al., *Livestock's Long Shadow*, 256.

62. Greenpeace Brazil, "Amazon Cattle Footprint," January 29, 2009, http://www.greenpeace.org/international/press/reports/amazon-cattle-footprint-mato.

63. Slaughter rates are from 1965 and 2007 and based on data available at FAOSTAT, http://faostat.fao.org/site/569/DesktopDefault.aspx?PageID = 569#ancor.

64. Kees Jansen and Sietze Vellema, *Agribusiness and Society: Corporate Responses to Environmentalism, Market Opportunities and Public Regulation* (London: Zed Books, 2004), 16.

65. "Coke vs. Coke: A Tale of Two Sweeteners," *Consumer Reports*, June 2009.

66. Anita Regmi, ed., *Changing Structure of Global Food Consumption and Trade* (Washington, DC: USDA ERS, May 2001), 47–51.

67. Personal communication, Steve Ettlinger, June 2009. See also Steve Ettlinger, *Twinkie, Deconstructed* (New York: Hudson Street Press, 2007).

68. Mark Gunther, "Eco-Police Find New Target: Oreos," *Money*, August 21, 2008.

69. USDA FAS, "Indonesia: Palm Oil Production Prospects Continue to Grow," December 31, 2007. http://www.pecad.fas.usda.gov/highlights/2007/12/Indonesia _palmoil.

70. USDA FAS, "Palm Oil: World Supply and Distribution," June 10, 2009.

71. Personal Communication, Lafcadio Cortesi, Rainforest Action Network, August 2009.

72. Wetlands International, http://www.wetlands.org/Whatwedo/Wetlandsand climatechange/Peatlandsandclimatechangemitigation/tabid/837/Default.aspx.

73. ———, "How the Palm Oil Industry is Cooking the Climate," 2.

74. Personal communication, Mohammed Ikhwan, Indonesian Peasant Union, May 2009.

75. "Palm Oil Firm Wilmar Harming Indonesia Forests-Group," Reuters, July 3, 2007, http://www.alertnet.org/thenews/newsdesk/SIN344348.htm.

76. Cargill-Malaysia, http://www.cargill.com.my/, and Cargill-Indonesia, http://www.cargill.com/news/issues/palm_current.htm.

77. See, for instance, Cargill's position statement: http://www.cargill.com/news/issues/palm_roundtable.htm#TopOfPage. See also Bunge: http://www.bunge.com/about-bunge/promoting_sustainability.html.

78. Herman E. Daly, *Ecological Economics and Sustainable Development: Selected Essays of Herman Daly*, (Cheltenham, UK, and Northampton, MA: Edward Elgar, 2007), 197–98.

79. *Food Miles: How Far Your Food Travels Has Serious Consequences for Your Health and the Climate* (Washington, DC: Natural Resources Defense Council, 2007).

80. From a Rutgers University study that found that 635,000 gallons of fuel was needed annually to import tomatoes into New Jersey, generating 6,616 metric tons of carbon dioxide.

81. *Urner Barry's Reporter* 3, no. 2 (Spring 2008): 50.

82. Peter Leo, "Cleveland Gets Testy over Bottled Water," *Pittsburgh Post Gazette*, July 20, 2006.

83. USDA ERS, "U.S. Cattle and Beef Industry, 2002–2007," http://www.ers.usda .gov/news/bsecoverage.htm. Most recent data available. Pounds noted here are measured by commercial carcass weight. U.S. Red Meat and Poultry Forecasts. Source: World Agricultural Supply and Demand Estimates and Supporting Materials. From USDA ERS. See also http://www.ers.usda.gov/browse/tradeinter nationalmarkets.

84. Personal communication, Michael McConnell, USDA ERS, November 2008.

85. Mary Hendrickson et al., *The Global Food System and Nodes of Power* (Social Science Research Network, 2008), 4, http://ssrn.com/abstract-1337273.

86. Stacey Rosen and Shahla Shapouri, "Obesity in the Midst of Unyielding Food Insecurity in Developing Countries," *Amber Waves*, 2008.

87. Ibid.

88. Ibid.

89. Ibid.

90. Juliette Jowit, "Supermarkets Come in from Cold as Part of Low Carbon Revolution," *Guardian*, October 25, 2008.

91. U.S. Department of Energy, Energy Information Administration, "1999 Commercial Buildings Energy Consumption Survey—Commercial Buildings Characteristics," www.eia.doe.gov/emeu/cbecs/char99/intro.html.

92. F. Walravens, Clare Perry, and Alexander von Bismarch, *Facing the F-Gas Challenge: The Need for a Global Phase-Out of HFCS* (London: Environmental Investigation Agency, 2007).

93. Emma Clarke, "HFCs: Ozone-Saving Gas Targeted for Climate Effect," ClimateChangeCorp, June 12, 2009, http://www.climatechangecorp.com/content.asp? contentid=6183.

94. *Fast Food Nation 2008: A Consumer Perspective on the Fast Food Industry* (Chicago: Research International USA, 2008).

95. Frazão, Meade, and Regmi, "Converging Patterns," xx.

96. U.N. Population Division, "World Urbanization Prospects: The 2007 Revision Population Database," http://esa.un.org/unup.

97. Regmi, *Changing Structure*, 24.

98. In Brazil, the Landless Workers Movements has helped more than a quarter of a million families build rewarding lives and sustainable communities in the countryside since its founding in the mid-1980s. In Niger, a farmer-led movement has re-greened 12.4 million acres of land, planting as many as 200 million trees, over the past two decades. For more inspiring examples, see my previous book, Frances Moore Lappé and Anna Lappé, *Hope's Edge: The Next Diet for a Small Planet* (New York: Tarcher/Penguin, 2002).

99. The EPA reports 12.5 percent of all municipal solid waste in the United States is food waste. http://www.epa.gov/waste/conserve/materials/organics/food/fd-basic .htm

100. ERS, *Nutrient Availability* (Washington, DC: USDA, 2008).

101. Smith et al., "Agriculture."

102. From Environmental Working Group data 1995 to 2006. Livestock Disaster/ Emergency, $1,456,101,626; Livestock Indemnity Program, $85,837,335; Total Dairy Program, $2,560,602,488. Total: $4,102,541,449. While I didn't analyze each recipient, I extrapolated that most were large-scale producers based on EWG's findings that nearly two thirds of farm subsidies were given to the top 10 percent—"the largest and generally wealthiest subsidized farming operations in the country"—of producers, http://farm.ewg.org/farm/regiondetail.php?fips= 00000&summlevel=2.

103. Data from Environmental Working Group, http://farm.ewg.org/sites/farmbill2007/ progdetail1614.php?fips=00000&progcode= otal&page=croptable.

104. Doug Gurian-Sherman, *CAFOs Uncovered: The Untold Costs of Confined Animal Feeding Operations* (Washington, DC: Union of Concerned Scientists, 2008), 2.

105. Timothy A. Wise, "Identifying the Real Winners from U.S. Agricultural Policies," ed. Global Development and Environment Institute (Medford, MA: Tufts University, 2005).

106. Timothy A. Wise and Elanor Starmer, "Feeding at the Trough: Industrial Livestock Firms Saved $35 Billion from Low Feed Prices," ed. Global Development and Environment Institute (Medford, MA: Tufts University, 2007).

107. Gurian-Sherman, "CAFOs Uncovered."

108. Office of U.S. senator Ken Salazar, press release, 2005, http://www.salazar.senate .gov/news/releases/050314embbeef.htm.

109. Switzer, *Environmental Activism*, 53.

110. See "Food and Agriculture Statistics Global Outlook" (as of June 2006), http:// faostat.fao.org/Portals/_Faostat/documents/pdf/world.pdf.

2. THE SHAPE OF THINGS TO COME

1. Coca-Cola Company, per-capita consumption data, http://www.thecoca-cola company.com/ourcompany/ar/percapitaconsumption.html.

2. FAO, press release, "Livestock a Major Threat to Environment, Remedies Urgently Needed," 2006, http://www.reuters.com/article/pressrelease/idus219553 +10-sep-2008+gnw20080910.

3. Rosegrant et al., *2020 Global Food Outlook*, "Trends, Alternatives, and Choices," 4.

4. Quoted in Steinfeld et al., *Livestock's Long Shadow*, xx (see introduction, n. 4).

5. Smith et al., "Agriculture," 500, 503–504 (see chap. 1, n. 26).

6. Elisabeth Rosenthal, "As More Eat Meat, a Bid to Cut Emissions," *New York Times*, December 3, 2008.

7. PepsiCo, press release, "PepsiCo Plans to Invest $1 Billion in China Over the Next Four Years," 2008, http://www.pepsico.com/PressRelease/PepsiCo-Plans-to-Invest-1-Billion-in-China-Over.th.html.

8. Ibid.

9. "Power Players," *Advertising Age*, October 13, 2008. Coca-Cola Company,

$776.8 million ad budget; PepsiCo, $473 million; McDonald's Corporation, $1.15 billion.

10. Betsy McKay, "Coke Bets on Russia for Sales Even as Economy Falls Flat," *Wall Street Journal*, January 28, 2009.
11. Ibid.
12. PepsiCo, "PepsiCo Plans."
13. Benjamin R. Barber, *Jihad vs. McWorld*, 1st Ballantine Books ed. (New York: Ballantine Books, 1996), 60.
14. Ibid., 69.
15. Ibid., 70.
16. Brent Berry and Taralyn McMullen, "Visual Communication to Children in the Supermarket Context: Health Protective or Exploitive?," *Agriculture and Human Values* 25, no. 3 (2008), 333–348.
17. Clive Thompson, "There's a Sucker Born in Every Medial Prefrontal Cortex," *New York Times*, October 26, 2003.
18. William Wallis and Javier Blas, "US Investor Buys Sudanese Warlord's Land," *Financial Times*, January 9, 2009.
19. William Wallis, Javier Blas, and Barney Jopson, "Quest to Create a New Sudan Bread Basket," *Financial Times*, January 9, 2009.
20. Ibid.
21. Devinder Sharma, "Land Grab for Food Security: Corporatising Agriculture," *Bangalore Deccan Herald*, November 13, 2008.
22. Deborah MacKenzie, "The 21st-Century Land Grab," *New Scientist*, December 6, 2008.
23. Sharma, "Land Grab."
24. Ibid. See also Santoosh Menon, "Enter the New Farmers," June 25, 2008, http://blogs.reuters.com/global/tag/ukraine.
25. Sharma, "Land Grab."
26. Ibid.
27. Ibid.
28. MacKenzie, "21st-Century Land Grab."
29. *Seized! GRAIN Briefing Annex* (GRAIN, October 2008), 8, http://www.grain.org/landgrab.
30. Ibid.
31. Alexandra Spieldoch, "Global Land Grab," Foreign Policy in Focus, 2009, http://www.fpif.org/fpiftxt/6201.
32. Ibid.
33. MacKenzie, "21st-Century Land Grab."
34. Central Intelligence Agency, the World Factbook, Poland, https://www.cia.gov/library/publications/the-world-factbook.
35. Smithfield Foods, Form 10-K, 2000.
36. ———, Form 10-K, 2004.
37. ———, Form 10-K, 2007.
38. Ibid.
39. USDA, Foreign Agricultural Service, Production Estimates, Crop Assessment Division, "Poland: Basic Agriculture: Past, Present, and Thoughts on Its Future in the European Union," December 1, 2003, http://www.fas.usda.gov/pecad2/highlights/2003/12/poland/index.htm.

40. Hendrickson et al., *Global Food System*, 8–9 (see chap. 1, n. 96).
41. Bankwatch Network, "Animex/Smithfield Operation, Poland," http://www .bankwatch.org/project-shtml?w/147579&s/153979.
42. Personal communication, Anna Witowska, Food & Water Watch Poland, August 2008.
43. Bankwatch Network, "Animex/Smithfield Operation, Poland."
44. Ibid.
45. Letter, from Hans Christian Jacobsen, director, Agribusiness, EBRD, to Polska Zielona Siec, sent February 24, 2004.
46. Hendrickson et al., *Global Food System*, 4.
47. Jeff Caldwell, "Vertical Integration Benefits Small Hog Producers, Says Farmland Foods CEO," *High Plains Journal*, April 7, 2005.
48. Mary Hendrickson and William Heffernan, "Concentration of Agricultural Markets," University of Missouri, Columbia, MO, April 2007.
49. Hendrickson et al., *Global Food System*, 1.
50. To learn more about Smithfield in Romania, see Terra Mileniul III, *Industrial Pig Farms and Their Environmental Impact: Case Study Smithfield in Romania* (Bucharest: Terra Mileniul III, 2006).
51. Personal communication, Anna Witowska, Food & Water Watch Poland, August 2008.
52. Smithfield, Form 10-K, 2004. See also Standard & Poor's, *Industry Surveys: Agribusiness* (Standard & Poor's, 2007), 13.
53. Ibid.
54. Tyson Foods, Form 10-K, 2007.
55. MacDonald, *Skillful Means* (see chap. 1, n. 57).
56. For a great overview of the expansion of industrial farming in China, see Danielle Nierenberg, WorldWatch Paper 171, *Happier Meals: Rethinking the Global Meat Industry*, "Country Study #3: China," 38. See also Mia MacDonald and Sangamithra Iyer, *Skillful Means: The Challenges of China's Encounter with Factory Farming* (New York: Brighter Green, 2008).

3. BLINDED BY THE BITE

1. Neff, Chan, and Smith, "Yesterday's Dinner," 80 (see introduction, n. 6).
2. Rosenthal, "As More Eat Meat" (see chap. 2, n. 7).
3. *MAP Report 2: Aspirational Environmentalism* (New York: Getty Images, 2007).
4. Elizabeth Kolbert, "The Catastrophist," *New Yorker*, June 29, 2009.
5. Globescan, "Greendex," *National Geographic*, June 2008, 10.
6. Jeffrey McNeely and Sara Scherr, *Ecoagriculture: Strategies to Feed the World and Save Wild Biodiversity* (Washington, DC: Island Press, 2003). See also Sara Scherr and Jeffrey McNeely, *Farming with Nature: The Science and Practice of Ecoagriculture* (Washington, DC: Island Press, 2007).
7. USDA ERS, "Food Security in the United States," 2007, http://www.ers.usda .gov/briefing/foodsecurity.
8. Christian Nellemann et al., *The Environmental Food Crisis: The Environment's Role in Averting Future Food Crises* (Nairobi, Kenya: United Nations Environment Programme, 2008).
9. Pachauri, "Global Warning" (see introduction, n. 8).

10. Juliette Jowit, "Hospitals Will Take Meat off Menus in Bid to Cut Carbon" *Guardian*, January 26, 2009.

11. Brook Lyndhurst, *London's Food Sector Greenhouse Gas Emissions* (London: Greater London Authority, February, 2008), http://www.london.gov.uk/mayor/publications/2009/02/food-emissions.jsp.

12. Curious to understand the extent to which climate change is considered a risk factor, liability, or opportunity across the food industry, a research assistant and I checked out the available 10-Ks of the world's thirty-two largest food companies over a four-year period, from 2004 to 2007. Twelve were food manufacturers; eight were meat producers and/or processors; twelve were agribusiness or agricultural-chemical companies. (Note: Many of these companies have operations that cut across all three sectors. We classified companies according to what they reported as their major source of earnings.) Reports were searched for frequency and context of key terms, including "climate change," "global warming," "emissions," "greenhouse gases," "carbon dioxide," "(CO_2)," "nitrous oxide," "methane," and "environment." In the process of reviewing these more than 125 reports, we found that the climate crisis went virtually unmentioned in all but a few cases. While we saw a small increase in the mention of global warming in reports starting in 2006, the crisis was otherwise out of the printed reports. (Special thanks to Catherine Dilley, who provided assistance with this research.) You can find all company reports filed with the SEC at www.secinfo.com.

13. Smithfield Foods, Form 10-K, 2007.

14. Ibid.

15. Peter Kilborn, "Hurricane Reveals Flaws in Farm Law as Animal Waste Threatens N. Carolina Water," *New York Times*, October 17, 1999.

16. Kilborn, "Hurricane Reveals Flaws."

17. Hormel, Form 10-K, Item 5, "Stockholder Proposal Requesting Disclosures," 2008.

18. Daniel C. Esty, "Transparency: What Stakeholders Demand," *Harvard Business Review*, October, 2007, 5–7.

19. Interview with Michel Santos, Bunge-Brazil, Corporate Marketing and Sustainability, by research assistant Laura Zaks, July 28, 2008.

20. TobaccoDocuments.org, Anne Landman's Collection, http://tobaccodocuments.org/landman/332506.html.

21. "Smoking and Health Proposal," http://legacy.library.ucsf.edu/tid/nvs40f00/pdf. This document is from the Brown & Williamson collection and is among the 9.7 million documents, adding up to a whopping 50-plus million pages, in the Legacy Tobacco Documents Library, a collection of the advertising, manufacturing, marketing, sales, and scientific-research activities of the tobacco industry. Brown & Williamson merged with R. J. Reynolds in 2004. Quoted in David Michaels, *Doubt Is Their Product: How Industry's Assault on Science Threatens Your Health* (Oxford and New York: Oxford University Press, 2008), xi.

22. "Luntz F. Memo: The Environment: A Cleaner, Safer, Healthier America," ca. 2003, http://www.ewg.org:16080/briefings/luntzmemo. Quoted in Michaels, *Doubt Is Their Product*.

23. National Cattlemen's Beef Association, https://www.beef.org/uDocs/issuesforum onenvissues-summerconf07.ppt.

24. Editorial, "The U.N.'s Meatless Drive: Our Appetite for Steaks and Burgers Is a Huge Contributor to Global Warming," *Los Angeles Times*, September 9, 2008.

25. Terry Stokes, audio news release, "CEO Terry Stokes Addresses Anti-Meat Activists' Claims That Methane Gas from Livestock Is Major Contributor to Global Warming," October 24, 2007, http://www.beefura.org/Docs/audiostokesweekly 10-24-07508.mp3.

26. Center for Consumer Freedom press release, March 25, 2009. For information about the Center for Consumer Freedom, see www.sourcewatch.org. Dr. Barry Popkin, "Reducing Meat Consumption Has Multiple Benefits for the World's Health," *Archives of Internal Medicine* 169, no. 6, (March, 2009), 543–545.

27. Stokes, "CEO Terry Stokes."

28. *US Emissions Inventory 2006: Inventory of U.S. Greenhouse Gas Emissions and Sinks: 1990–2006* (Washington, DC: Environmental Protection Agency, 2008), http://www.epa.gov/climatechange/emissions/downloads/08_CR.pdf.

29. David Pimentel and Marcia Pimentel, *Food, Energy, and Society*, (Boca Raton, FL: CRC Press, 2008), 188.

30. U.S. Department of Energy, Carbon Dioxide Information Analysis Center, cited in *Who Is Heating Up the Planet? A Closer Look at Population and Global Warming* (Sierra Club, 2008). Figures based on IPCC reporting and analyzed by the World Resources Institute. Personal communication, Thomas Damassa, World Resources Institute, February 2009. Other estimates peg our emissions at about 18 percent.

31. Julian Borger, "Half of Global Car Exhaust Produced by U.S. Vehicles," *Guardian*, June 29, 2006. The source cited in the *Guardian* article is John DeCiccio, Freda Fung, and An Feng, *Global Warming on the Road: The Climate Impact of America's Automobiles* (Environmental Defense Fund, 2006), http://www.edf.org/documents/5301_globalwarmingontheroad.pdf.

32. Terry Stokes.

33. Nierenberg and Koneswaran, "Global Farm Animal Production" (see chap. 1, n. 14). The sources cited by Nierenberg and Koneswaran include: C. Cederberg et. al. "System Expansion and Allocation in Life Cycle Assessment of Milk and Beef Production," *International Journal of Life Cycle Assessment*, vol. 8, 2003, 350–356; D. Fanelli, "Meat is Murder on the Environment," *New Scientist*, July 18, 2007, 15. http://environment.newscientist.com/article.ns?id=mg19526134 .500&feedId=online-news_rss20; A. Ogino, "Evaluating Environmental Impacts of the Japanese Beef Cow-Calf System by the Life Cycle Assessment Method," *Animal Science Journal*, vol. 78, 2007, 424–432.

34. Alex Avery and Dennis Avery, letter to the editor, *Environmental Health Perspectives* 116, no. 9 (October, 2008), 374–375.

35. Ibid.

36. Dennis T. Avery, *Saving the Planet with Pesticides and Plastic: The Environmental Triumph of High-Yield Farming*, 2nd ed. (Indianapolis: Hudson Institute, 2000), 138.

37. Ibid, 132.

38. Avery and Avery, letter.

39. Ibid.

40. Leopold Center, "Organic, Natural and Grass-fed Beef: Profitability and Constraints to Production in the Midwestern United States," (Ames, Iowa:

Leopold Center, 2008), http://www.leopold.iastate.edu/research/grants/2008/M2005-30.pdf.

41. Personal communication, Professor John Lawrence, Iowa State University, September 2008.
42. Personal communication, Allen Baker, USDA, September 2008.
43. Personal communication, Professor Timothy Searchinger, Princeton University, September 2008.
44. Timothy Searchinger et. al, "Use of U.S. Croplands for Biofuels Increases Greenhouse Gases Through Emissions from Land-Use Change," *Science*, 319, no. 5867, (February 2008), 1238–1240.
45. *US Emissions Inventory 2005: Inventory of U.S. Greenhouse Gas Emissions and Sinks: 1990–2003: Nitrous Oxide Emissions by Source (TgCO2 Equivalents)* (Washington, DC: Environmental Protection Agency, 2005), http://www.epa.gov/nitrousoxide/sources.html.
46. Sara Scherr and Sajal Sthapit, "Chapter 3: Farming and Land Use to Cool the Planet," *State of the World 2009* (Washington, DC: WorldWatch, 2009), 30–49.
47. Personal communication, Christel Cederberg, September 2008.
48. IRS Form 990, publicly available. Find the 990 for the Hudson Institute and any other 501(c)(3) at Guidestar.com or contact the organization directly. All funding sources are listed in the Hudson Institute's annual report. The 2003 report, posted in March 2005, is the most recent report available on its Web site, http://www.hudson.org/files/publications/2003_annual%20report.pdf.
49. Examples of Hudson Institute funders with ties to the livestock industry from the 2003 annual report include, from the Trustees' Circle, Eli Lilly, Monsanto, John M. Olin Foundation, PotashCorp, Sarah Scaife Foundation, and Syngenta Crop Protection; from the Chairman's Circle, Pioneer Hi-Bred International, DuPont, and Dow AgroSciences; from the President Circle, American Feed Industry Association; and the corporate sponsors of the Doolittle Award Luncheon, Archer Daniels Midland Foundation and Bayer Corporation.
50. Yahoo! Finance company profile, http://finance.yahoo.com/q/pr?s=lly.
51. Cattle Network, "Eli Lilly & Company Announces Acquisition of Ivy Animal Health," June 25, 2007.
52. Bayer HealthCare Portal: http://www.viva.vita.bayerhealthcare.com/index.php?id=36&tx_ttnews%5btt_news%5d=10883&chash=e0874c3c0c.
53. PotashCorp, http://www.potashcorp.com/about_potashcorp.
54. Roberta Rampton, "Update 2: Potash Corp Says Fertilizer Outlook Still Strong," Reuters, September 17, 2008.
55. John M. Olin Foundation, http://www.jmof.org.
56. Olin Corporation, http://www.olin.com and http://www.chloralkali.com.
57. Monsanto, "Biotechnology Trait Acreage: Fiscal Years 1996–2007," June 28, 2007, http://www.monsanto.com/pdf/pubs/2007/q32007acreage.pdf. For market percentages see Mary Hendrickson and William Heffernan, "Concentration of Agricultural Markets," http://www.nfu.org/wp-content/2007-heffernanreport.pdf.
58. AFIA, http://www.afia.org/afia/home.aspx.
59. Sheldon Rampton and John C. Stauber, *Mad Cow U.S.A.: Could the Nightmare Happen Here?*, 1st. ed. (Monroe, ME: Common Courage Press, 1997).
60. Press release, "Alliance Announces First East Coast Anti-Terrorism Training

Course," January 12, 2006, http://www.animalagalliance.org/main/home.cfm? Section=2006_0111_Terrorism&Category=ConferencesEvents.

61. PowerPoint presentation: http://www.gmaonline.org/events/2008/sustainability/presentations/kahn%20gma%20fwo1_friday%20general%20session.pdf.
62. Dow Chemical, Form 10-K, 2007.
63. ———, Form 10-K, 2004.
64. DuPont, Form 10-K, 2006.
65. Thanks to Carolyn Daly, who provided excellent research assistance.
66. Larry Aylward, "And Now for the Weather: Mother Nature's Impact on the Business Climate Looms Large," *Meat & Poultry*, December 2003.
67. Joanna Peot, "New Products Annual: Salads and Salad Dressings," *Prepared Foods*, March 2008.
68. Editorial, "Packaged Food Trends U.S.: The Growing Green Movement," *Prepared Foods*, March 2008.
69. Ibid.
70. William A. Roberts Jr., "Gluten-Free to Nutrient-Rich—Trendspotting at ExpoWest," *Prepared Foods*, June 2008.
71. Bob Sperber, "Renovating for Energy Efficiency," *Food Processing*, June 2008.
72. Esty, "Transparency."
73. Ibid.
74. Andrew Hoffman, "Regulation: If You're Not at the Table, You're on the Menu," *Harvard Business Review*, 2007.
75. Ibid.
76. Sperber, "Renovating for Energy Efficiency."

4. PLAYING WITH OUR FOOD

1. I attended five industry marketing conferences: the Grocery Manufacturers Association's Environmental Sustainability Summit (Washington, D.C., January 2008); the Meat Conference, sponsored by the Food Marketing Institute, among other groups (Nashville, March 2008); *Advertising Age*'s Green Conference (NYU, New York City, June 2008); American Strategic Management Institute's Green Marketing workshop (Washington, D.C., April 2008); BDI's Green Communications 2008 Case Studies conference (CUNY, New York City, June 2008). Research assistants attended an additional two: the Food Marketing Institute's Sustainability Summit (Minneapolis, June 2008) and the Biotechnology Industry Organization's annual summit (San Diego, July 2008).
2. Quoted in Michael Skapinker, "Virtue's Reward? Companies Make the Business Case for Ethical Initiatives," *Financial Times*, April 28, 2008. Original source: Milton Friedman, *Capitalism and Freedom* (Chicago: University of Chicago Press, 1962).
3. Henry I. Miller, "Firms Need to Focus on Profits: CEOs Are Often Distracted by Corporate Social Responsibility and Other Forms of Social Activism," *Genetic Engineering & Biotechnology News* 28, no. 3 (February 1, 2008), http://www.genengnews.com/articles/chitem.aspx?aid/2353.
4. *The Future of the Corporate Brand* (New York: Euro RSCG Biss Lancaster Worldwide, 2008). The study was based on a survey of 1,851 adults in the United Kingdom, the United States, and France.

5. Ibid.
6. Source for revenues: "The Global 2000," Forbes, April 2, 2008, http://www .forbes.com/lists/2008/18/biz_2000global08_The-Global-2000_Rank.html. Source for GDPs: CIA, the World Factbook, 2008, http://www.cia.gov/library/ publications/the-world-factbook.
7. Source for S&P 500 revenues: CompuStat Research Insight, 2008. Source for GDP for countries: CIA, the World Factbook, 2008, http://www.cia.gov/library/ publication/the-world-factbook.
8. "Engine Charlie," Time, October 6, 1961.
9. Lobbying total: "Lobbying Database," Center for Public Integrity, http://www .opensecrets.org/lobbyists.
10. Lobbyists: "Lobbying Database," Center for Public Integrity, http://www .opensecrets.org/lobbyists. In 2008, there were 15,138 registered lobbyists in the United States, according to the center.
11. Future of the Corporate Brand (Euro RSCG Biss Lancaster Worldwide).
12. Courtney Barnes, "Sustainability Reporting: Ensuring Long-Term Notoriety in the Marketplace" (paper, at the ASMI Green Marketing workshop, Washington, DC, April 22, 2008).
13. Personal communication, Carol Somody, stewardship manager, Syngenta, July 28, 2008.
14. Economist/YouGov/Polimetrix poll, quoted in "Deflating a Myth: Consumers Aren't as Devoted to the Planet as You Wish They Were," Adweek, May 12, 2008.
15. Stuart Hart, Capitalism at the Crossroads: The Unlimited Business Opportunities in Solving the World's Most Difficult Problems, (Wharton School Publishing, 2005).
16. Adam Werbach, "Seeing Green? Maybe It's Time to Go Blue," Advertising Age, May 2008.
17. "Half-Price Big Mac to Fight Global Warming Proves Big Hit in Japan," AFP, September 4, 2007.
18. Ibid.
19. McDonald's press release, "McDonald's 'Summer of Happy Meal Fun' Concludes in Style with Miniature Fashion and Big Off-Road Adventure," August 3, 2006.
20. Daniel C. Esty and Andrew S. Winston, Green to Gold: How Smart Companies Use Environmental Strategy to Innovate, Create Value, and Build Competitive Advantage (New Haven: Yale University Press, 2006), 78.
21. Ibid.
22. Ibid., 137.
23. Kenny Bruno, "BP: Beyond Petroleum or Beyond Preposterous?," CorpWatch, December 14, 2000, http://www.corpwatch.org/article.php?id=219%20see %20for%20info%20on%20bp%20renewables.
24. Ibid.
25. BP press release, "BP Amoco Invests $45 Million in Solarex Stake to Create World's Biggest Solar Company," April 6, 1999, http://www.bp.com/genericarticle .do?categoryId=2012968&contentId=2001268. See also Agis Salpukas, "It's Official: BP Is Planning to Buy ARCO," New York Times, April 2, 1999, http://www .nytimes.com/1999/04/02/business/it-s-official-bp-is-planning-to-buy-arco .html.

26. Jad Mouawad, "Oil Giants Loath to Follow Obama's Green Lead," *New York Times*, April 7, 2009. Elizabeth Bluemink, "BP Cost Cuts Threaten Alaska's Oil Field Contractors," *Anchorage Daily News*, September 2, 2009.

27. Esty and Winston, *Green to Gold*.

28. Ibid., 140.

29. Laurel Brubaker Calkins and Margaret Cronin Fisk, "Victims of BP's Texas Refinery Explosion Seek $2 Billion," *International Herald Tribune*, November 21, 2007.

30. "BP Settles More Claims from a Texas Refinery Fire," *International Herald Tribune*, February 23, 2007.

31. Felicity Barringer, "Large Oil Spill in Alaska Went Undetected for Days," *New York Times*, March 15, 2006.

32. Ibid.

33. U.S. Chemical Safety Board (CSB), "BP American Refinery Explosion," March 23, 2005, http://www.csb.gov/investigations/detail.aspx?ISID=20.

34. Esty and Winston, *Green to Gold*, 140.

35. Ibid., 141.

36. Cargill, "Our Businesses," http://www.cargill.com/about/organization/business_list.htm.

37. Felicity Lawrence, "Should We Worry About Soya in Our Food?," *Guardian*, July 25, 2006.

38. "Special Report: The Global 2000," Forbes.com, April 2, 2008, http://www.forbes.com/lists/2008/18/biz_2000global08_The-Global-2000_Company_12.html.

39. Roderick Boyd, "Agricultural Giant to Launch Hedge Fund Next Month," *New York Sun*, December 9, 2003.

40. "SunEdison Closes $161 Million in Financing; Six Investment Partners Participate in Solar Energy Services Provider's Equity and Debt Financings," Business Wire, May 23, 2008. Nicole Garrison-Sprenger, "CarVal Growing Beyond Cargill: Equity Group Draws Investors," *St. Paul Pioneer Press*, March 16, 2007.

41. Cargill, "Cargill Global Emissions, Euro Power & Gas Trading," http://www.cargill.com/about/organization/emissions_power_trading.htm.

42. For more about Cargill I highly recommend Felicity Lawrence, *Eat Your Heart Out: Why the Food Business Is Bad for the Planet and Your Health* (London and New York: Penguin Books, 2008). A British journalist, Lawrence travels to Brazil and pieces together the story of the controversial Cargill operation there.

43. Cargill, "Financial Information," http://www.cargill.com/company/financial/index.jsp.

44. *MAP Report 2: Aspirational Environmentalism* (Getty Images).

45. Letter, Joe Bonanno, Nestlé Waters North America, to Joe Holtz, April 14, 2008.

46. "Perdue Farmhouse: Embracing the Future by Rebuilding the Past," *Urner Barry's Reporter*, Spring 2008.

47. Perdue, "Perdue Farms: Who We Are," http://www.perdue.com/company/about/who_we_are.html.

48. See, for instance, *Factory Farm Offender* (Horsham, PA: Farm Sanctuary, 2008).

49. For clients, see http://www.osborn-barr.com.

50. Lisa Rathke, "Ben & Jerry's Opposes Monsanto's Move in Several States to Ban rBGH-Free Labels," Associated Press, February 5, 2008.

51. Donors can be found in the Ducks Unlimited annual report. A selection of donors from 2006: Gold Legacy ($500,000 to $749,999), Bayer CropScience, Dow Chemical, and ExxonMobil; Legacy ($250,000 to $499,999), Monsanto, Penzoil Products, ChevronTexaco, and Coors Brewing; Benefactor ($100,000 to $249,999), Shell Oil Company; Diamond Heritage ($75,000 to $99,999), Cargill; and Heritage ($50,000 to $74,999), Syngenta, Tyson Foods, and Dow AgroSciences.

52. "Syngenta Donates Herbicide to Ducks Unlimited," Ducks Unlimited, http://www.ducks.org/states/25/news/pub/article1424.html.

53. National Agricultural Statistics Services, Agricultural Chemical Use Database, (Washington DC: USDA, 2005).

54. Carl T. Hall, "From Boyhood Curiosity to Scientific Discovery," *San Francisco Chronicle*, November 4, 2002.

55. Professor Tyrone Hayes interviewed by Steve Curwood on Living on Earth, National Public Radio, April 26, 2006, http://www.loe.org/shows/segments.htm?programID=06-P13-00016&segmentID=1.

56. Charles Duhigg, "Debating How Much Weed Killer Is Safe in Your Water Glass," *New York Times*, August 22, 2009.

57. Ibid.

58. Syngenta Global, "Ensuring There is Honey Still for Tea," June 1, 2006, http://www.syngenta.com/en/media/newstopics.01.06.2006.html.

59. Ibid.

60. Tyson Foods, *Sustainability Report: Living Our Core Values*, 2005, http://www.tyson.com/corporate/pressroom/docs/s-2005.pdf.

61. *Summary of Litigation Accomplishments* (Washington, DC: U.S. Department of Justice, Environment and Natural Resources Division, 2003).

62. Tyson Foods, multiple Form 10-Ks, 1999 to 2002, http://www.secinfo.com.

63. *Summary of Litigation Accomplishments* (U.S. Department of Justice).

64. Tyson Foods, *Sustainability Report*, 32.

65. Ibid, 35.

66. Sierra Club, press release, "Tyson on the Hook for Factory Farm Pollution," November 7, 2003, http://www.sierraclub.org/pressroom/releases/pr2003-11-07.asp.

67. Syngenta Global, "Environmental Performance," http://www.syngenta.com/en/corporate_Fresponsibility/hse_environment.html.

68. Ibid.

69. Hoffman, "Regulation" (see chap. 3, n. 87).

70. Ibid.

71. Smithfield Foods, "Smithfield Foods, Inc. 2007 Environmental Excellence Awards," *Smithfield News* 5, no. 1 (2007), http://www.smithfieldfoodsnews.com/volumev_numberi/pageiv.html.

72. Ibid.

73. EPA Toxic Release Inventory data from the EPA TRI Program Web site, http://epa.gov/TRI/.

74. Ibid.

75. Ibid.

76. For information about the Forbes-Ethisphere awards, see http://ethisphere.com/worlds-most-ethical-companies-rankings.

77. Esty and Winston, *Green to Gold*, 13.

78. Ipsos Reid poll conducted from April 19 to April 23, 2007. A randomly selected sample of 1,236 adult home owners was interviewed online.

79. Tom Wright, "False 'Green' Ads Draw Global Scrutiny," *Wall Street Journal*, January 30, 2008.

80. Malaysian Palm Oil Council, http://www.mpoc.org.my/main_coprofile.asp.

81. Wright, "False 'Green' Ads."

82. Advertising Standards Authority, http://www.asa.org.uk/asa.

83. Ibid.

84. Liz Gorman and Jonathan Pocius, "Launch Pad: Communicating Your Green Initiatives," *PRNews*, August 25, 2008.

85. J. Thomas Rosch, "Responsible Green Marketing" (American Conference Institute's Regulatory Summit for Advertisers and Marketers, Washington, DC, June 18, 2008).

86. Personal communication, James Kohm, FTC, summer 2008.

87. The 2007 *GfK Roper Green Gauge Study* is based on findings from two thousand American adults ages eighteen and up surveyed via the GfK Online Consumer Panel in May 2007, http://www.csrwire.com/news/9473.html.

88. Rosch, "Responsible Green Marketing."

89. Ibid.

90. "Ad Groups Tell FTC to Go Slow on Green Marketing Guidelines," Environmental Leader, February 13, 2008, http://www.environmentalleader.com/2008/02/13/ad-groups-tell-ftc-to-go-slow-on-green-marketing-guidelines.

91. Jim Hanna, FTC Green Guide Hearings, Washington, DC, April 30, 2008, http://www.vodium.com/vs_data/transcript/pn100383_ftc81p8sr5y.txt. For more information, see http://www.ftc.gov/bcp/workshops/packaging/index.shtml.

92. Lisa Manley, presentation, Green Communications 2008: The Case Studies Conference, New York City, July 15, 2008.

93. Urs Niggli, Jane Earley, and Kevin Ogorzalek, *Issue Paper: Organic Agriculture and Environmental Stability of the Food Supply* (Rome: FAO, 2007), 4. See also, U.N. Educational, Scientific and Cultural Organization (UNESCO), "World Water Assessment Program," http://www.unesco.org/water/wwap/facts_figures/basic_needs.shtml.

94. Stacy Mitchell, "Wal-Mart Takes Greenwashing to a New Level," Beacon Broadside, April 25, 2008, http://www.newrules.org/retail/article/walmart-takes-greenwashing-new-level. See also, Stacy Mitchell, *Big-Box Swindle: The True Cost of Mega-Retailers and the Fight for America's Independent Businesses*, (Beacon Press, 2006).

95. Ibid.

5. CAPITALIZING ON CLIMATE CHANGE

1. Sergejus Lebedevas, "Use of Waste Fats of Animal and Vegetable Origin for the Production of Biodiesel Fuel," *Energy and Fuels* 20, no. 5 (2006), 2274–2280.

2. Tyson Foods, Form 10-K, 2007.

3. Ibid, 5.

4. Ibid., 13.

5. Ibid. Biofuels production figures based on e-mail communication with Jessica Robinson at the National Biodiesel Board.
6. "AOM Plots Biodiesel Future," *Biodiesel Magazine*, January 2007, http://www.biodieselmagazine.com/article.jsp?article_id=1349.
7. Livestock production in the United States is estimated to be responsible for 55 percent of soil and sediment erosion and roughly one third of nitrogen and phosphorus loading in our drinking water. Pew Commission on Industrial Farm Animal Production, *Putting Meat on the Table: Industrial Farm Animal Production in America* (Baltimore, MD: Johns Hopkins School of Public Health and Pew Charitable Trusts, 2008), 25.
8. Personal communication, Jeff Plowman, Institute for Agriculture and Trade Policy.
9. Personal communication, Jessica Robinson, National Biodiesel Board, January 2009.
10. Pew Commission, "Putting Meat," 23.
11. *Summary of Litigation Accomplishments*, fiscal year 2003 (Washington, DC: U.S. Department of Justice).
12. "Syntroleum & Tyson Get Tax-Free Bond Status for Dynamic Fuels Venture," 247wallst.com, June 20, 2008, http://www.247wallst.com/2008/06/20/syntroleum-tyso.
13. Personal communication, Phelps Dunbar, a lawyer who represents this project. Because the bonds are tax-exempt, they can be offered at interest rates that are 25 to 30 percent lower than the market rate.
14. Personal communication, Kristina Batulis, director of retention and small business development, Ascension Economic Development Corporation, February 20, 2009.
15. Glenn Hess, "Tyson and Syntroleum Partner for Fat-Based Fuel," *Chemical & Engineering News*, June 26, 2007, http://pubs.acs.org/cen/news/85/i27/8527news5.html.
16. Warwick HRI, University of Warwick, *AC0401: Direct Energy Use in Agriculture: Opportunities for Reducing Fossil Fuel Inputs* (Warwick, UK: Department for Environment, Food and Rural Affairs, 2007), 38.
17. Ibid.
18. EPA, AgSTAR Program, http://www.epa.gov/agstar/index.html. In the U.S. in 2008, there were 121 operational digesters, 77 percent on dairy farms, 17 percent on swine farms, 2.4 percent on farms with laying hens.
19. Pew Commission, "Putting Meat." 23.
20. Greenhouse Gas Inventory Summary (2000–2006), California Environmental Protection Agency, Air Resources Board, http://arb.ca.gov/app/ghg/2000-2006/ghg_sector_data.php.
21. Ibid.
22. Janelle Hope Robbins, *Understanding Alternative Technologies for Animal Waste Treatment: A Citizen's Guide to Manure Treatment Technologies* (Irvington, NY: Waterkeeper Alliance, 2005), 68.
23. EPA, press release, "U.S. EPA Celebrates Sonoma County's First Methane Digester," September 25, 2007, http://www.epa.gov/agstar/resources/press.html.
24. EPA, "U.S. EPA Celebrates."

278 NOTES TO PP. 123–146

25. Dennis Frame et al., "Anaerobic Digesters and Methane Production," (Madison: University of Wisconsin, 2001).
26. Pew Commission, "Putting Meat," 53.
27. Robbins, *Understanding Alternative Technologies*, 1.
28. Personal communication, Janelle Hope Robbins, Waterkeeper Alliance.
29. Robbins, *Understanding Alternative Technologies*, 1.
30. Ibid., 11.
31. Personal communication, Robbins, Waterkeeper Alliance. June 2009.
32. Personal communication, Brian Depew, Center for Rural Affairs, August 2008.
33. Dairyland climate-change statement: http://www.dairynet.com/environment/climate_position.php.

6. COOL FOOD: FIVE INGREDIENTS OF CLIMATE-FRIENDLY FARMING

1. "About 90 percent of US cropland is currently losing soil above the sustainable rate." From "Soil and Sediment Erosion," Geoindicators, http://www.lgt.lt/geoin/doc.php?did=cl_soil.
2. J. Russell Smith, *Tree Crops: A Permanent Agriculture* (Washington, D.C.: Island Press, 1987), from the introduction by Wendell Berry. Originally published in 1929. http://journeytoforever.org/farm_library/smith/treecrops1.html.
3. Masanobu Fukuoka, *The One-Straw Revolution: An Introduction to Natural Farming* (Emmaus, PA: Rodale Press, 1978).
4. Smith, *Tree Crops*.
5. Flannery, *The Weather Makers*, 256 (see introduction, n. 9).
6. Paustian, Antle, and Sheehan, *Agriculture's Role*, (see chap. 1, n. 5).
7. Tim J. LaSalle and Paul Hepperly, "Regenerative Agriculture: A Solution to Global Warming," (Kutztown, PA: Rodale Institute, 2008), 3.
8. Paul Hepperly, *Organic Farming Sequesters Atmospheric Carbon and Nutrients in Soils* (Kutztown, PA: Rodale Institute, 2008).
9. Jules Pretty, *Agroecological Approaches to Agricultural Development* (Essex, UK: University of Essex, 2006). http://www.rimsp.org/getdoc.php?docid=6440.
10. Ibid.
11. Ibid.
12. D. G. Hole et al., "Does Organic Farming Benefit Biodiversity?," *Biological Conservation* 122, no. 1 (March, 2005) 113–130. Quote from James Randerson, "Organic Farming Boosts Biodiversity," *New Scientist*, October 11, 2004.
13. Nadia El-Hage Scialabba and Caroline Hattam, *Organic Agriculture, Environment and Food Security* (Rome: FAO, 2002), 90.
14. Rodale Institute, "Organic Crops Perform up to 100 Percent Better in Drought and Flood Years," November 7, 2003, http://www.newfarm.org.
15. Fukuoka, *One-Straw Revolution*, 58.
16. Ken Ausubel and J. P. Harpignies, *Nature's Operating Instructions: The True Biotechnologies* (San Francisco: Sierra Club Books, 2004); Janine M. Benyus, *Biomimicry: Innovation Inspired by Nature*, (New York: Morrow, 1997).
17. Fukuoka, *One-Straw Revolution*.
18. IAASTD, "Summary Report," *Executive Summary of the Synthesis Report* (International Assessment of Agricultural Knowledge, Science and Technology for Development, Johannesburg, South Africa, April 2008), 9.

19. Greenpeace, press release, "Urgent Changes Needed in Global Farming Practices to Avoid Environmental Destruction," April 15, 2008, http://www.greenpeace.org/international/press/releases/changes-to-global-farming.

20. Pesticide Action Network, "The Future of Food and Farming: UN Debate Concludes in Johannesburg," http://www.panna.org/jt/agAssessment.

21. IAASTD press release, "Civil Society Statement from Johannesburg, South Africa: A New Era of Agriculture Begins Today," April 12, 2008, http://www.agassessment.org/docs/civil_society_statement_on_iaastd-28apr08.pdf.

7. MYTH-INFORMED: ANSWERING THE CRITICS

1. La Vía Campesina, http://viacampesina.org/main_en.

2. R. Douglas Hurt, *American Agriculture: A Brief History* (West Lafayette, IN: Purdue University Press, 2002), 405.

3. Estimates of farmers worldwide vary widely, from 2.8 billion (according to La Via Campesina) to 1.3 billion (according to the IPCC's Fourth Assessment).

4. Louis A. Ferleger, "A World of Farmers, but Not a Farmer's World," *Journal of the Historical Society*, Winter 2002.

5. Pesticides: World Health Organization, "The Impact of Pesticides on Health," June 2004, http://www.who.int/mental_health/prevention/suicide/en/Pesticides Health2.pdf. Dead zones: According to a new study in *Science*, there are now 405 identified dead zones worldwide, up from 49 in the 1960s. David Biello, "Oceanic Dead Zones Continue to Spread," *Scientific American*, August 15, 2008, http://www.scientificamerican.com/article.cfm?id=oceanic-dead-zones-spread.

6. "Position of the American Dietetic Association: Agricultural and Food Biotechnology," *Journal of the American Dietetic Association* 106, no. 2 (2006), 285–293.

7. Clive James, "ISAAA Brief 2008," International Service for the Acquisition of Agri-Biotech Applications, 2008, http://www.isaaa.org/resources/publications/briefs/39/pptslides/default.html.

8. Ibid.

9. Ibid.

10. Ibid. Figure calculated from ISAAA data and USDA fact sheet on Chinese agricultural land, www.ers.usda.gov/publications/aib775/aib775e.pdf.

11. *2002 Census of Agriculture*, vol. 1 (Washington, DC: USDA, National Agricultural Statistics Service, 2003), Table 8.

12. For more on La Via Campesina, see Annette Aurelie Desmarais, *La Vía Campesina: Globalization and the Power of Peasants* (Halifax: Fernwood, 2007).

13. Mars, Inc., http://www.mars.hu/global/who+we+are/cocoa+sustainability.htm.

14. Euan Rocha, "Dow Sees Bright Future in Biotech," *Forbes*, June 5, 2008.

15. Editor, "Chairman of Syngenta's Board High on Modern Agriculture," *Better Farming, USA*, April 6, 2008.

16. Ibid.

17. David Lees, "Food by Design: Giant Monsanto Thinks It's Got the Answer to the World's Food Problems. Its Critics Argue That Genetic Engineering Can Be Dangerous," *Financial Post*, October 1, 1998.

18. Jeffrey Sachs, *The End of Poverty: Economic Possibilities for Our Time* (New York: Penguin Press, 2005), 18.

19. *Rural Poverty Report 2001—The Challenge of Ending Rural Poverty* (International Fund for Agricultural Development, 2001), 15–16. See also *World Development Report 2008: Agriculture for Development* (Washington, DC: World Bank, 2007), 95.

20. CIA, the World Factbook, 2007, http://www.cia.gov/library/publications/the-world-factbook/geos/ks.html.

21. *Dumping Without Borders: How US Agricultural Policies Are Destroying the Livelihoods of Mexican Corn Farmers*, briefing paper, no. 50 (Oxfam, 2003). See also "Mexico: NAFTA Corn," *Migration News* 6, no. 4 (February 2000).

22. Desmarais, *La Vía Campesina*, 33.

23. Ted Nordhaus and Michael Shellenberger, *Break Through: From the Death of Environmentalism to the Politics of Possibility* (Boston: Houghton Mifflin, 2007), 6.

24. Ibid., 27.

25. Ibid.

26. U.S. Department of Energy, "Making Coal Cleaner for the Future," http://www.energy.gov/discovery/making_coal_cleaner.html.

27. Elizabeth Economy, "The Great Leap Backward," *Foreign Affairs*, September 1, 2007.

28. For more information about the lawsuit, see the documentary *Crude: The Real Price of Oil* and visit http://www.chevrontoxico.com.

8. THE HUNGER SCARE

1. BIO International Convention workshop, "Organic Agriculture and Biotechnology: Won't You Be My Neighbor," Philadelphia, 2005.

2. Andrew Pollack, "In Lean Times, Biotech Grains Are Less Taboo," *International Herald Tribune*, April 21, 2008.

3. Deborah Keith of Syngenta, "Comment and Analysis," *New Scientist*, April 5, 2008.

4. Clancy Gebler Davies, "Twenty Questions: Michael Pragnell, Chief Executive Officer of Syngenta," *Independent*, April 11, 2001.

5. Ibid.

6. Jonathon Riley, "GM Crops Greener Than Organic Ones, Says Chem Maker," *Farmers Weekly*, May 29, 1998.

7. Ibid.

8. See, for instance, National Association of Wheat Growers, "Wheat Industry Biotechnology Principles for Commercialization," November 2008, http://www.wheatworld.org/userfiles/file/wheat%20industry%20biotech%20principles%20for%20commercialization.pdf.

9. Catherine Badgley et al., "Organic Agriculture and the Global Food Supply," *Renewable Agriculture and Food Systems* 22, no. 2 (2007): 86–108, 90, table 3.

10. Badgley et al., "Organic Agriculture," 86.

11. Ibid.

12. Pretty, *Agroecological Approaches* (see chap. 6, n. 9).

13. Bryan Walsh, "Can Slow Food Feed the World?," *Time*, September 4, 2008.

14. Ibid.

15. Ibid.

16. Personal communication, Christopher Matthews, FAO Media Relations, November 2008.

17. Eric Reguly, "No Organic for Me, Please," *Globe and Mail*, August 29, 2008.

18. Ibid.

19. Scott DeCarlo, "The World's Biggest Companies," Forbes.com, April 2, 2008, www.forbes.com/2008/04/02/worlds-largest-companies-biz-2000global08-cx_sd_0402global_land.html.

20. Reguly, "No Organic."

21. Ibid.

22. Ibid.

23. Personal communication, Niels Halberg, International Centre for Research in Organic Food Systems, September 9, 2008.

24. Niels Halberg et al., "The Impact of Organic Farming on Food Security in a Regional and Global Perspective," in N. Halberg et al., eds., *Global Development of Organic Agriculture: Challenges and Promises* (CAB International, 2005).

25. Halberg et al., "Impact of Organic Farming," 2.

26. Ibid., 6. Sub-Saharan Africa is the only region in the world in which the number and proportion of malnourished children have been rising consistently over the years, according to analysts at IFPRI. Rosegrant et al., *2020 Global Food Outlook*.

27. Personal communication, Halberg.

28. Christine Zundel and Lukas Kilcher, "Issues Paper: Organic Agriculture and Food Availability," *International Conference on Organic Agriculture and Food Security* (Rome: FAO, 2007), 17–18.

29. Personal communication, Catherine Badgley, University of Michigan, February 2009.

9. THE BIOTECH BALLYHOO

1. Martin Brookes and Andy Coghlan, "Live and Let Live," *New Scientist*, October 31, 1998.

2. Editorial, "New Crop Is Said to Aid Nutrition," *New York Times*, December 10, 1999.

3. Robert Shapiro, "Agriculture and Biotechnology: Considerations for the Future," speech, Fourth Annual Greenpeace Business Conference, London, October 6, 1999, http://news.bbc.co.uk/2/hi/science/nature/468147.stm.

4. Data on acreage: ISAAA, http://www.isaaa.org.

5. African Agricultural Technology Foundation, "Project 4: Water Efficient Maize for Africa (WEMA)," personal communication, Grace Wachoro, AATF, January 14, 2009. See also http://www.monsanto.com/pdf/droughttolerantcorn/wema_project_brief.pdf.

6. Funding information: AATF, http://www.aatf-africa.org.

7. Eric James Vettel, *Biotech: The Countercultural Origins of an Industry* (Philadelphia: University of Pennsylvania Press, 2006), 8–12.

8. WEMA, press release, "African Agricultural Technology Foundation to Develop Drought-Tolerant Maize Varieties for Small-Scale Farmers in Africa," March 19, 2008, http://www.aatf-africa.org/newsdetail.php?newsid=95.

9. Kristi Heim, "Want to Work for the Gates Foundation?" *Seattle Times*, October 17, 2006.

10. Anuradha Mittal and Melissa Moore, *Voices from Africa: African Farmers and Environmentalists Speak Out Against a New Green Revolution in Africa* (Oakland, CA: Oakland Institute, 2009), 2.

11. AATF, http://www.aatf-africa.org/about_aatf.php?subcat=3&sublev=5&staff_id=1&mode=more. According to its detractors, ISAAA's purpose "is to facilitate the delivery of proprietary biotechnologies from the corporate labs of the industrialized world into the food and farming systems of the [Global] South." Devlin Kuyek, "ISAAA in Asia: Promoting Corporate Profits in the Name of the Poor," GRAIN, October 2000, http://www.grain.org/briefings/?id=137#2.

12. Among other funding, Rockefeller supported the *2007 ISAAA Report on Global Status of Biotech/GM Crops*, according to Clive James, ISAAA Board of Directors. http://www.isaaa.org/resources/publications/briefs/37/pptslides/briefs-37-flashpaper.swf.

13. AATF, "Water Efficient Maize." See also Irma Venter, "Kenyan Group Moves Ahead with Drought-Tolerant Maize Innovation, *Creamer Media's Engineering News*, April 25, 2008.

14. Salamander Davoudi, "Monsanto: Giant of the $6.15bn GM Market," *Financial Times*, November 15, 2006.

15. Richard Weiss, "BASF Sees $2 Billion Value From Monsanto Seed Venture," Bloomberg News, August 4, 2009, http://www.bloomberg.com/apps/news?pid=20601100&sid=alMaAZmg56w8.

16. Personal communication, Wachoro, January 14, 2009.

17. David Adam, "GM Will Not Solve Current Food Crisis, Says Industry Boss," *Guardian*, June 27, 2008.

18. Clive James, "ISAAA Brief 37-2007: Executive Summary," International Service for the Acquisition of Agri-Biotech Applications, 2007, http://isaaa.org/resources/publications/briefs/37/executivesummary/default.html.

19. Denise Caruso, *Intervention: Confronting the Real Risks of Genetic Engineering and Life on a Biotech Planet* (San Francisco: Hybrid Vigor Institute, 2006).

20. H. S. Chawla, *Introduction to Plant Biotechnology*, (Enfield, NH: Science Publishers, 2002), 153.

21. Barry Commoner, "Unraveling the DNA Myth: The Spurious Foundation of Genetic Engineering," *Harpers*, February 2002. See also Denise Caruso, "RE:FRAMING: A Challenge to Gene Theory, a Tougher Look at Biotech," *New York Times*, July 1, 2007.

22. Personal communication, Chapela.

23. Ignacio Chapela, presentation, "Things Are Often Not What They Appear," Academic Senate of the University of California, Berkeley Division, March 8, 2007.

24. Ignacio Chapela and David Quist, "Transgenic DNA Introgressed into Traditional Maize Landraces in Oaxaca, Mexico," *Nature* 414, (2001) 541–543.

25. Coverage of this incident can be found in the *Guardian*. See George Monbiot, "Corporations Are Inventing People to Rubbish Their Opponents on the Internet," *Guardian*, May 14, 2002.

26. Jack Heinemann, *A Typology of the Effects of (Trans)gene Flow on the Conservation and Sustainable Use of Genetic Resources* (Rome: FAO, Commission on Genetic Resources for Food and Agriculture, 2007).

27. Patrick Walter, "Anti-Gas Grass: Climate-Change-Ready Grasses Promise to Up Milk Production and Cut Methane Emissions," *Chemistry and Industry*, May 5, 2008.

28. Ibid.

29. " 'Burpless' Grass Cuts Methane Gas from Cattle, May Help Reduce Global Warming," ScienceDaily, May 8, 2008, http://www.sciencedaily.com/releases/2008/05/080506120859.htm.

30. Personal communication, Doug Gurian-Sherman, Union of Concerned Scientists, April 2009. See also Doug Gurian-Sherman, *Contaminating the Wild? Gene Flow from Experimental Field Trials of Genetically Engineered Crops to Related Wild Plants* (Washington, DC: Center for Food Safety, 2006).

31. Jill Carroll, "Reviews of Crops Altered by Genetics Are 'Superficial,' " *Wall Street Journal*, February 21, 2002.

32. Biotech detractors have also raised human- and animal-health concerns about genetically modified crops. For an overview, see Jeffrey M. Smith, *Genetic Roulette: The Documented Health Risks of Genetically Engineered Foods* (Fairfield, IA: Yes! Books, 2007).

33. Paul Brown, "GM Crops Created Superweed, Say Scientists," *Guardian*, July 25, 2005.

34. Personal communication, Gurian-Sherman.

35. See details about weeds and herbicide resistance here: http://www.weedscience.org/summary/uspeciesmoa.asp?lstmoaid=12&fmhracgroup=go.

36. D. N. Shepherd et al., "Novel Sugarcane Streak and Sugarcane Streak Reunion Mastreviruses from Southern Africa and La Réunion," *Archives of Virology* 153 (2008).

37. Steve Connor, "Farmers Use As Much Pesticide with GM Crops, US Study Finds," *Independent*, July 27, 2006; Shengui Wang, David Just, and Per Pinstrup-Andersen, "Tarnishing Silver Bullets: Bt Technology Adoption, Bounded Rationality, and the Outbreak of Secondary Pest Infestations in China," in *American Agricultural Economics Association Annual Meeting* (Long Beach, CA: 2006).

38. Wang, Just, and Pinstrup-Andersen, "Tarnishing Silver Bullets," 6.

39. William Underhill and Marisa Katz, "High Tech Harvests: Some Europeans Fear Biotech Food," *Newsweek International*, July 13, 1998.

40. For an analysis on GMO and yields, see Doug Gurian-Sherman, *Failure to Yield* (Washington, DC: Union of Concerned Scientists, 2008).

41. Chuck Benbrook, *Evidence of the Magnitude and Consequences of the Roundup Ready Soybean Yield Drag from University-Based Varietal Trials in 1998* (Sandpoint, ID: Ag BioTech InfoNet, 1999).

42. Ibid.

43. A. Turrini, C. Sbrana, and M. Giovannetti, "Experimental Systems to Monitor the Impact of Transgenic Corn on Keystone Soil Microorganisms" (paper, IFOAM Organic World Congress, Modena, Italy, June 16–20, 2008).

44. Bill Freese, *The StarLink Affair: A Critique of the Government/Industry Response to Contamination of the Food Supply with StarLink Corn and an Examination of the Potential Allergenicity of StarLink's Cry9C Protein* (Washington, DC: FIFRA Scientific Advisory Panel Considering Assessment of Additional Scientific Information Concerning StarLink™ Corn, 2001).

45. James, "ISAAA Brief 37-2007."

46. A. J. Haughton et al., "Invertebrate Responses to the Management of Genetically Modified Herbicide-Tolerant and Conventional Spring Crops," *Philosophical Transactions: Biological Sciences* 358, no. 1439 (2003).

47. Suzanne J. Clark, Peter Rothery, and Joe N. Perry, "Farm Scale Evaluations of Spring-Sown Genetically Modified Herbicide-Tolerant Crops: A Statistical Assessment," *Philosophical Transactions: Biological Sciences* 358, no. 1439 (2003).

48. "Tracing the Trend Towards Market Concentration," presentation, U.N. Conference on Trade and Development, April 2006.

49. Matthew Dillon, "Monsanto Buys Seminis," *Organic Broadcaster*, March/April 2005.

50. Monsanto and De Ruiter Seeds, press release, "Monsanto Company Announces Agreement to Acquire De Ruiter Seeds, a Leading Global Vegetable Seed Company," March 31, 2008, http://www.monsanto.com/deruiterseeds/default.asp.

51. F. William Engdahl, " 'Doomsday Seed Vault' in the Arctic: Bill Gates, Rockefeller and the GMO Giants Know Something We Don't," Global Research, December 4, 2007, http://www.globalresearch.ca/index.php?context=va&aid=7529; Centre for Genetic Resources, "Svalbard Global Seed Vault: Frequently Asked Questions," February 22, 2008, http://www.cgn.wur.nl/uk/newsagenda/archive/news/2008/cgn_seeds_in_svalbard_global_seed_vault.htm.

52. Adam, "GM Will Not Solve."

53. Fifty-seven governments approved the *Executive Summary of the Synthesis Report*. An additional three governments—Australia, Canada, and the United States—did not fully approve the document, and their reservations are entered in the Annex. IAASTD, "Summary Report," *Executive Summary of the Synthesis Report*.

54. Editorial, "Deserting the Hungry?," *Nature* 451, no. 7176 (2008), 223–24.

55. Keith, "Comment and Analysis," 18 (see chap. 8, n. 4).

56. Personal communication, Martin Clough and Anne Birch, Syngenta, September 9, 2008.

57. Robert L. Paarlberg, *Starved for Science: How Biotechnology Is Being Kept Out of Africa* (Cambridge, MA: Harvard University Press, 2008).

58. Ibid.

59. Mittal and Moore, *Voices from Africa*, 4.

60. Sue Edwards et al., *The Impact of Compost Use on Crop Yields in Tigray, Ethiopia, 2000–2006 Inclusive* (Rome: FAO, 2008).

61. Personal communication, Sue Edwards, Tigray Project, February 2009.

62. Quoted in Mittal and Moore, *Voices from Africa*, 5.

63. Edwards et al., *Impact of Compost Use*.

64. Environment and Development UNEP-UNCTAD Capacity-Building Task Force on Trade, *Organic Agriculture and Food Security in Africa* (Geneva: United Nations, 2008).

65. Thomas Hargrove, "World Fertilizer Prices Soar as Food and Fuel Economies Merge," International Center for Soil Fertility and Agricultural Development, February 19, 2008, http://www.ifdc.org.

66. AATF, http://www.aatf-africa.org/aatf_projects.php?sublevelone=30&subcat=5.

67. Nicholas Sitko, "Maize, Food Insecurity, and the Field of Performance in Southern Zambia," *Agriculture and Human Values* 25 no. 1 (January 2008): 4.

68. National Academy of Sciences, *Lost Crops of Africa*, vol. 3, *Fruits*; *Lost Crops of Africa*, vol. 2, *Vegetables*; *Lost Crops of Africa*, vol. 1, *Grains* (Washington, DC: National Academy of Sciences, 2008, 2006, 1996).

10. EAT THE SKY: SEVEN PRINCIPLES OF A CLIMATE-FRIENDLY DIET

1. "Estimated Annual Sales and Market Share of the Top 15 Supermarket Chains in 2005," from *Progressive Grocer* 2006.
2. Marion Nestle, *What to Eat*, (New York: North Point Press, 2006). See also Marion Nestle, *Food Politics: How the Food Industry Influences Nutrition and Health* (Berkeley: University of California Press, 2002).
3. For more information on farmers' markets, visit USDA, http://www.ams.usda.gov.
4. Personal communication, Gurian-Sherman (see chap. 9, n. 40).
5. Steinfeld et al., *Livestock's Long Shadow*, xxi (see Introduction, n. 4). See also Smith et al., "Agriculture," 510 (see chap. 1, n. 26).
6. Steinfeld et al., *Livestock's Long Shadow*, xxi.
7. Pachauri, "Global Warning" (see introduction, n. 8). The USDA has slightly different figures, claiming that at least half of all corn and 80 percent of all soy is diverted from human consumption to the livestock industry. USDA ERS, *Feed Grains Database* (see chap. 1, n. 38).
8. Steinfeld et al., *Livestock's Long Shadow*.
9. Naylor et al., "Effect of Aquaculture."
10. L. Reijnders and S. Soret, "Quantification of the Environmental Impact of Different Dietary Protein Choices," *American Journal of Clinical Nutrition* 78, supp. (2003).
11. The Cornell study focused on farming and food consumption in New York State. The researchers found that if every New Yorker adopted a low-fat, plant-centered diet, Empire State farms could feed roughly 50 percent more people—about a third of the state's population. Christian J. Peters, Jennifer L. Wilkins, and Gary W. Fick, "Testing a Complete-Diet Model for Estimating the Land Resource Requirements of Food Consumption and Agricultural Carrying Capacity: The New York State Example," *Renewable Agriculture and Food Systems* 22, no. 2 (2007).
12. L. Baroni, et. al., "Evaluating the Environmental Impact of Various Dietary Patterns Combined with Different Food Production Systems," *European Journal of Clinical Nutrition*, vol. 61, October 2006, 279–286.
13. On the importance of upping our vegetable intake, see, for example, Walter Willett et al., *Eat, Drink, and Be Healthy: The Harvard Medical School Guide to Healthy Eating* (New York: Free Press, 2005). See also Mollie Katzen and Walter Willett, *Eat, Drink, and Weigh Less* (New York: Hyperion, 2006); T. Colin Campbell and Thomas M. Campbell, *The China Study: The Most Comprehensive Study of Nutrition Ever Conducted and the Startling Implications for Diet, Weight Loss and Long-Term Health*, (Dallas: BenBella Books, 2006).
14. ERS, "*Agricultural Baseline Projections: U.S. Livestock, 2009–2018*," (Washington, DC: USDA, 2009); McMichael et al., "Food, Livestock Production."
15. The workshop was called "Health, Wellness & the Meat Department: Turning a Negative Rap into a Good Wrap!" Meat Conference, Gaylord Opryland Resort and Convention Center, March 9–11, 2008.

16. Data are based on ERS estimates of per-capita quantities of food available for consumption, on imputed consumption data for foods no longer reported on by the ERS, and on estimates from the USDA.

17. *Food, Nutrition, Physical Activity, and the Prevention of Cancer: A Global Perspective* (Washington, DC: World Cancer Research Fund, 2007). In addition, a study published last year, researchers at the National Institutes of Health found that both "red and processed meat intakes were positively associated with cancers of the colorectum and lung; furthermore, red meat intake was associated with an elevated risk for cancers of the esophagus and liver." Amanda Cross et al., "A Prospective Study of Red and Processed Meat Intake in Relation to Cancer Risk," *PLoS Medicine* 4, no. 12 (2007). In a 2006 meta-study, researchers at Sweden's National Institute of Environmental Medicine surveyed fifteen studies of red-meat consumption and fourteen studies of processed-meat consumption. They found that "consumption of red meat and processed meat was positively associated with risk of both colon and rectal cancer, although the association with red meat appeared to be stronger for rectal cancer." Susanna C. Larsson and Alicja Wolk, "Meat Consumption and Risk of Colorectal Cancer: A Meta-Analysis of Prospective Studies," *International Journal of Cancer* 119, no. 11 (2006).

18. *Food, Nutrition.* Not everyone agreed with the fund's recommendations. The American Meat Institute responded with a press release that claimed the recommendations reflected the fund's "well-known anti-meat bias and should be met with skepticism." The AMI's only counter-evidence, though, was a reference to an unpublished 2004 study from the Harvard School of Public Health of 725,000 men and women that allegedly "showed no relationship between" meat consumption and cancer. My research assistant and I were initially unable to locate the study, nor could the HSPH's communications office when we first contacted it. I followed up with Dr. Walter Willett, chair of the Department of Nutrition at the School of Public Health, and he could only guess that the AMI was referring to an abstract from a preliminary analysis. The study has since concluded, with more data collected and a paper on its way, and its findings also raise concerns about a diet of heavy meat consumption.

19. Cross et al., "Prospective Study." See also Rashmi Sinha et al., "Meat Intake and Mortality: A Prospective of Over Half a Million People," *Archives of Internal Medicine* 169, no. 6 (2009).

20. The organic regulations were first authorized under the Organic Foods Production Act of 1990, and they regulate the domestic marketing of organically produced fresh and processed food. The final rule was published in December 2000 but didn't go into effect until October 21, 2002.

21. David Pimentel, *Impacts of Organic Farming on the Efficiency of Energy Use in Agriculture* (Ithaca, NY: Organic Center, 2006), 9.

22. Wenonah Hauter and Mark Worth, *Zapped: Irradiation and the Death of Food* (Washington, DC: Food & Water Watch, 2008).

23. Meredith Niles, "Sustainable Soils: Reducing, Mitigating, and Adapting to Climate Change with Organic Agriculture," *Sustainable Development Law & Policy,* 2008: 20. See also Pimentel and Pimentel, *Food, Energy, and Society* (see chap. 3, n. 29).

24. See, for instance, D. A. Boadi et al., "Effect of Low and High Forage Diet on En-

teric and Manure Pack Greenhouse Gas Emissions from a Feedlot," *Canadian Journal of Animal Science* 84 (2004); H. A. DeRamus et al., "Methane Emissions of Beef Cattle on Forages: Efficiency of Grazing Management Systems," *Journal of Environmental Quality* 32 (2003). See also Pimentel and Pimentel, *Food, Energy, and Society.*

25. Joanna Pearlstein, "Surprise! Conventional Agriculture Can Be Easier on the Planet," *Wired*, June 19, 2008.

26. *Behind the Bean: The Heroes and Charlatans of the Natural and Organic Soy Foods Industry* (Cornucopia Institute, 2009). The USDA doesn't track volume of organic-food imports, so there is no official record confirming, or challenging, this figure.

27. James McWilliams, "Food That Travels Well," *New York Times*, August 6, 2007. Less than a year after the study praising New Zealand lamb and other products was published, one of its authors, Professor Caroline Saunders of Lincoln University, was quoted in a University National Lamb Day press release trumpeting that lamb she had so praised. "The story of New Zealand's sheepmeat export industry is a marvelous one," said Saunders. "It contains all the ingredients of personal initiative, enterprise and persistence that are seen in so many commercial successes. It well deserves celebrating." And her study celebrated it well, giving the industry a boost, from the pages of the Gray Lady to the online home of the World Trade Organization.

28. World Trade Organization, "The Impact of Trade Opening on Climate Change," http://www.wto.org/english/tratop_e/envir_e/climate_impact_e.htm.

29. Energy Information and Modeling Group of the Ministry of Economic Development, "New Zealand Energy Data File—2009," 2009, http://www.med.govt.nz/upload/68617/1_Energy%20Data%20File%202009LR.pdf, 98.

30. Department of Energy and Climate Change, "The UK Renewable Energy Strategy 2009—Executive Summary," August, 27, 2009, 4, http://www.decc.gov.uk/en/content/cms/what_we_do/uk_supply/energy_mix/renewable/res/res.aspx.

31. U.N. Environment Programme, Climate Neutral Network, http://www.unep.org/climateneutral/default.aspx?tabid=154.

32. Natural Resources Defense Council, "Food Miles: How Far Your Food Travels Has Serious Consequences for Your Health and the Climate," (Washington, D. C.: NRDC, 2007).

33. Matthew Mariola, "The Local Industrial Complex? Questioning the Link Between Local Foods and Energy Use," *Agriculture and Human Values* 25 (2008).

34. Natural Resources Defense Council, "Food miles," 4.

35. Barry Wallerstein, South Coast Air Quality Management District, quoted in "EPA Pressured to Cut Ship Pollution," Forbes.com, February 13, 2008.

36. American Farmland Trust, Fact Sheet, http://www.farmland.org/news/media/documents/aftfactsheet.pdf.

37. Martin Heller and Gregory Keoleian, *Life Cycle-Based Sustainability Indicators for Assessment of the U.S. Food System* (Ann Arbor, MI: Center for Sustainable Systems, University of Michigan, 2000), 14.

38. Elizabeth Royte, *Bottlemania: How Water Went on Sale and Why We Bought It* (New York: Bloomsbury, 2008).

39. Charlie Goodyear, "S.F. First City to Ban Plastic Shopping Bags," *San Francisco Chronicle*, March 28, 2007.

40. Sean Alfano, "Big Mac Hits the Big 4-0," CBSNews.com, August 24, 2007.
41. Goodyear, "S.F. First City." Jared Blumenfeld, director of the city's Department of the Environment.
42. "Irish Bag Tax Hailed Success," BBC News, August 20, 2002.
43. "Enact Global Plastic Bags Ban, Says UN Environment Chief," NowPublic.com, June 9, 2009.
44. http://www01.smgov.net/cityclerk/council/agendas/2007/20070109/s200701007 -a.htm.

11. BEYOND THE FORK

1. Jonathan Tirone, " 'Dead-end' Austrian Town Blossoms with Green Energy," Bloomberg News, August 28, 2007.
2. James M. Jasper, *The Art of Moral Protest: Culture, Biography, and Creativity in Social Movements* (Chicago: University of Chicago Press, 1997), 251–53.
3. Brook Lyndhurst, *London's Food Sector*.
4. Ibid.
5. Ibid., 29–30.
6. Learn more about the policy here: http://www.seattleglobaljustice.org/wp -content/uploads/Local%20Food%20Action%20Initiative%20April%202009 .pdf.

CONCLUSION

1. Kolbert, "Catastrophist."
2. Kathleen Merrigan, speech, All Things Organic, June 23, 2009.
3. "Agency Says Germans Should Eat Less Meat," *The Local*, January 22, 2009, http://www.thelocal.de/national/20090122-16931.html.
4. "Death Toll in Peru Violence Rises to 34: Official," *China Post*, June 9, 2009, http://www.chinapost.com.tw/international/americas/2009/06/09/211432/death -toll.htm.

SELECTED BIBLIOGRAPHY

Ausubel, Ken, and J. P. Harpignies, *Nature's Operating Instructions: The True Biotechnologies.* (San Francisco: Sierra Club Books, 2004).

Baldwin, Cheryl, *Sustainability in the Food Industry.* (Ames, IA: Wiley-Blackwell, 2009).

Barber, Benjamin R., *Jihad vs. McWorld.* (New York: Ballantine Books, 1996).

Barker, Rodney, *And the Waters Turned to Blood: The Ultimate Biological Threat.* (New York, NY: Simon & Schuster, 1997).

Bender, Daniel E., and Richard A. Greenwald, *Sweatshop USA: The American Sweatshop in Historical and Global Perspective.* (New York: Routledge, 2003).

Benyus, Janine M., *Biomimicry: Innovation Inspired by Nature.* (New York: Morrow, 1997).

Berry, Wendell, *The Way of Ignorance: And Other Essays.* (Emeryville, CA: Shoemaker & Hoard, 2005).

Bové, José, and François Dufour, *Food for the Future: Agriculture for a Global Age.* (Malden, MA: Polity Press, 2005).

Campbell, T. Colin, and Thomas M. Campbell, *The China Study: The Most Comprehensive Study of Nutrition Ever Conducted and the Startling Implications for Diet, Weight Loss and Long-Term Health.* (Dallas, TX: BenBella Books, 2006).

Caruso, Denise, *Intervention: Confronting the Real Risks of Genetic Engineering and Life on a Biotech Planet.* (San Francisco, CA: Hybrid Vigor Institute, 2006).

Clay, Jason W., *World Agriculture and the Environment: A Commodity-by-Commodity Guide to Impacts and Practices.* (Washington, D.C.: Island Press, 2004).

Connor, John M., *Global Price Fixing: Our Customers Are the Enemy.* (Boston: Kluwer Academic, 2001).

Davis, Mike, *Planet of Slums.* (London: Verso, 2007).

Desmarais, Annette Aurelie, *La Vía Campesina: Globalization and the Power of Peasants.* (Halifax: Fernwood, 2007).

Esty, Daniel C., and Andrew S. Winston, *Green to Gold: How Smart Companies Use Environmental Strategy to Innovate, Create Value, and Build Competitive Advantage.* (New Haven: Yale University Press, 2006).

Ettlinger, Steve, *Twinkie, Deconstructed.* (New York, NY: Hudson Street Press, 2007).

Fukuoka, Masanobu, *The One-Straw Revolution: An Introduction to Natural Farming.* (Emmaus: Rodale Press, 1978).

Halweil, Brian, *Eat Here: Reclaiming Homegrown Pleasures in a Global Supermarket.* 1st ed. (New York: W.W. Norton, 2004).

Halweil, Brian, Thomas Prugh, and Worldwatch Institute, *Home Grown: The Case for Local Food in a Global Market.* (Washington, D.C.: Worldwatch Institute, 2002).

Ho, Mae-Wan, Sam Burcher, and Lim Li Ching, *Food Futures Now: Organic, Sustainable, and Fossil Fuel Free*. (Third World Network and Institute of Science and Society, 2008).

IPCC, *Climate Change 2007: Fourth Assessment Report of the Intergovernmental Panel on Climate Change*. (New York: Cambridge University Press, 2007).

Jansen, Kees, and Sietze Vellema, *Agribusiness and Society: Corporate Responses to Environmentalism, Market Opportunities and Public Regulation*. (London: Zed Books, 2004).

King, F. H., *Farmers of Forty Centuries*. (Madison, WI: Mrs. F.H. King, 1911).

Kolbert, Elizabeth, *Field Notes from a Catastrophe: Man, Nature, and Climate Change*. (New York: Bloomsbury, 2006).

Lappé, Anna, and Bryant Terry, *Grub: Ideas for an Urban Organic Kitchen*. (New York: Jeremy P. Tarcher/Putnam, 2004).

Lappé, Frances Moore, *Diet for a Small Planet*. Twentieth anniversary edition. (New York: Ballantine Books, 1991).

Lappé, Frances Moore, Joseph Collins, and Cary Fowler, *Food First: Beyond the Myth of Scarcity*. (Boston: Houghton-Mifflin, 1977).

Lappé, Frances Moore, Joseph Collins, Peter Rosset, Luis Esparza, *World Hunger: Twelve Myths*. (San Francisco: Grove Press, 1998).

Lappé, Frances Moore, and Anna Lappé, *Hope's Edge: The Next Diet for a Small Planet*. (New York: Jeremy P. Tarcher/Putnam, 2003).

Lawrence, Felicity, *Eat Your Heart Out: Why the Food Business is Bad for the Planet and Your Health*. (New York: Penguin Books, 2008).

McKibben, Bill, *Deep Economy: The Wealth of Communities and the Durable Future*. (New York: Times Books, 2007).

McNeely, Jeffrey A., and Sara J. Scherr, *Ecoagriculture: Strategies to Feed the World and Save Wild Biodiversity*. (Washington: Island Press, 2003).

Michaels, David, *Doubt is their Product: How Industry's Assault on Science Threatens Your Health*. (New York: Oxford University Press, 2008).

Micheletti, Michele, Andreas Føllesdal, and Dietlind Stolle, *Politics, Products, and Markets: Exploring Political Consumerism Past and Present*. (New Brunswick, NJ: Transaction Publishers, 2004).

Nestle, Marion, *Food Politics: How the Food Industry Influences Nutrition and Health*. (Berkeley: University of California Press, 2002).

———, *What to Eat*. (New York: North Point Press, 2006).

Patel, Raj, *Stuffed and Starved: The Hidden Battle for the World Food System*. (Brooklyn, NY: Melville House, 2008).

Pollan, Michael, *The Omnivore's Dilemma: A Natural History of Four Meals*. (New York: Penguin Press, 2006).

Princen, Thomas, Michael Maniates, and Ken Conca, *Confronting Consumption*. (Cambridge, MA: MIT Press, 2002).

Richardson, Jill, *Recipe for America: Why Our Food System is Broken and What We Can Do to Fix It*. 1st ed. (Brooklyn, NY: Ig, 2009).

Roberts, Paul, *The End of Food*. (Boston: Houghton Mifflin Company, 2008).

Rogers, Heather, *Gone Tomorrow: The Hidden Life of Garbage*. (New York: New Press, 2005).

Rosenzweig, Cynthia, and Daniel Hillel, *Climate Change and the Global Harvest: Po-*

tential Impacts of the Greenhouse Effect on Agriculture. (New York: Oxford University Press, 1998).

Royte, Elizabeth, *Bottlemania: How Water Went on Sale and Why We Bought It.* (New York: Bloomsbury, 2008).

Sachs, Jeffrey, *The End of Poverty: Economic Possibilities for Our Time.* (New York: Penguin Press, 2005).

Scherr, Sara J., and Jeffrey A. McNeely, *Farming with Nature: The Science and Practice of Ecoagriculture.* (Washington, D.C.: Island Press, 2007).

Shiva, Vandana, *Earth Democracy: Justice, Sustainability, and Peace.* (Cambridge, MA: South End Press, 2005).

———, *Manifestos on the Future of Food and Seed.* (Cambridge, MA: South End Press, 2007).

———, *Monocultures of the Mind: Perspectives on Biodiversity and Biotechnology.* (Dehra Dun: Natraj Publishers, 1993).

———, *Soil Not Oil: Environmental Justice in a Time of Climate Crisis.* (Cambridge, MA: South End Press, 2008).

———, *Stolen Harvest.* (Cambridge, MA: South End Press, 2000).

Smith, J. Russell, *Tree Crops: A Permanent Agriculture.* (New York: Harcourt, Brace, 1929).

Steinfeld, Henning, Pierre Gerber, T. D. Wassenaar, Vincent Castel, Mauricio Rosales, Cees de Haan, Food and Agriculture Organization of the United Nations. *Livestock's Long Shadow: Environmental Issues and Options.* (Rome: Food and Agriculture Organization of the United Nations, 2006).

Stern, N. H., *The Economics of Climate Change: The Stern Review.* (Cambridge: Cambridge University Press, 2007).

Tal, Alon, *Speaking of Earth: Environmental Speeches That Moved the World.* (New Brunswick, NJ: Rutgers University Press, 2006).

Tannahill, Reay, *Food in History.* (New York City: Three Rivers Press, 1988).

Vettel, Eric James, *Biotech: The Countercultural Origins of an Industry.* (Philadelphia: University of Pennsylvania Press, 2006).

Weber, Karl, ed., *Food, Inc.: How Industrial Food is Making us Sicker, Fatter and Poorer—And What You Can Do About it.* 1st ed. (New York: PublicAffairs, 2009).

Weis, Tony, *The Global Food Economy: The Battle for the Future of Farming.* (London: Zed Books, 2007).

Willett, Walter, P. J. Skerrett, Edward L. Giovannucci, and Maureen Callahan, *Eat, Drink, and Be Healthy: The Harvard Medical School Guide to Healthy Eating.* (New York: Free Press, 2005).

Winne, Mark, *Closing the Food Gap: Resetting the Table in the Land of Plenty.* (Boston: Beacon Press, 2009).

ACTION & LEARNING RESOURCES

I. ORGANIZATIONS

You've read about many of these organizations throughout the book. Here they are in one place for easier reference. Find more online at www .takeabite.cc.

You can find out more about my work at www.smallplanet.org and www.smallplanetfund.org.

350.ORG
(International)
Launched by environmentalist Bill McKibben, 350.org is an international campaign building grassroots support for real solutions to the climate crisis. 350.org has connected concerned citizens in at least 181 countries.
www.350.org

AGRICULTURE AND PUBLIC HEALTH GATEWAY
(Johns Hopkins University, Baltimore, Maryland)
Lots of good resources on the impact of agriculture on climate change and climate change on agriculture. Check out the sections on the environment and farming.
www.aphg.jhsph.edu

BON APPETIT MANAGEMENT COMPANY FOUNDATION-EAT LOW CARBON CALCULATOR
(USA)
Discover the ecological foodprint of your next meal. Play around with the "carbon calculator" on this Web site and learn more about how to green your plate.
www.eatlowcarbon.org

CALIFORNIA CLIMATE AND AGRICULTURE NETWORK
(California)
Formed in 2009, the Network is a coalition of California-focused organizations developing policy solutions at the nexus of climate change and sustainable agriculture.
www.calclimateag.org

CENTER FOR FOOD SAFETY—COOL FOODS CAMPAIGN
(Washington, D.C.)
A great resource for all of us interested in choosing more climate-friendly food, the Cool Foods Campaign includes educational resources and consumer information. Join the Center to stay abreast of policy developments related to climate-friendly farming.
www.coolfoodscampaign.org

CENTER FOR LIVABLE FUTURE
(Johns Hopkins University, Baltimore, Maryland)
The Center promotes research and dialogue about the interconnections between diet, the environment, food production, and health.
www.jhsph.edu/clf

CORNUCOPIA INSTITUTE
(Cornucopia, Wisconsin)
The Institute educates consumers, family-scale farmers, and the media about the economic and environmental benefits of organic and sustainable agriculture. Cornucopia also produces "scorecards" rating organic food companies on their environmental stewardship and more.
www.cornucopia.org

ENVIRONMENTAL WORKING GROUP
(Washington, D.C.)
Great resources on toxic contaminants in our food and water and on replacing environmentally-harmful federal policies with ones that foster sustainability. Check out EWG for resource guides about climate-friendly food choices.
www.ewg.org

FARM SANCTUARY
(USA)
Farm Sanctuary works to end cruelty to farm animals through animal rescue, education, and advocacy. As part of its advocacy efforts, Farm Sanctuary helped to spearhead the NYC Foodprint Alliance—a coalition of organiza-

tions working to promote local and plant-based foods and to encourage New Yorkers to eat lower on the food chain. Following the introduction of the NYC Foodprint, green resolutions have become a nationwide initiative for Farm Sanctuary and its advocacy team.
www.farmsanctuary.org

FOOD & WATER WATCH
(International/Washington, D.C.)
A nonprofit consumer organization that works to ensure clean water and safe food in the United States and around the world.
www.foodandwaterwatch.org

FOOD CLIMATE RESEARCH NETWORK
(UK)
An excellent resource for the latest research about food and climate change. The Network is a fantastic one-stop shop for your burning food-and-climate-change questions.
http://www.fcrn.org.uk

FOOD FIRST
(Oakland, California)
Since 1975, the Institute for Food and Development Policy/Food First (co-founded by my mother, Frances Moore Lappé) has helped expose the root causes of global hunger, poverty, and ecological degradation and share solutions in partnership with global movements.
www.foodfirst.org

GREENPEACE—COOL FARMING
(International)
Greenpeace is one of the world's preeminent environmental organizations, using peaceful direct action and creative communication to expose global environmental crises and to promote solutions.
www.greenpeace.org

HUMANE SOCIETY OF THE UNITED STATES—LIVESTOCK AND CLIMATE CHANGE
(USA)
The nation's largest animal protection organization, the Humane Society has great resources to help you learn more about the connection between livestock

and climate change and ways to get involved in promoting more humane, and climate-friendly, animal production systems.
www.hsus.org

Institute for Agriculture and Trade Policy
(Minneapolis, Minnesota)
IATP's advocacy and research focuses on clean-energy economies, analysis of the impact of global trade agreements on agricultural policies, and more. Their studies are top-notch. See, especially, their policy papers on climate and agriculture.
www.iatp.org/climate

International Commission on the Future of Food and Agriculture
(International)
The commission was founded by Claudio Martini, president of the region of Tuscany and Dr. Vandana Shiva, executive director of the research foundation for technology, science, and ecology. The commission is composed of leading activists, academics, scientists, politicians, and farmers around the world working to shape more socially and ecologically sustainable food systems. Check out their "Manifesto on Climate Change and the Future of Food Security."
www.futurefood.org

Just Food
(New York, New York)
Since 1994, Just Food has been working to create a food system in the city that expands access to local and sustainable foods for all New Yorkers. Their work helps build new opportunities for regional, rural family farms in New York State and establish more resources for the city's communities and community gardeners.
www.justfood.org

National Family Farming Coalition
(Washington, D.C.)
The Coalition represents twenty-four grassroots organizations working on family farm issues in thirty-two states.
www.nffc.net

NATIONAL ORGANIC COALITION
(USA)
A coalition of organizations across the country, the NOC is working to provide a "Washington voice" for farmers, ranchers, environmentalists, consumers, and progressive industry members to strengthen the organic movement. The Coalition is working to maintain the integrity of the organic label, promote the environmental benefits of organic agriculture, encourage diverse access to organic foods, and overall, ensure the long-term viability of organic family farmers and businesses.
www.nationalorganiccoalition.org

NATIONAL SUSTAINABLE AGRICULTURE COALITION
(Washington, D.C.)
A national alliance of family farm, food, conservation, rural and urban organizations advancing policies for sustainable agriculture.
www.sustainableagriculture.net

THE OAKLAND INSTITUTE—VOICES FROM AFRICA PROJECT
(Oakland, California)
This Oakland-based think tank works to increase public participation and promote fair debate on critical social, economic and environmental issues. Check out the Voices from Africa project, with its interactive Web site, that serves as an online clearinghouse on genetic engineering in African agriculture and as a space to explore true solutions for food sovereignty across the continent.
www.oaklandinstitute.org

THE ORGANIC CENTER
(USA)
The Center produces peer-reviewed studies that ground the benefits of organic farming and organic products in scientific research.
www.organic-center.org

OXFAM INTERNATIONAL—CLIMATE CHANGE CAMPAIGN
(International)
Oxfam International's Climate Change Campaign is focused on helping poor communities adapt to the impact of global warming. Oxfam is also advocating for resources to help those most affected by climate change, including many of the world's small-scale farmers.
www.oxfam.org/en/climatechange

Rainforest Action Network (RAN)—Agribusiness Campaign
(San Francisco, California)
RAN is dedicated to campaigning for environmental protection around the world, from fighting tar sands exploration in Canada to addressing unsustainable palm oil production in Indonesia and Malaysia. Visit RAN's Web site to learn more about the organization's Agribusiness Campaign and to get involved through direct action and advocacy.
www.ran.org

Real Food Challenge
(USA)
A national network of students promoting locally grown, sustainably raised and fair food on college and university campuses across the country.
www.realfoodchallenge.org

Rodale Institute
(Kutztown, Pennsylvania)
A leading researcher and promoter of sustainable farming practices. The Institute conducts research on the ground and their findings inspire the organization's trainings with farmers in Africa, Asia, and the Americas.
www.rodaleinstitute.org

Slow Food USA
(National)
The U.S. branch of an international phenomenon, Slow Food USA promotes good, clean, fair food through school and campus-based initiatives and community programs safeguarding food biodiversity and connecting eaters with their food and the people who grow it.
www.slowfoodusa.org

Sustainable Table
(New York, New York)
The brains behind the international Web video sensation *The Meatrix*, Sustainable Table produces creative education materials to educate people about sustainability. Their Web site also houses a robust database including farms, CSAs, and more.
www.sustainabletable.org

UNITED NATIONS FOOD AND AGRICULTURE ORGANIZATION
(International)
The FAO is an excellent source of data about food and farming around the
world. Visit the Web site for reports and analysis as well as raw data sets to help
you learn more about food and agriculture.
www.fao.org

II. BLOGS

> *From laptops across the country—near brussels sprout fields in
> Santa Cruz and tomato patches in Toledo—bloggers are weigh-
> ing in on the most important food politics questions of the day,
> including food and climate change. You can weigh in, too. Here
> are some of my favorites. Check them out, follow them on Twit-
> ter, and add to the conversation.*

> Find the *Diet for a Hot Planet* blog at *www.takeabite.cc/blog*

CHEWSWISE
Run by longtime journalist Samuel Fromartz (author, *Organic Inc.*), Chewswise, says Fromartz, provides commentary on "big" issues—like pesticides and
GMOs—as well as the ins and outs of a farm sale or a peek at artisanal bread
making.
www.chewswise.com

CIVIL EATS
Promoting critical thought about sustainable agriculture and food systems as
part of building economically and socially just communities, the blog encourages dialogue among local and national leaders about the U.S. food system
and its impact abroad.
www.civileats.com

COOKING UP A STORY
Want to know how to can fresh pears? Learn about the origins of corn in Mexico? Discover how to raise chickens in your backyard? Cooking Up a Story
showcases short videos answering these questions, and more, helping you discover the hands-on ways to choose a more climate-friendly diet.
www.cookingupastory.com

Ethicurean

Frequent topics include news, food safety, food politics, eating ethics, and cooking—all served up with a big helping of humor.
www.ethicurean.com

Green Fork

The official blog of the Eat Well Guide, check out the Green Fork for insightful commentary and news about local foods.
www. blog.eatwellguide.org

Grist

Check out food editor Tom Philpott's "food kingdom" on Grist.org. Philpott and guest writers provide excellent insight to national food news alongside tantalizing recipes for healthy, delicious meals.
www.grist.org

La Vida Locavore

Started by Daily Kos blogger Jill Richardson, this blog covers not only the hands-on (planting, growing, weeding, fertilizing, raising, picking, harvesting, processing, cooking, baking, making, serving, buying, selling, distributing, transporting, and composting of food), but also the politics of food, with insightful analysis of food policy.
www.lavidalocavore.org

III. FILMS

> These films explore our food chain in celluloid. You'll discover why kids in the Bronx care about basil, get inspired by the miracle of fertility (of soil, that is), and learn how to make high-fructose corn syrup. Find these documentaries on Netflix, your local video store, or directly at the Web sites listed below.

What's On Your Plate?, a film by Catherine Gund

Follow two eleven-year-old city kids as they explore their place in the food chain. With youthful curiosity, the girls visit supermarkets, fast food chains, and school lunchrooms as well as sustainable farms, greenmarkets, and community supported agriculture programs. Through their journey, the two friends develop a sophisticated and compassionate view of the state of food and what they can do about it. Funny, engaging, and ultimately inspiring.
www.whatsonyourplateproject.org

DIRT, A FILM BY BILL BENENSON AND GENE ROSOW
Dirt brings to life the environmental, economic, social, and political impact of soil, telling the story of the earth's most valuable and underappreciated source of food.
www.dirtthemovie.org

FRESH, A FILM BY ANA SOFIA JOANES
Beautifully shot with a sonorous soundtrack, *Fresh* is a surprisingly uplifting critique of industrial agriculture. It juxtaposes the woes of industrial agriculture—told through the voices of the farmers themselves—with the pleasure and pride of sustainable farmers. With clips from a composting workshop in one of the country's most innovative urban farms, the film makes you want to get out of your seat and dig into the dirt.
www.freshthemovie.com

FOOD, INC., A FILM BY ROBERT KENNER (PRODUCER/DIRECTOR) AND ERIC SCHLOSSER (CO-PRODUCER)
Featuring interviews with Eric Schlosser (*Fast Food Nation*), Michael Pollan (*The Omnivore's Dilemma*), and food entrepreneurs like Stonyfield's Gary Hirshberg and Joel Salatin of Polyface Farm, *Food, Inc.* reveals surprising—and sometimes shocking—facts about what we eat and how it's produced. The film does a particularly impressive job explaining the impact of Monsanto's practices on farmers.
www.foodincmovie.com

KING CORN, A FILM BY IAN CHENEY AND CURT ELLIS
Watch what happens when two friends see what it takes to grow an acre of corn in Iowa. The two get a firsthand look at the genetically modified foods industry, nitrogen fertilizers, and how to make high-fructose corn syrup (clue: wear gloves). As the friends follow their corn from the farm into the food system, they uncover troubling truths about what we eat—and how we farm.
www.kingcorn.net

THE FOOD AND CLIMATE CONNECTION: FROM HEATING THE PLANET TO HEALING IT, A FILM BY WORLD HUNGER YEAR
The film highlights the impact of today's global food system on the climate and how a community-based food movement around the world is bringing to life a way of farming and eating that's better for our bodies and the planet. Featuring interviews with farmers, community leaders, and sustainability advocates, the film highlights how the industrial food system is among the greatest contributors to global warming and how sustainable farming practices can pose a powerful solution to the crisis.

INDEX

A Note on the Author

Anna Lappé is a national bestselling author recognized for her work on food politics, sustainability, and social change. Named one of *Time*'s "eco" Who's Who, Anna has been featured in the *New York Times, Gourmet, Natural Health Yoga Journal*, and *Food & Wine*, among many other publications. Anna is a founding principal of the Small Planet Institute and Small Planet Fund, a volunteer-led initiative that has raised more than $750,000 for democratic social movements worldwide since 2002.

She is the coauthor of *Grub: Ideas for an Organic Kitchen* (with eco-chef Bryant Terry) and *Hope's Edge* (with her mother, Frances Moore Lappé). Her writing has been published in the *Washington Post, Los Angeles Times, International Herald Tribune*, and Canada's *Globe and Mail*. She is also a contributing author to numerous books, including *Food Inc., WorldChanging*, and *Feeding the Future*. She can be seen on the Sundance Channel's *Big Ideas for a Small Planet* on the PBS special *Nourish* and as a co-host of the public television series *The Endless Feast*.

A board member of Rainforest Action Network, Anna is a graduate of Brown University and earned her M.A. at Columbia University's School of International and Public Affairs. From 2004 to 2006, she was a Food and Society Policy Fellow, a national program of the W. K. Kellogg Foundation. She lives in Brooklyn's Boerum Hill neighborhood with her husband and their daughter.

www.takeabite.cc

www.smallplanet.org

www.smallplanetfund.org

QUESTIONS FOR DISCUSSION

These questions are designed to enhance your group's conversation about *Diet for a Hot Planet*. To find other resources, visit www.takeabite.cc.

1. Anna Lappé begins *Diet for a Hot Planet* with a passage from the environmental philosopher Susan Griffin, who writes, "Like artistic and literary movements, social movements are driven by imagination" (xi). What do you think Griffin means by this and why do you think Lappé begins the book this way?

2. Lappé focuses her opening chapter on the connections between the climate crisis and the food system. Were you aware of the connection between global warming and food before reading the book? Were there facts that surprised you? In what way, if any, has your understanding or opinion changed?

3. In "The Climate Crisis at the End of Our Fork," one focus is the connection between livestock production and climate change. Why is industrial livestock such a big contributor to the crisis?

4. In "The Shape of Things to Come," Lappé argues that the expansion of the American-style fast food and processed food diet is driven by three forces, including the food industry's explicit push to change the tastes of consumers around the globe. She writes, "Our food future is being forged by specific policies, unquestioned assumptions, and corporate decisions" (43). Do you agree? Can you think of

specific examples of how the food industry may have influenced your choices as a consumer?

5. In "Blinded by the Bite," Lappé details the lack of media coverage of the role the global food system plays in climate change. Do you think the media has historically missed this story? Do you think the media is covering this angle now? Why or why not? Lappé offers several possible reasons why people are not more aware of the connection between food and climate. Which of these reasons do you think is the most significant and why? What other explanations do you have for why we've missed this story?

6. Lappé draws a parallel between the food industry and the tobacco industry's approach to questioning science. Do you think this is a fair comparison? Why or why not?

7. In "Playing with Our Food," Lappé dissects corporate greenwashing, and on page 90, she identifies the six "plays" from the industry spin book. Which one of these do you think is the most common and why? Can you think of any of these strategies you've personally seen in action? Lappé says she is hoping to foster more savvy, not more cynical, consumers. On the spectrum of savvy to cynical, where do you fall?

8. Henry Miller of the Hoover Institution writes that "neither free enterprise nor the human condition is likely to experience net benefit from companies pursuing corporate responsibility" (87). Do you think corporations have a social responsibility? Do you think that food companies should be held to a higher social standard than other types of corporations? In "Beyond the Fork," Lappé details activists who are pushing food corporations to be more socially responsible. Did you think their actions are justified? Which kinds of campaigns do you think are most successful?

9. In the beginning of "Cool Food," Lappé describes discussing with farmer Mark Shepard what "progress" really means. What's your definition of progress? Do you feel that Mark's farm, as described in this chapter, represents progress? Why or why not?

10. In her discussion of the motivations for social change, Lappé quotes the authors of *Break Through* who write, "Ecological concern remains far weaker in Brazil, India, and China than in the United States, Japan, and Europe. And it explains why, when environmentalism does emerge in developing countries, such as Brazil, it does so in Rio De Janeiro's most affluent neighborhoods, where people have met their basic material needs, and not in its slums, where people live in fear of hunger and violence" (162). Does this statement seem logical? What argument does Lappé give that this idea is a myth?

11. In "The Hunger Scare," Lappé explores one of the most contentious debates about food and hunger. Do you think we can feed the world with climate-friendly food? Why or why not?

12. In "Eat the Sky," Lappé shares nuanced definitions of "local food" and "locavores." How do you define a locavore, and do you consider yourself one? Why or why not?

13. What are some barriers to following the seven principles of a climate-friendly diet? Are they attitudinal barriers or are they structural ones? Do you think we can most effect change by transforming how people think or do we need to change policy, or both?

14. On page xxii of the introduction, Lappé writes that "by turning our sights to food, we may just find the integrating lens—and grounding source—for bringing to life the real solutions already before us." What do you think she means by this? How do you feel after reading *Diet for a Hot Planet*? Did the book inspire you to make changes in your diet, or to take other action? In what ways could you make a difference?